Operative Mitral and Tricuspid Valve Surgery

Narain Moorjani • Bushra S. Rana
Francis C. Wells

Operative Mitral and Tricuspid Valve Surgery

Springer

Narain Moorjani
Department of Cardiothoracic Surgery
Royal Papworth Hospital
Cambridge
UK

Bushra S. Rana
Department of Cardiology
Royal Papworth Hospital
Cambridge
UK

Francis C. Wells
Department of Cardiothoracic Surgery
Royal Papworth Hospital
Cambridge
UK

ISBN 978-1-4471-4203-4 ISBN 978-1-4471-4204-1 (eBook)
https://doi.org/10.1007/978-1-4471-4204-1

Library of Congress Control Number: 2018952092

Printed on acid-free paper

This Springer imprint is published by the registered company Springer-Verlag London Ltd. part of Springer Nature.
The registered company address is: The Campus, 4 Crinan Street, London, N1 9XW, United Kingdom

For Vanessa, Sam and Rohan,
and Lada

Foreword

I thoroughly enjoyed reading *Operative Mitral and Tricuspid Valve Surgery* by Narain Moorjani, Bushra Rana and Francis Wells, from the Royal Papworth Hospital, Cambridge, UK. The authors present the topics in 18 separate chapters, each one written in a consistent and comprehensive style. This book covers all aspects of the mitral and tricuspid valves, from basic sciences and imaging to an extensive surgical armamentarium of operative techniques to treat the entire range of pathologies of both valves.

The authors give the reader a wonderful historical perspective on the anatomy of the atrioventricular valves. The chapter on echocardiography contains numerous pearls for the student of both valves. Indications for surgery for mitral and tricuspid valve disease continue to evolve, and practitioners need to stay abreast of current information regarding the timing of surgery. The literature has plenty of guidelines that are frequently updated to incorporate newer knowledge. The next chapter deals with operative approaches to the mitral and tricuspid valves, detailing surgical 'tips and tricks' that can significantly enhance the surgeons' view of the valve, the most important aspect of surgery being 'vision'.

The other 13 chapters are written in an innovative and unique style, where a patient is presented with diagnostic images and other tests, and the authors discuss the operative procedure used and alternative methods in a very comprehensive and complete way. The format enables surgeons to reach a better understanding of the multiple considerations involved in the evaluation and management of these complex patients. All of the techniques are beautifully explained, and one cannot add much to what they have described. The text is supported by the important references from the literature.

A picture is worth a thousand words and this is true for the chapters on operative techniques making the text easy to interpret, with the presence of exceptional illustrations and operative images. One of the key messages of this book is for the surgeon operating on the mitral and tricuspid valves to have a great understanding of the pathophysiology of the valve disease process and to be well versed in the different options available to obtain a durable repair.

In summary, this book succinctly presents an overview of the surgical therapeutic options used for patients presenting with a wide variety of mitral and tricuspid valve pathologies. *Operative Mitral and Tricuspid Valve Surgery* is a book for all novice and experienced surgeons who operate on the mitral and tricuspid valves.

Tirone David
Melanie Munk Chair of Cardiovascular Surgery
Peter Munk Cardiac Centre at Toronto General Hospital
Professor of Surgery, University of Toronto
Toronto, ON, Canada

Preface

The field of mitral and tricuspid valve surgery continues to evolve and is recognised as a subspecialty of cardiac surgery, with dedicated groups of surgeons, cardiologists who are expert in imaging and clinical diagnosis, radiologists and electrophysiologists bringing to bear their expertise to the benefit of the patient with mitral and tricuspid valve disease. The specialist heart valve team is now the gold standard for care of these often highly complex patients.

The surgical approach to mitral and tricuspid valve disease has significantly evolved, and the challenge for surgeons is to maximise repair rates in the context of the highest standards of clinical care and stringent outcome measures. No longer is it acceptable for one to 'simply replace the valve'. There is continued development of new techniques and operations, as well as the refinement of established surgical procedures. In parallel with this, the demand for knowledge regarding how these new procedures are performed is increasing.

In the context of actual clinical cases, *Operative Mitral and Tricuspid Valve Surgery* sets out to describe the gamut of surgical techniques that are currently available as a guide and aid to surgeons wishing to develop their experience and skill sets in the real world. This book provides a contemporary text that systematically covers all the surgical techniques in the field of mitral and tricuspid valve surgery. Each chapter contains detailed echocardiographic imaging, a pathophysiological description of the underlying disease process and a surgical strategy on management of the common mitral and tricuspid valve pathologies. Each surgical procedure is accompanied by photographical images and drawings to illustrate the surgical technique, supported with important references for further reading and a greater depth of knowledge. In addition, there are individual chapters on anatomy and physiology, echocardiographic imaging and evidence-based indications for surgery of the mitral and tricuspid valves.

It is our hope that *Operative Mitral and Tricuspid Valve Surgery* will be a valuable contribution to the training of the next generation of surgeons and as an aid to practising surgeons who wish to expand their clinical care for patients with often complex underlying pathologies.

Cambridge, UK

Narain Moorjani
Francis C. Wells

Contents

1 Anatomy and Physiology of the Mitral Valve

Keywords
Anatomy · Physiology · Embryology · Leaflet · Chordae tendinae · Papillary muscle · Commissure · Annulus · Cleft · Trigone

Introduction

The heart is a dynamic living pump that has evolved in such a way that the whole organ functions as a holistic unit, which can adapt to the constantly changing demands of flow and pressure. Efficient function of this pump requires the presence of unidirectional valves. Nature has evolved valves that both operate under the highest pressure that the heart can generate and that also maintain the structural integrity of the muscle chambers that house them. Of all the cardiac valves, the mitral has the biggest task. It has to withstand the highest closing pressure and support the left ventricle, the powerhouse of the heart.

In framing our thoughts about the mitral valve, it may be constructive to think of the valve unit as a machine. Whilst this may initially sound somewhat nonsensical, consideration of the definition will illustrate the point. A machine is an apparatus using or applying mechanical power, having several parts, each with a definite function and together performing certain kinds of work. With respect to the atrioventricular valves and in particular the mitral valve, although of course the same applies to the tricuspid valve, the particular function of valve competence cannot be separated from its unitary function as the 'linchpin' of normal ventricular function. The ventricle and valve components work together to give valve competence and ventricular stability under all working conditions. Any surgical interference with the valve must be cognisant of this relationship if disorder of either valve or ventricular function is not to result.

The dynamic nature of the valve is revealed by the way it responds to maximal exercise. As oxygen demands of the body rise, the cardiac output increases in response, and at maximal cardiac output, the atrioventricular valve orifices can exceed the natural surface areas of the leaflets that close them. To achieve this, the left ventricular basal muscle, which acts as a sphincter at the base of the heart, will open widely in diastole to allow maximum flow through the valve. The valve orifice can change by up to 40% of the resting area through the cardiac cycle (Fig. 1.1).

This dynamic orifice area is enhanced by the presence of the normal clefts in the posterior leaflet, which extend for about 30% of the height of the leaflet. Exaggerated clefts extending to the annulus are very frequently found in regurgitant valves, the relevance of which will be discussed later.

Synchronised ventricular muscular relaxation allows the valves to open and diastolic ventricular filling to occur, partially passively but also

N. Moorjani et al., *Operative Mitral and Tricuspid Valve Surgery*,
https://doi.org/10.1007/978-1-4471-4204-1_1

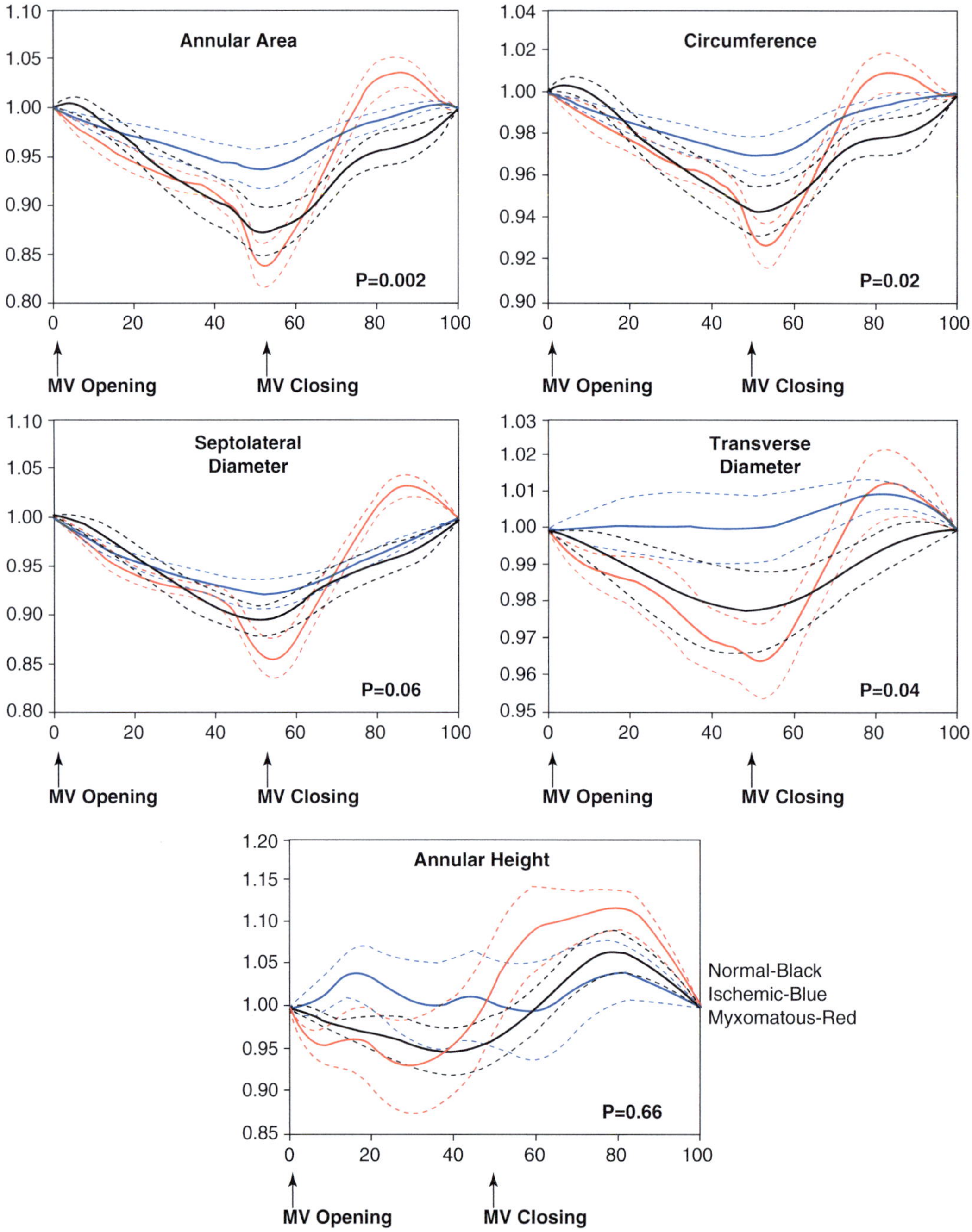

Fig. 1.1 Dynamic changes of the mitral valve during the cardiac cycle. (Reproduced with permission from Levack et al. Three-dimensional echocardiographic analysis of the mitral annular dynamics. Implications for annuloplasty selection. Circulation. 2012;126(suppl 1):S183–8)

partially actively with a suction component. The untwisting of the relaxing complex, conically shaped ventricular chamber generates the suction. The momentum of the entering blood is augmented at the end of the diastolic phase by atrial contraction, the 'atrial kick'. The synchronization of these complex motions is electromechanical. The electrical component is the synchronised polarisation and depolarisation of the myocytes. The mechanical component is

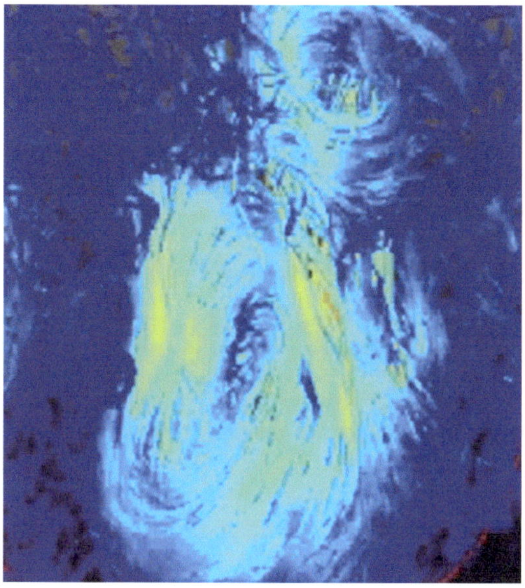

Fig. 1.2 Magnetic resonance imaging (MRI) blood flow scan showing the swirling vortex within the left ventricle

enhanced by the connection between the base of the heart and the ventricular walls by the atrioventricular valves, with the chordal connections preventing abnormal distortion of the ventricular walls and chamber.

In early diastole, blood entering the ventricular chamber encounters the apex of the left ventricle and flows back along the curved walls of the ventricle forming vortices that circulate beneath the leaflets of the atrioventricular valves and begin the return motion of the valve leaflets (Fig. 1.2).

The presence of the papillary muscles, as projections from the ventricular wall with the chordal attachments along their upper surfaces, prevent the fully open leaflets from being forced against the ventricular wall enhancing the ease with which they float back into the inflow tract of the ventricle which is the first part of closure. The increasing pressure within the ventricle then pushes the returning leaflets towards each other more forcibly. Systolic ventricular contraction also narrows the orifice of the valve and the muscular projections within the ventricles, the papillary muscles, draw the leaflets together and down into the ventricular cavity. This motion ensures maximum coaptation of the leaflets.

Disruption of any part of this mechanism will interfere with normal valve function and, equally importantly, normal ventricular function. Therefore, retention of the subvalvar apparatus during valve replacement is vital for optimal cardiac function post-operatively. A full appreciation of atrioventricular valve structure and function therefore is essential for anyone working in this field.

Historical Oversight

The heart valves were recognised as important entities in some of the earliest anatomical descriptions of the heart. The first recognizable reference that is known is from the writings of Erasistratus (304–250 BC), the physician to King Selenicus Nicator of Syria. Among Erasistratus's achievements was the founding of the school of anatomy in Alexandria with Herophilus (335–280 BC). Not only did he describe the valves of the heart but also correctly characterised the heart as a pump and stated that the brain was the seat of sensation and not the heart.

Aristotle (384–322 BC) seems to have had little to say about the anatomy of the heart in general or the valves in particular, focussing on the heart as the emotional centre. On the other hand, Hippocrates (460–370 BC) described the valves in some detail. His description of the atrioventricular valves holds resonance with modern interpretation of valve function. Writing in 1964, Lillehei stressed the vital importance of the mitral valve as an integral part of the left ventricular functional apparatus; excise the whole valve and the heart will fail quite quickly despite a functioning prosthetic mitral valve, with 50% mortality at 5 years. Two millennia before Lillehei expressed the vital nature of this interaction, Hippocrates wrote about the atrioventricular valves as the '*hidden membranes*'. His words are prescient; *"membranes and fibres spread throughout the chambers (of the heart), like cobwebs especially around the orifices. There are filaments implanted into the walls of the chambers as well. The author believes these to be 'guy ropes' and stays of the heart as well as the foundation of the arteries"*.

Truth is truth expressed in any age and the gift of the original thinker is important to be noted from any period of history.

Galen (first century AD; 129-c200/c216) wrote specifically but incorrectly on the flow of the blood within the body. He described the movement of the blood in the body in a way that would fit his version of events. In Galenic terms, the blood ebbed and flowed within the arteries passing out to the periphery and then returning to the heart in reverse manner. In addition, he postulated that the blood passed back and forth across the heart valves allowing the 'sooty vapours' formed in the periphery to pass back to the heart and thence back to the lungs where they were exhaled. He said that the lungs had a direct connection with the atria allowing this to happen. This explanation called for a connection between the right and left ventricles, the "ventricular pores". Despite their non-existence, their presence was proclaimed by practically every major voice in the field of anatomy and medicine for the next 1.6 millennia.

In Galenic terms, the blood needed to be able to flow in both directions across the atrioventricular valves, the 'membranes' of the heart. In a way therefore, the presence of functional one-way non-return valves were a nuisance for his philosophy of cardio-vascular function. His voice was so powerful that he inhibited meaningful thought until the work of Vesalius and Harvey in the sixteenth and seventeenth centuries.

The first *published* appropriate visual representation of the heart valves appeared in "*De humani corporis fabrica*" written by Andreas Vesalius. Published in 1543, this magnum opus, often referred to simply as the 'de Fabrica', revolutionised the known world's view of anatomy. Whilst no discussion of the development of anatomical thinking could be complete without the work of Andreas Vesalius, his contribution to the understanding of cardiac, and in particular valve function, is relatively small and constrained by the Galenic theory of the 'to and fro' of blood from the heart, as opposed to the continuous circulation proposed by William Harvey in *de Motu Cordis*. Galen's model of cardio-pulmonary function relied upon fictitious connecting pores between the right and left ventricles. Vesalius could not find them in his dissections and wrote cautiously of his observations thus:

> *In explaining the construction of the heart and the function of its parts, I have to a great extent made my account agree with the views of Galen. This is not because I believe ...everywhere consonant with the truth...it was because for a long time I lacked the courage to depart in the least way from the view of Galen, prince of physicians. Students of anatomy must carefully investigate the septum .... which is as heavy compact and dense as the rest of the heart. I therefore do not know how the slightest amount of blood can be taken through the substance of this septum from the right into the left ventricle.*

It was the Renaissance anatomist Benedetti who first published a description of the unidirectional nature of valve function. Benedetti first used the term *valvulae* (little valves) taken from the Latin term valvar, which means *a leaf of a door*, conjuring up the important and correct concept of the importance of opening and closing of the valve. These recorded observations were made in physiological isolation.

Before these accounts, Leonardo da Vinci had been working on the detailed functional anatomy of the heart. Sadly, his work cannot be considered in the pantheon of contemporary acknowledged work, as he did not publish any of it. Leonardo's anatomical work was known about during his lifetime. Antonio de Beatis, travelling chaplain and secretary to Cardinal Luigi of Aragon, wrote of the "great deal of anatomy" written about and illustrated by Leonardo. The Cardinal's retinue called on Leonardo when housed at the Manor house at Clous, where Leonardo was the guest of King Francis I, having left Rome under something of a cloud. Other than Leonardo's own words, no other commentary on his anatomical work exists. His extensive anatomical research lay hidden for over 200 years before coming to light, being publicised to some degree by the great eighteenth century anatomist William Hunter. Among Leonardo's achievements, now recognised, was the description of the heart as a four chambered structure, that the cardiac muscle was just that and had its own blood and nerve supply, the bronchial arteries, that the trachea had no connection

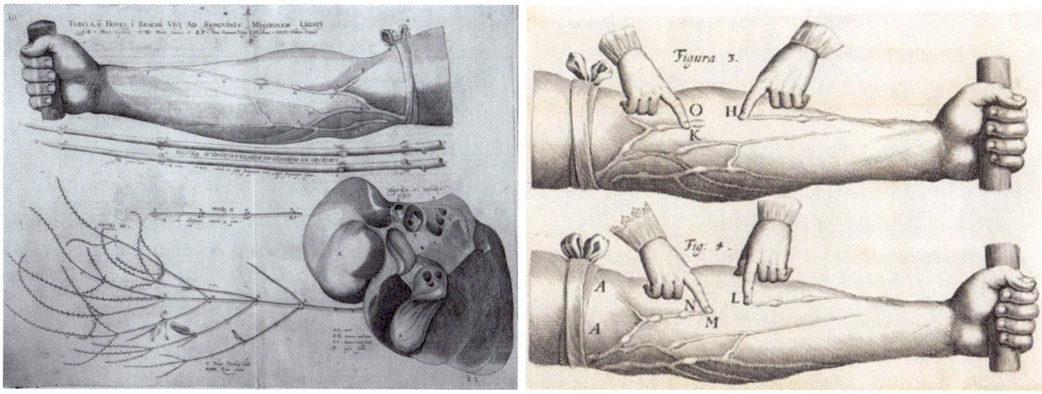

Fig. 1.3 Venous valves directing flow of blood to the heart. (Illustrations from *Valves of the veins* by Fabricius, 1603 and *de Motu Cordis* by William Harvey, 1628)

with the atria as suggested by Galen and the moderator band in the right ventricle attributing the correct function to it. We are unlikely to ever know if Vesalius and others, such as Harvey, were made familiar with his work, although it is possible as Leonardo's anatomy was celebrated after his death by Giorgio Vasari (1511–1574) in 'The lives of the most eminent painters, sculptors and architects', which was published first in 1550.

On reading his notes, you find Leonardo struggling with the Galenic description of valve function, as did Vesalius, particularly in the detailed research that he carried out on the aortic and pulmonary valves. As an engineer, Leonardo would have appreciated the implications of valve function on the flow of a fluid. Whilst it has become well appreciated that his description of the normal closure mechanism of the aortic and pulmonary valves was correct, it is less well recognised that he had appreciated the importance of the mitral and tricuspid valve ventricular interdependence in a thoroughly modern way. He likened the mitral valve and its connection to the ventricle through the tendinous chords to the relationship between the sails on a ship (the leaflets) and the ropes (the chordae) that attached them to the capstan on the deck (the papillary muscles).

Although it is commonly thought that the beginning of meaningful cardio-vascular physiology was the suggestion of William Harvey that blood circulated around the body, the foundation of this hypothesis was first suggested by Harvey's Professor in Padua, Hieronymus Fabricius (1537–1569). It was he who first described the venous valves and it was from an original drawing to be found in his work that Harvey derived the now famous drawing in *de Motu Cordis* (Fig. 1.3).

The impetus for postulating the circulation of the blood was dependent upon the acceptance and effectiveness of the valves of the heart acting as one-way non-return valves in exactly the same way as that postulated by Leonardo in his unpublished work. On Windsor sheet RL 19081 recto he writes "*The cusps of the greater valves of the heart are closed by the percussion of the blood which escapes from the lower ventricles of the heart. They are reopened by the influx of blood pushed from the upper ventricles (atria) into the lower.*" He continues on RL 19045 recto, "*The movement of the liquid (blood) from one direction proceeds in the original direction as long as the force remains in it which was given to it by the first mover (the heart).*"

Harvey's second condition for the need for a circulation was the necessary mass of blood expelled from the heart (ventricular volume x heart rate per minute) was the same one as that recorded by Leonardo. In Harvey's case, the argument was strengthened by the observable effect of onward progression of blood through the subcutaneous venous valves with visible prevention of return. Leonardo had demonstrated the true mechanism of valve closure and calculated the cardiac output also commenting upon the great weight of blood that left the heart each minute.

It seems almost inconceivable that such a great mind would not have considered the now obvious continuous circulation of the blood, anticipating the great contribution of William Harvey by over 100 years. Sadly, there is no extant record that supports this thought.

It is interesting that one of the major driving forces towards mitral valve surgical reconstruction, the physiological importance of the interdependency of the atrio-ventricular valves and their related ventricles, first suggested by Leonardo, took another 400 years to be spelt out by Dr. Walt Lillehei. The slow realisation of the physiological thinking behind this concept is perhaps understandable, as it requires a sophisticated appreciation of heart function in a somewhat abstract way. Perhaps that is why it took the disconnection of the valve from the ventricle and its removal from the living heart in the modern era of cardiac surgery to appreciate the profound nature of this relationship. It also serves to remind us that many of the greater truths are ignored or overlooked in the teaching and learning of a didactic society. It takes true greatness to diverge from the thinking of the herd and realise the importance of a simple observation, as witnessed by Harvey's distinguished place in the history of science.

Anatomy

Before describing the anatomy of the mitral valve, let us first consider the origin of the word valve. It is derived from the Latin word 'valvar', which, as mentioned before, in direct translation means 'the leaflets of a door'. Cardiac valve leaflets, like the leaflets of a door, have to both open and close and each movement is important. Restricted opening of the valve leaflet will lead to valve stenosis and imperfect closure will lead to valve regurgitation. This, however, is where the analogy ends, as cardiac valve leaflets do not close in the same way as a door where the edge of the door meets the door frame in perfect edge to edge closure. The leaflets come together and meet over a portion of the surface of the leaflet referred to as the coaptation zone (Fig. 1.4). This broad area of contact (usually 0.3–0.5 cm) allows a perfect seal in the normal valve. As we shall see, loss of this coaptation area completely disrupts valve and ventricular function.

Whilst diseases of the valve, such as rheumatic fever, leading to mitral stenosis were rare in countries that can afford sophisticated health care systems, it is increasing for a variety of reasons beyond the scope of this book. Regurgitant valves in an ageing population with ready access to health screening is becoming ever more commonly discovered and reparative procedures for such valves are now very common. The over-riding importance of post-operative competence has resulted in a somewhat blinkered vision of post-operative valve function. This approach has led to the tendency towards a restriction of valve orifice area and hence cardiac function in the diastolic phase of the cardiac cycle. This has occurred at the same time as a keener appreciation of the importance of

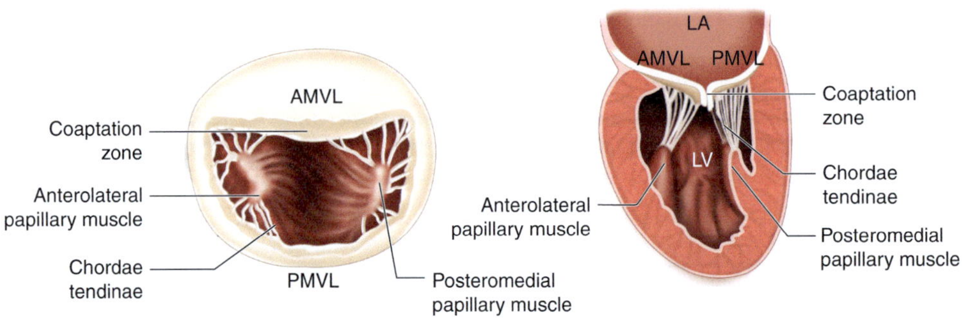

Fig. 1.4 Coaptation zone of the mitral valve. AMVL anterior mitral valve leaflet, PMVL posterior mitral valve leaflet, LA left atrium, LV left ventricle

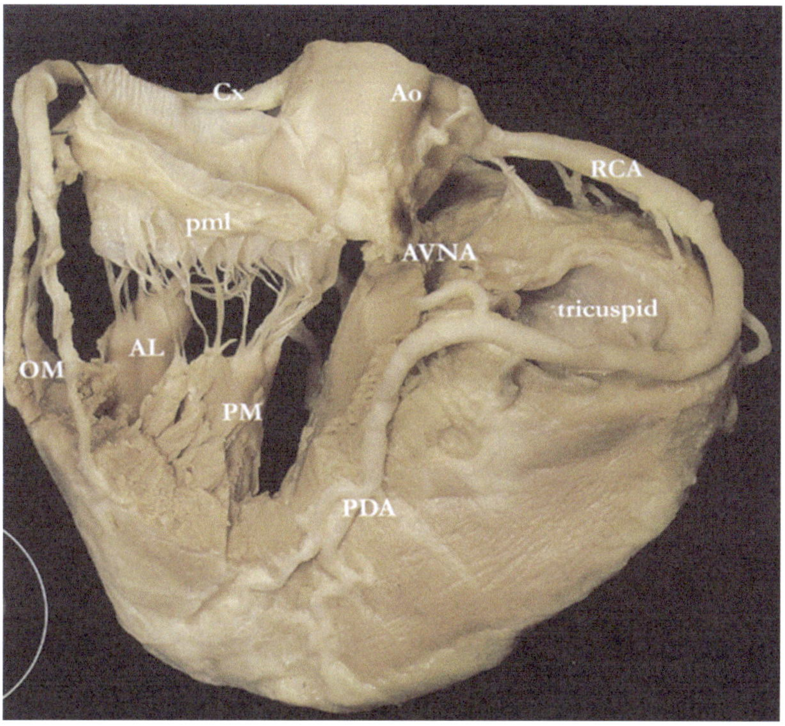

Fig. 1.5 Anatomical specimen depicting the annuloventricular loop, consisting of the left ventricular muscle, papillary muscles, chordae tendineae, mitral valve leaflet and mitral valve annulus. OM obtuse marginal artery, AL anterolateral papillary muscle, PM posterior medial papillary muscle, pml posterior mitral valve leaflet, Cx circumflex coronary artery, AVNA atrioventricular nodal artery, RCA right coronary artery, PDA posterior descending artery, Ao aorta. (Reproduced with permission from Dr. Horia Muresian, University Hospital of Bucharest, Romania)

diastolic function that has been developing, especially in the failing heart. Whilst this is perhaps of less importance in the elderly population, the move to earlier surgery in the younger population makes this something that needs to be considered. The surgeon and the cardiologist would do well to keep these dual functions in mind when considering the analysis of any valve lesion and the potential solution.

The valve has the following components: two leaflets, tendinous chords and papillary muscles, which are connected in a loop via the ventricular wall to the basal orifice of the ventricle (Fig. 1.5).

This anatomical or mechanical loop forms a functional unit but each component will be considered separately.

The Chordae Tendineae and Papillary Muscles

The atrioventricular valve leaflets are suspended from tendinous chords that arise from muscular ventricular projections, the papillary muscles (Fig. 1.6).

These chordae are described as being arranged in three arcades, primary, secondary and tertiary chords (Fig. 1.7). Whilst this description is functionally useful as each group have different roles, their separation is not as clear as the literal description implies. Close inspection reveals that apparent secondary chords can be branches of primary chords and vice versa. It is their point of insertion that governs their behaviour and the forces that are acting upon them as they develop determine this behaviour and form.

The primary chords insert into the leading edges of the leaflets. These act as 'guy ropes' preventing prolapse of the leaflet during the early part of valve closure, ensuring that the edges meet in coaptation. They are not load-bearing chords.

The secondary chords are the important load-bearing chords (Fig. 1.8). Their vaulting insertion forming chordal arcades reveals their fundamental role in load sharing. Like the radiating beams of the ceilings of King's College, Cambridge, and La Sagrada Familia, Barcelona, these secondary chordal projections spread the systolic load of closure evenly across the leaflets.

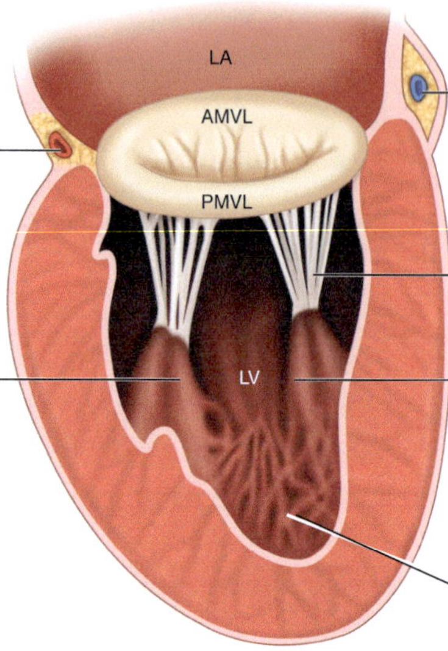

Fig. 1.6 The papillary muscles with chordal insertion into the leaflets. AMVL anterior mitral valve leaflet, PMVL posterior mitral valve leaflet, LA left atrium, LV left ventricle

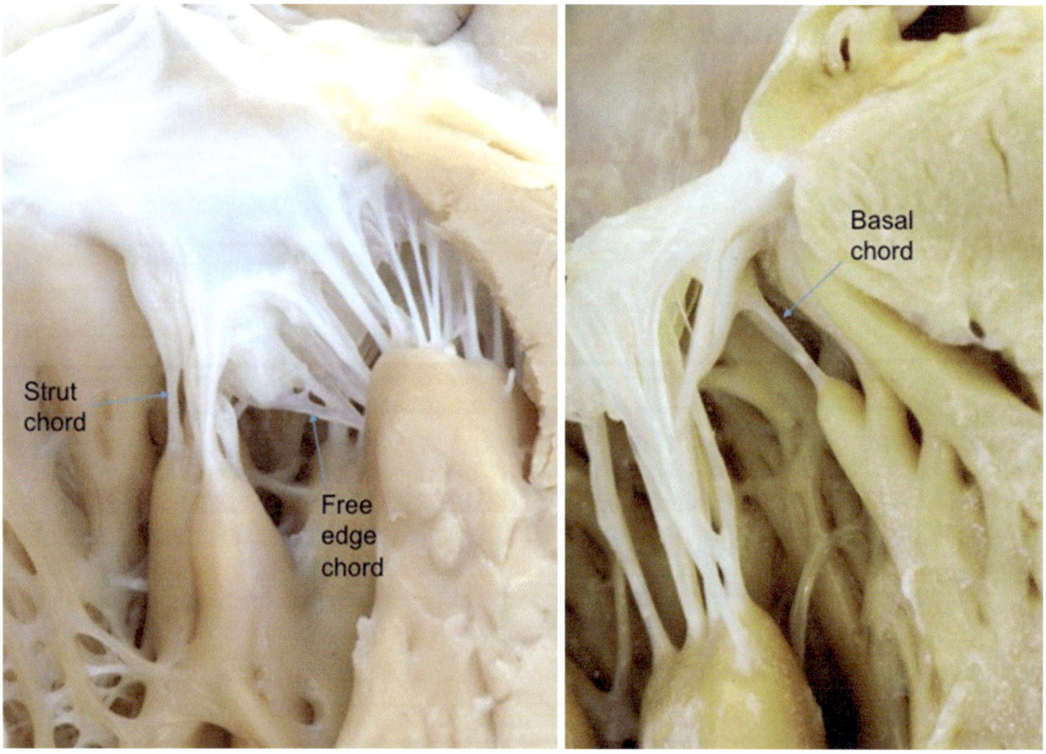

Fig. 1.7 Mitral valve chordae tendineae. (Reproduced with permission from Dr. Robert Anderson)

The leaflets are composed of two layers and the secondary chords become an integral part of the ventricular layer (Fig. 1.9).

The tertiary chords insert into both the base of the leaflets and the ventricular wall close to the base of the leaflet. These chords are tensioned throughout the cardiac cycle giving resilience to the ventricular-leaflet/atrial connection.

The shape and arrangement of the papillary muscles determine the arrangement and dispo-

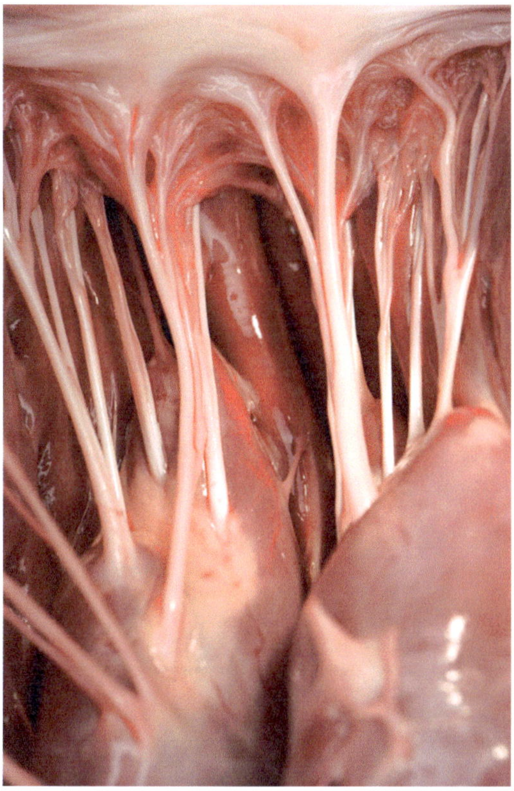

Fig. 1.8 Secondary chordae tendineae of the mitral valve. (Reproduced with permission of ben@erproductions.co.uk)

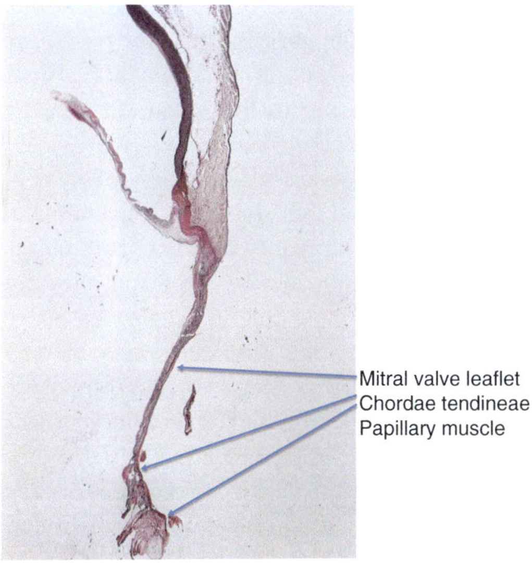

Fig. 1.9 Histology of the mitral valve leaflet in cross-section

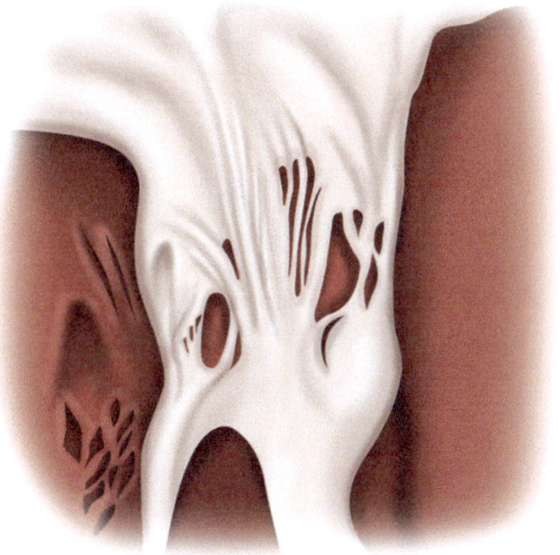

Fig. 1.10 Horseshoe shape of the papillary muscles within the left ventricle

sition of the chordae because they are formed together as the trabecular myocardium differentiates from the compact part of the myocardium.

There are usually two principal papillary muscle projections that form an approximate horseshoe shape (Fig. 1.10).

In the strictest anatomical context, they lie anterolaterally and inferomedially with reference to the mid-sagittal and coronal planes. The chordae arising from them reach both leaflets at the corresponding end of the leaflet commissures (Fig. 1.11).

Their arrangement has evolved to allow maximal efficiency in load bearing. The ends of each commissure are supported by chordae that arise from the tips of the papillary muscles at the centre of the 'horseshoe'. Chords reaching the leaflet edges away from the commissural ends arise from further along the papillary muscle body and are longer, more so as they reach towards the mid-line. The chords that arise from the posteromedial papillary muscle spread out more than those from the anterolateral muscle.

Where there are clefts in the posterior leaflet, the chordal extension spreads into the depths of the cleft and even to its deepest part. This is the case regardless of the depth of the cleft. These may be referred to as the cleft chordae. Some

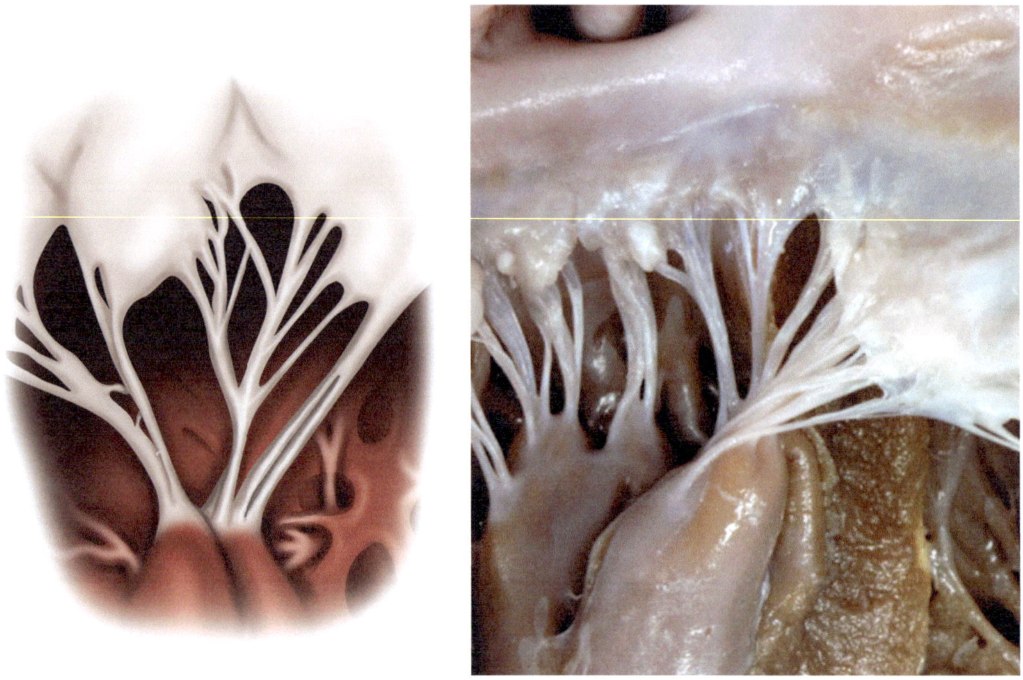

Fig. 1.11 Commissural chords. (Photographical image reproduced with permission from Dr. Robert Anderson)

basal chords meet the leaflet in the depths of the clefts that reach the annulus.

As described above, the secondary chords often arise in parallel with, or as branches from, the primary chords but in general, they tend to be behind them further from the ventricular cavity. Muscle fibres originating from the basal portion of the ventricular muscle run towards the apex and from there run towards, and then enter the papillary muscles. This interconnection is very important in normal left ventricular function as well as that of the mitral valve.

Considerable variation in papillary muscle shape exists (Fig. 1.12).

The posteromedial complex shows the greatest variability. Patients with mitral regurgitation appear to have the greatest tendency to variation, with multiple papillary muscle heads that in some cases arise from the ventricular wall very close to the underside of the valve (Fig. 1.13).

It appears that this variation contributes to the development of valve insufficiency in later life through insufficient support. This will be discussed in more depth in the next section. The muscular part of the papillary muscle usually, but not exclusively, has a fibrous tip that in turn gives rise to the tendinous chords.

It is common to find muscular bridges extending from one papillary muscle body to another or between elements of one papillary muscle. As the papillary muscles are projections from the trabecular portion of the ventricular muscle, this is perhaps not surprising. Their formation is a considerable natural achievement and it is not at all surprising to find great variation in their form.

Reading the very early descriptions of the papillary muscles and their function (Leonardo and Lower), where the reader will find pure observation with no influence of didactism, they are described as having a role in keeping the valve leaflets away from the ventricular walls thereby being in a position to float back into the closing position. If they were pinned against the ventricular wall in end diastole, then it is likely that they would not achieve the competence that is needed for full closure. Just like the aortic valve leaflets that if left to close by simple reflux of the blood will simply fold up and be incompetent as is sometimes seen when administering antegrade cardioplegia.

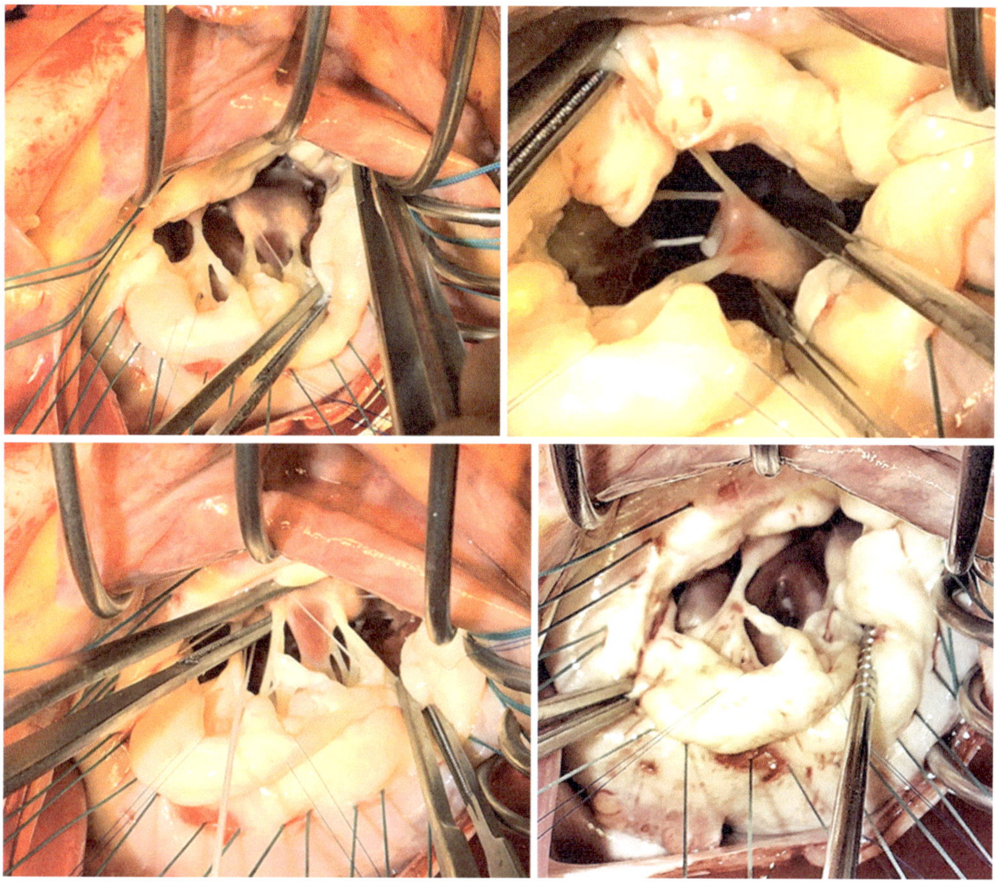

Fig. 1.12 Anatomical variation in papillary muscle configuration

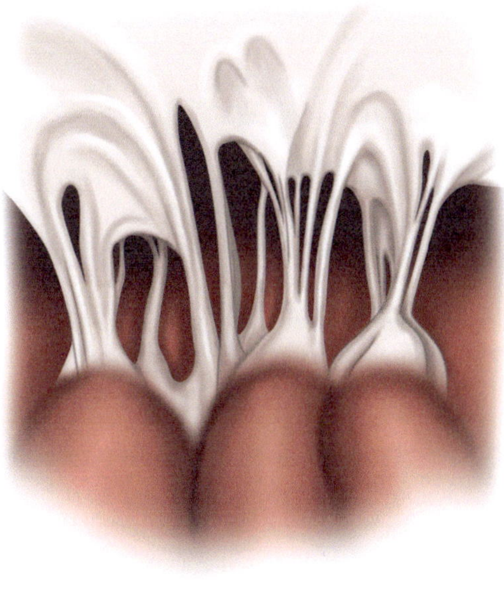

Fig. 1.13 Separate heads of the posteromedial papillary muscle

Interesting studies from the time of Richard Lower (1669) to Buckberg, more recently, have suggested that the gross anatomy of the ventricles is arranged as a muscle spiral that commences at the base of the heart and terminates at the tips of the papillary muscles. The boiling of the muscle and then peeling apart of the layers can produce this apparent muscular spiral. This appearance gives the impression of a single broad elastic band (Fig. 1.14).

With the base of the leaflets of the mitral valve forming one end of the band and the chordae tendinae at the tip of the papillary muscles, it becomes easy to imagine the continuous mechanical loop, the atrioventricular loop so often referred to in any discussion on this subject.

Anderson, Yen Ho and others find this work artificial and do not agree with this account of the anatomy. They point out that there is a very

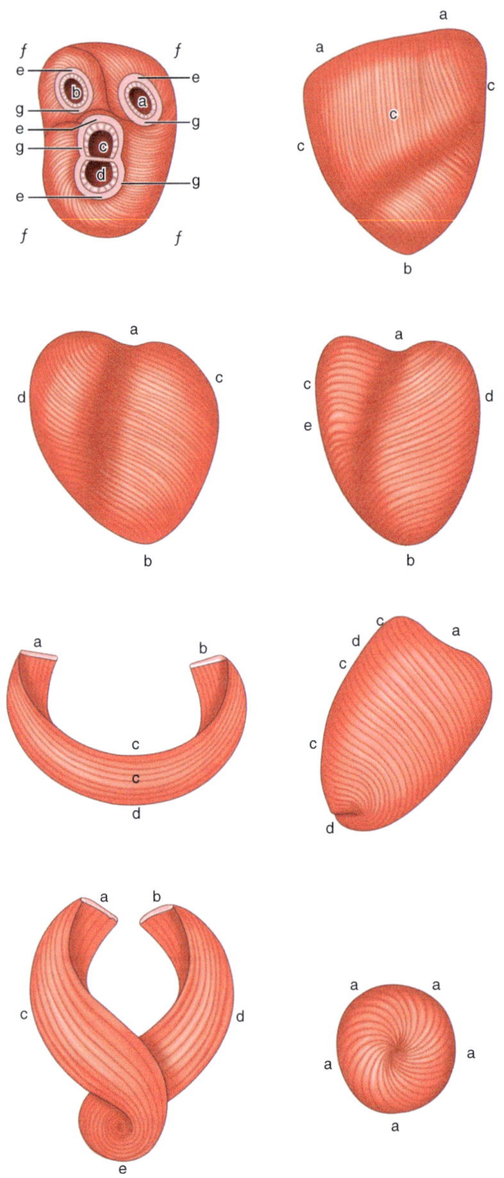

Fig. 1.14 Composition of the heart muscle. (Illustrations from *Tractatus de Corde* by Richard Lower, 1640)

complex relationship at myofibrillar level with tangential association between myocytes that cannot be explained by this simplistic approach. Whatever the truth of this relationship, it is clear that the papillary muscles are the point of transmission of left ventricular forces to the valve via the chordae and vice versa.

The mitral valve is found in the inflow of the left ventricle with the anterior leaflet forming a partial boundary between the inflow and outflow components of the ventricle (Fig. 1.15).

The valve leaflets form a funnel shaped opening into the ventricle, the edge of which is the orifice of the atrioventricular junction along two-thirds to three-quarters of the valve orifice. There is an apparent hinge between the two fibrous trigones along which the septal portion of the anterior leaflet opens. The portion of anterior leaflet above this geometric chord is small (Fig. 1.16).

During systole, as the ventricular cavity becomes pressurized, the outflow tract becomes cylindrical. This has the effect of forming the anterior leaflet into a 'saddle shape' between the two fibrous trigones. Hence, this configuration is a dynamic one and an example of the functional integration of the whole valve-ventricular unit. There has been a lot of discussion about the shape of annuloplasty rings to create this inherent saddle shape. In fact, the best way to achieve the desired shape is to leave the septal portion alone and to use partial rings or bands reaching from trigone to trigone. The pressurised outflow tract will do the rest. This complex 3-D anatomy is important to allow the full deployment of the anterior leaflet, similar to a ship's sail filled with wind. If it is compromised, it can cause the anterior leaflet to fold abnormally, which in turn could prevent normal coaptation of both leaflets and hence regurgitation.

The 'Annulus'

Much is made of the notion of an encircling structure around the orifice of the mitral valve that is termed the annulus. The orifice of the valve lies at the atrioventricular junction and the valve leaflets form an integral part of this. There is condensation of fibrous tissue particularly at the trigones, more so in the anterolateral one. This forms part of the fibrous skeleton of the heart and in some species, such as the dog, is commonly calcified forming the *Os Cordis*. The atrioventricular origin of the mitral valve is commonly referred to as the annulus, in such a way so as to imply that it exists as a definitive

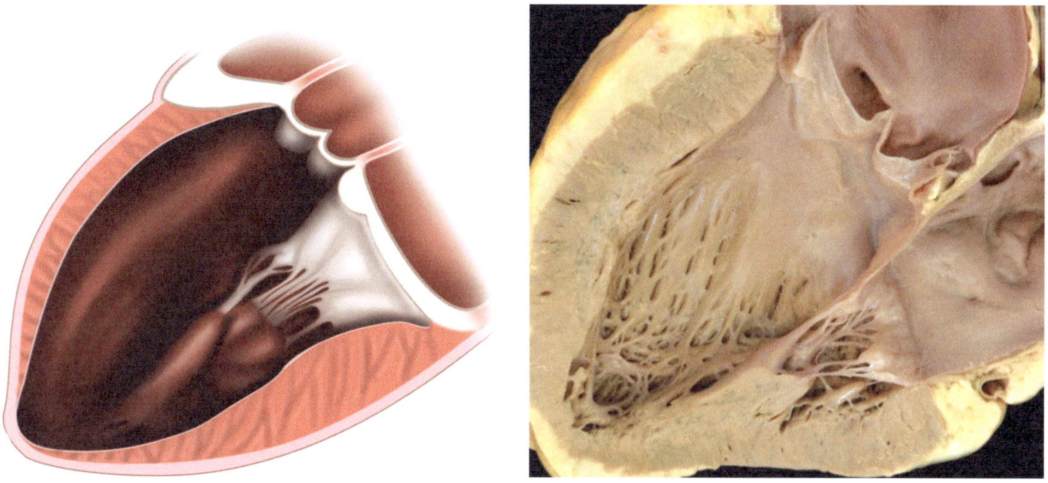

Fig. 1.15 Cross-section long-axis view of the left ventricle demonstrating the inflow and outflow chambers are separated by the anterior mitral valve leaflet. (Photographical image reproduced with permission from Dr. Robert Anderson)

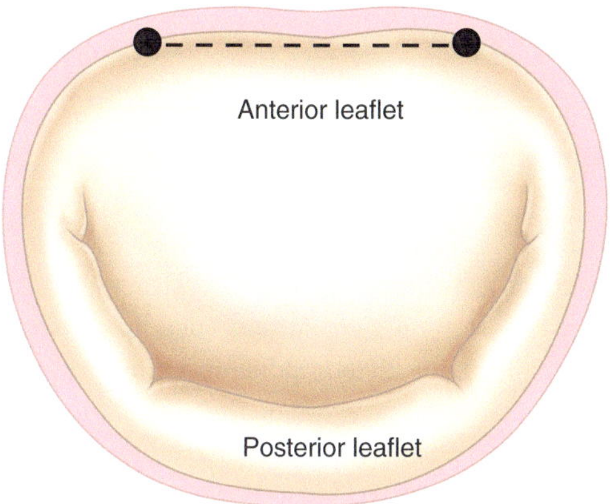

Fig. 1.16 Hinge point of the anterior mitral valve leaflet along a line between the two fibrous trigones

structure. In fact, the only parts of the atrioventricular margin of the valve that reliably contains a fibrous skeleton are the two trigones and a variable extension from the anterolateral trigone along the superior aspect of the valve, as far as the first part of the posterior leaflet. The extension of fibrous tissue along the perimeter of the mitral valve is very variable but can only reliably be found for up to one third of the circumference. There may be islands of scattered fibrous tissue around the orifice but certainly not enough to allow the description of a definite and reproducible entity. For most of the ventricular circumference, there is simply a fat pad with initially the circumflex coronary artery and latterly the coronary sinus. Beyond that point in the majority of valves, there is just a fat pad filling in the gap between the epicardium and the atrioventricular junction (Fig. 1.17).

Within this space lies a part of the circumflex coronary artery superiorly and a part of the coronary sinus inferiorly (Fig. 1.18).

Anteriorly is the junction with the membranous septum. In close proximity to the right fibrous trigone is the atrioventricular bundle of conduction tissue. It is very important for the surgeon to be aware of these relationships to minimize the chance of damaging them when placing sutures for annuloplasty rings or valve prostheses.

The mitral leaflet consists of four distinct histological layers (Fig. 1.19), which are covered by a layer of endothelial cells that are continuous with the endothelial cells of the atrium and the ventricle.

(a) Atrialis – which is the uppermost layer that lies adjacent to the left atrium and is composed of elastic and collagen fibres
(b) Spongiosa layer – which consists of collagen, elastic fibres and an extracellular matrix of proteoglycans and glycosaminglycans

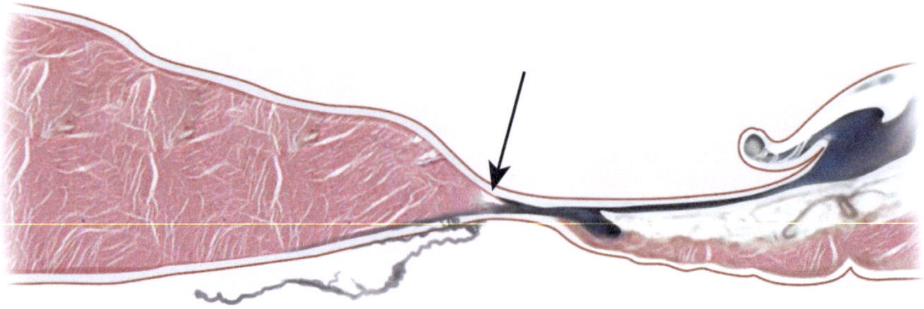

Fig. 1.17 Histological image demonstrating a fat pad (arrow) in the gap between the epicardium and the atrioventricular junction

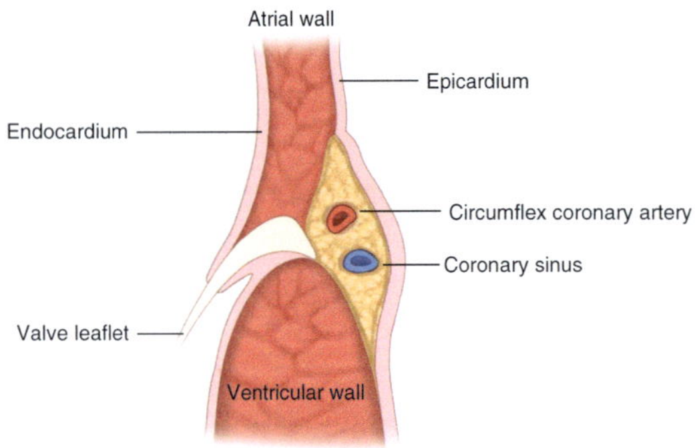

Fig. 1.18 Circumflex coronary artery and coronary sinus lying at the atrioventricular junction

(c) Fibrosa layer – which consists of dense collagen and represents the major load-bearing layer
(d) Ventricularis – which is the lowermost layer adjacent to the left ventricle and contains collagen and elastic fibres

The important structures that are related to the orifice have already been discussed. The most important thing about the atrioventricular orifice is that it is normally highly dynamic and constantly alters in size and shape considerably throughout the cardiac cycle. The orifice area can change by up to 40% between systole and diastole. In addition, the planar shape alters considerably. There is an inherent saddle shape to the anterior leaflet and septal annulus that is formed by the pressurised blood in the outflow tract behind it. The surface area of the anterior leaflet has accommodated this atrial bowing. If the septal portion is flattened out with a complete rigid ring that does not accommodate this form, the coaptation surface at the commissure will be irregular and can produce regurgitation.

There are many types of annuloplasty rings many of which impose an unnatural shape on the annulus. A fuller discussion of this subject will follow in Chap. 6.

Abnormal Anatomy

In reviewing the normal anatomy of the mitral valve, the enormous potential for structural variation is clear. Yet normal and sustainable function relies upon all components being properly formed and properly aligned. Any or all components of the valve can deviate from the ideal for optimal function. This enormous complexity means therefore that the lines between what can be regarded as normal and abnormal anatomy are easily blurred.

Surgeons operating upon the valve encounter a malfunctioning unit. We do not operate upon normal valves! In addition, we have been taught that the valve has been subject to a disease process that has altered the structural integrity of the valve. If the normally functioning valve is compared with those that we regularly see, we find some frequently occurring structural differences. Closer inspection reveals that these lesions probably originate from the embryological development.

Before considering this further, it is perhaps a help to get a clearer understanding of the valve as a load-bearing structure sharing the forces of

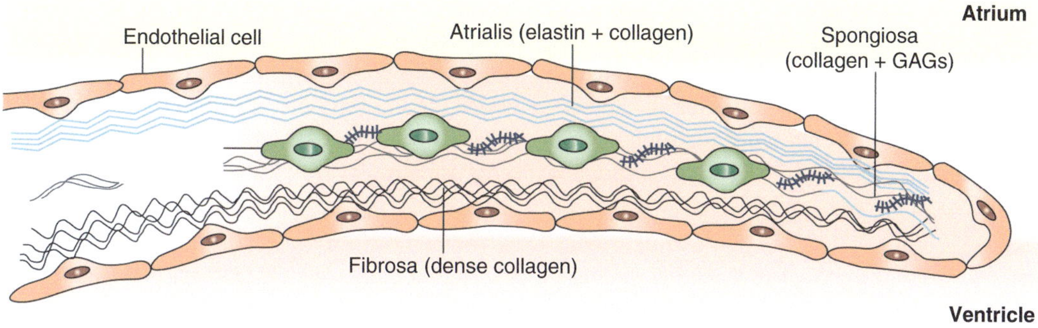

Fig. 1.19 Histological layers of the mitral valve leaflet. *GAGs* glycosaminoglycans. (Reproduced with permission from Levine et al. Mitral valve disease – morphology and mechanisms. Nat Rev Cardiol. 2015;12(12):689–710)

systole with the rest of the ventricle. If the leaflets of the valve and their supporting chords are seen as a 'force field', then the structures begin to take on a relevance that simple anatomical description fails to achieve. The use of the term force field in this context refers to a surface that is distributing the forces applied to the surface so as to achieve minimal energy at every point. Where this is not possible, the surface is strengthened with increased thickness and the array of connective tissue condensation that spreads the load. A review of the anatomy in these terms follows but first let us remind ourselves that the valve has to serve two functions. The first is to allow ventricular filling with the minimum of impedance and the second is to prevent backflow during systole. To achieve the perfect balance between these two diametrically opposed actions within a fully flexible context is a true wonder of nature and biological evolution.

Optimal ventricular filling under all physiological conditions requires a big dynamic flux in the shape and size of the orifice, as well as the complex interaction with ventricular and atrial motion, all beyond the scope of this book. Ventricular emptying requires a stable and resilient platform preventing the retrograde egress of blood. The forces that the valve experiences in this phase of the cardiac cycle are the greatest that the heart can generate.

Let us examine the features of the valve that are key to these functions that lead to problems if not perfectly formed. First, the features that allow maximum flow through the valve. These can be listed as the dynamic and flexible nature of the orifice (annulus), the presence of clefts in the posterior leaflet and the leaflet morphology that allows rapid opening. With ventricular filling, the orifice is capable of opening to a surface area that is greater than the surface area of the fully closed valve. This depends upon the absence of a rigid annular structure, the presence of clefts and the very long commissure. Without clefts, the opening would be relatively more restricted and the valve could only open as far as the down-folding of the leaflets would allow. With the clefts and the flexible annulus, the orifice can dilate as well as the leaflets falling open. Hence, clefts that are up to 30–40% of the depth of the leaflet are normal. In failing regurgitant valves with posterior leaflet prolapse, however, it is almost the rule to find clefts that extend all the way to the annulus. This is a congenital lesion, as the chordae can be seen to extend to the base of the cleft. Put plainly, the valve has developed in this way. In the classical mid-portion prolapse (P2) of the posterior leaflet, the regurgitant part of the posterior leaflet usually has a deep cleft on either side of the lesion. If we now return to the idea of the closed and pressurised valve as a force field that is designed to spread the load evenly, it can be seen clearly that this interruption of posterior leaflet continuity will isolate the vulnerable segment, preventing it from properly sharing the stress imposed upon it. In the normal load sharing arrangement, the force per unit area is the same throughout the valve. Load is passed from the anterior to the posterior leaflet by the end commissural bridging leaflets. The commissural chords that are shortest and most abundant in this area support these load sharing bridging leaflets. The net effect of complete interruption of the posterior leaflet by complete clefts is to unevenly load this area of the valve that inevitably will cause the leaflet to stretch. Long-term excessive load may cause the leaflet to thicken with disruption of collagen and mucoid deposition. These are the hallmarks of myxomatous degeneration. The associated chords will stretch and may eventually rupture.

In addition, this area of prolapse, most commonly P2/P3, overlies the portion of the annulus that is unsupported. The dilating effect of volume overload that accompanies the chronic valve regurgitation will cause this portion of the ventricular wall to stretch, worsening coaptation of this part of the commissure. Reduced coaptation leads to a further reduction of leaflet support.

It is also common to find that the prolapsing portion is commonly obtended by chordae from each papillary muscle head. If the papillary muscles are widely separated one from the other, which is commonly the case, the chords obtend an obtuse angle to the leaflets rather than a more acute one, thereby increasing the strain upon them. As regurgitation develops, further distraction of papillary muscle heads will occur, thereby worsening the situation.

All of these factors create a situation that reduces the ability of the posterior leaflet to withstand strain over many years. This is likely to be why, in the majority of cases, patients present with significant mitral regurgitation later in life.

The majority of lesions occurs at the P2/P3 region of the mural leaflet but can occur at the P1 region, next to the anterolateral end of the commissure. If this is the case, then there is almost always a deep cleft between P1 and P2, and the bridging leaflet at the anterolateral commissure is abnormally narrow. This arrangement mimics the most common findings at P2/P3. If there are multiple areas of prolapse, then multiple clefts of varying depth are commonly found.

In some valves with posterior leaflet prolapse, there may be only one complete cleft, usually to the left of the prolapsing area from the surgeon's viewpoint. In this situation, there is usually a quite abnormal posteromedial papillary muscle. It is common to find multiple heads to the papillary muscle that are commonly very highly placed in the ventricle. It is also common to find that the proximate P3 area of the leaflet is markedly shallow. These structural variations lead to reduced support for the isolated segment.

The patients who have the anatomical variant 'Barlow's valve' have very exaggerated anatomical variation from the norm. Multiple deep clefts are found in both the posterior and anterior leaflets. This has the effect of rendering the valve into multiple series of isolated segments that cannot load share. It is likely then that the process described above are amplified throughout the valve leading to the complex lesions found in this condition.

The Leaflets

There are two principal leaflets, the aortic (commonly referred to as the anterior leaflet but with strict reference to the defined anatomical planes is antero-inferior) and the mural (similarly styled the posterior leaflet but lies in the postero-superior plane) leaflets. The posterior leaflet has a series of clefts in its leading edge. These usually coincide with the junction of the leaflet when divided into thirds. Carpentier proposed this in his functional characterisation of the posterior leaflet into P1, P2 and P3 segments (Fig. 1.20).

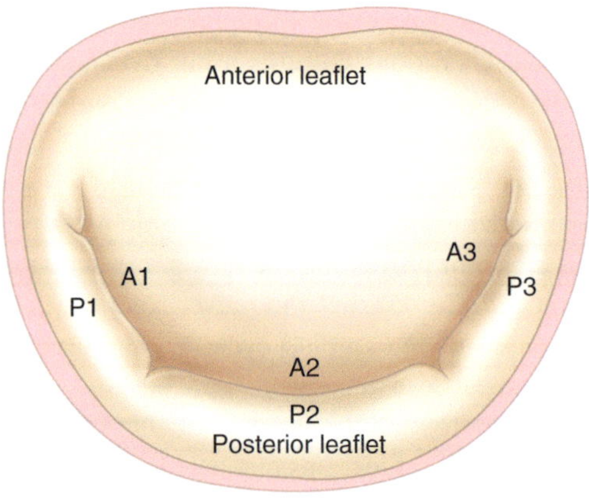

Fig. 1.20 Mitral valve leaflets

This is helpful to cardiologists and surgeons who communicate over valve anatomy. Whilst very useful, it is not strictly correct, as the clefts (indentations in the leaflet) are quite variable in placement and depth (Fig. 1.21). These clefts (indentations) are present to allow maximal ease of opening of the leaflets rather like the use of pleats in a long skirt that allows opening of the material for free movement of the legs in striding out. They also mark the end of outward growth and development of the leaflets as they mature from the foetal atrio-ventricular cushions. Hence, the variability in their depth and number reveals the variability in their embryological genesis. Unlike the normal mitral valve, the clefts in regurgitant valves commonly extend to the atrio-ventricular orifice or annulus. The implications of this will be discussed in the section on the morbid anatomy of the valve.

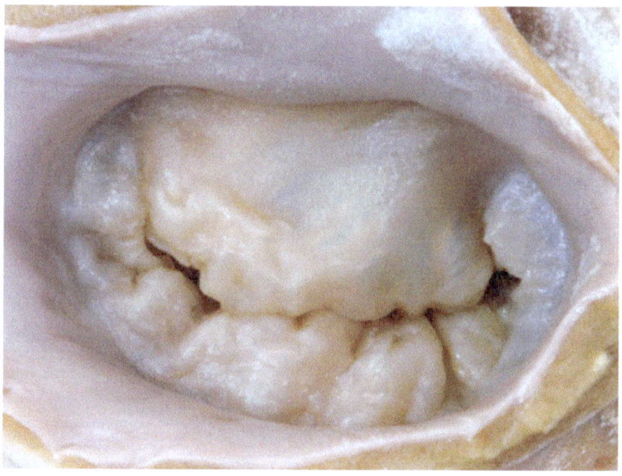

Fig. 1.21 Variable placement and depth of the clefts and indentations in the mitral valve leaflets. (Reproduced with permission from Dr. Robert Anderson)

The posterior leaflet has the greatest surface area by virtue of the fact that it is significantly longer than the anterior leaflet. Its length from the junction with the anterior leaflet at the anterolateral and the posteromedial commissures represents approximately two-thirds of the circumference of the valve orifice. The anterior leaflet is roughly the shape of a broad semi-ellipse with its base being continuous with the septum.

The leaflets are supported by the tendinous chords that arise from the papillary muscle projections of the left ventricular trabecular muscle. On either side of the leading edge, there are strut chords from each of the principal papillary muscle heads. Their distribution will be described later.

The continuous line of coaptation between the two leaflets is called the commissure (Fig. 1.22).

The commissures do not reach the annulus but have bridging leaflets that are usually 5–10 mm in height. The anterior and posterior leaflets continue with each other at the lateral limits of the commissures. These bridging leaflets serve to allow the sharing of the systolic load between the leaflets, thereby ensuring lateral competence of the valve. These bridging leaflets are often incorrectly referred to as the commissures and this practice is unlikely to change.

The overall shape of the valve in ventricular systole tends towards a 'D' shape with the anterolateral to posteromedial length being

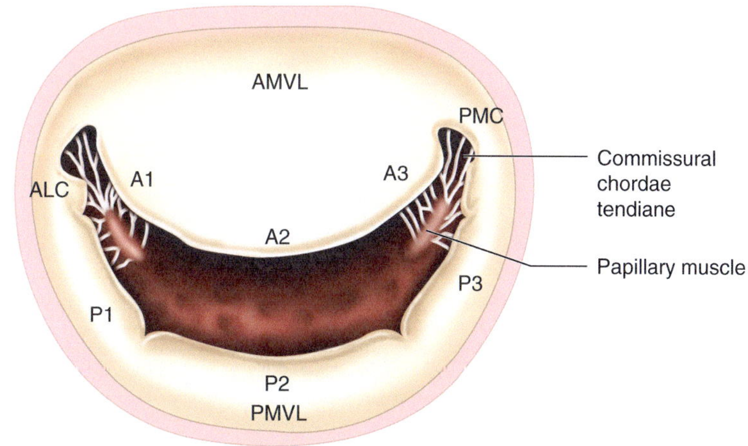

Fig. 1.22 Anterolateral and posteromedial commissures of the mitral valve, with attached commissural chords. AMVL anterior mitral valve leaflet, PMVL posterior mitral valve leaflet, ALC anterolateral commissure, PMC posteromedial commissure

longest at a ratio of 3:4. The leaflets quite frequently have uneven marginal heights. In some valves, the commissural margin of the anterior leaflet will not approximate to a smooth curve but will have parts that project further than the expected curve and matching these projections where they occur will be a reciprocal deficiency in the posterior leaflet. This anomaly is usually to be found this way around but sometimes, there will be advancement of the posterior leaflet and foreshortening of the anterior leaflet. This natural balancing of surfaces should be acknowledged when repairing the valve as if this relationship is ignored, unnatural coaptation may result with a persistence in regurgitation or the creation of a newly regurgitant area.

The circumference of the valve has many important structures arranged around it (Fig. 1.23).

The trigones are condensations of fibrous tissue and form part of the fibrous skeleton of the heart. The left trigone lies' above the anterolateral commissural extremity and is related to the non-coronary leaflet of the aortic valve. It is important to bear this in mind when placing annuloplasty or valve sutures in this area as the aortic valve may be damaged by too deep placement. In a clockwise direction, the anterior leaflet is in continuity

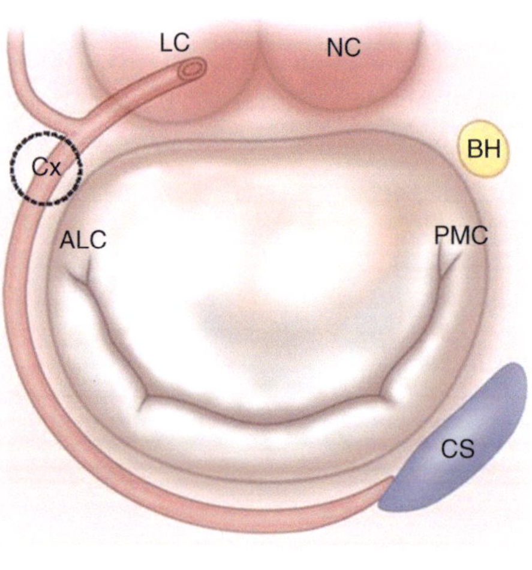

Fig. 1.23 Anatomical relations of the mitral valve orifice. NC non-coronary sinus, LC left coronary sinus, Cx circumflex coronary artery, ALC anterolateral commissure, PMC posteromedial commissure, CS coronary sinus, BH bundle of His

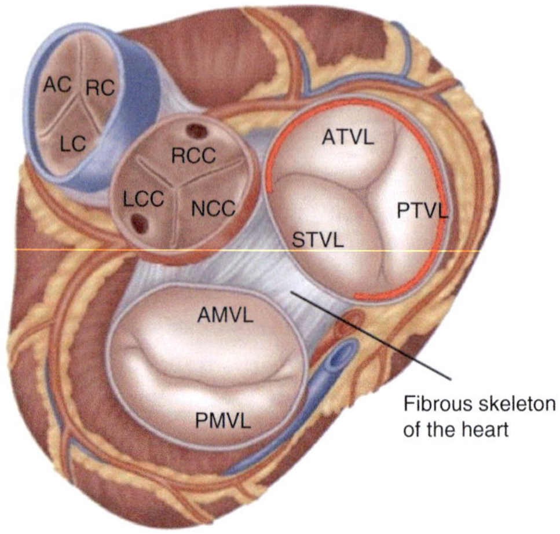

Fig. 1.24 Fibrous skeleton of the heart. AC anterior cusp of the pulmonary valve, LC left cusp of the pulmonary valve, RC right cusp of the pulmonary valve, NCC non-coronary cusp of the aortic valve, LCC left coronary cusp of the aortic valve, RCC right coronary cusp of the aortic valve, AMVL anterior mitral valve leaflet, PMVL posterior mitral valve leaflet, ATVL anterior tricuspid valve leaflet, PTVL posterior tricuspid valve leaflet, STVL septal tricuspid valve leaflet

with the aorto-mitral curtain, a fibro-membranous sheet of continuity forming one third of the left ventricular outflow tract. The atrioventricular node lies close to the right fibrous trigone above the posteromedial commissural extension. Again, deep misplacement of sutures in this area will result in heart block. The left or superior fibrous trigone forms the centre of the fibrous skeleton of the heart that links the base of the aorta, the atria and the ventricles together (Fig. 1.24).

Embryological Development of the Atrioventricular Valves

The heart begins to form at the stage that simple diffusion of nutrients and removal of waste products can no longer support the organism. Thus, it is the first organ in the forming foetus to function. The first indication of valve formation is when endocardial cushions form in the outflow tract and the atrioventricular canal regions of the primitive heart tube. The initial endocardial cushions function as valves to drive unidirectional flow in the primitive heart tube. The development of the

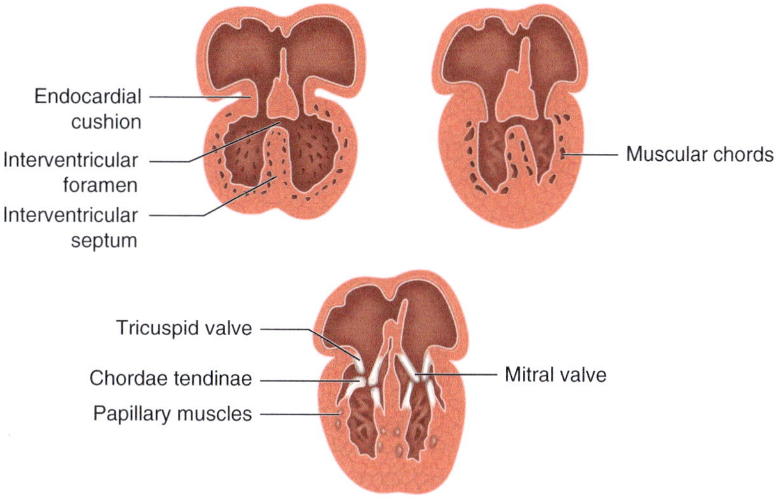

Fig. 1.25 Embryological development of the atrioventricular cushions

tissue of the valve leaflet involves complex signalling mechanisms, inducing epithelial to mesenchymal transformation. Valve leaflet formation is characterised by thinning and elongation of the valve primordia, as well as the remodelling of the extracellular matrix into layers rich in elastin, fibrillar collagen and proteoglycans. It is thought that the atrioventricular cushions develop as rounded projections, which link up at their bases as the leaflets extend (Fig. 1.25).

It is easy to imagine how the evolving leaflets will develop the clefts in their leading edges as they progress when the thinning and extension of the leaflets is uneven. The deep clefts seen in the regurgitant posterior leaflets can easily be explained by insufficient growth at those points. This also explains the presence of the chordal attachments to the base of the clefts which have not grown up.

As the leaflets are developing, the papillary muscles are being formed from the trabecular ventricular myocardium and form into discrete muscle groups, the papillary muscle heads. Again, as this process is such a complex system of signalling and tissue response, it is not surprising to find variations in the result.

All the time, these structures are developing under the stresses and strains of the functioning heart tube. Valve tissue experiences exceptionally high strain because the tissues cycle from a completely loaded state into a completely unloaded one with each and every heartbeat. These changing, deforming forces result in compensatory changes in the cellular matrix. Over the average lifetime, the heart beats approximately three billion times handling 5 litres of blood per minute or in excess of 210 million litres of blood!

It is not at all surprising therefore that valve failure will result from an underlying predisposing genotype and valve malformation that alters the response to physiological stresses. The long-held appreciation of age-related degeneration and latent valve disease almost certainly represents subtle defects in valvular tissue development and maintenance as regulated by developmental pathways.

The most common lesion in patients with mitral valve prolpase is of P2 prolapse. In these patients with fibro-elastic deficiency, the bluish thinned areas of the valve (the anterior leaflet and the P1 and P3 regions of the posterior leaflet) are are not commonly prolapsing. The prolpased P2 region is thickened and stretched. This suggests that there must be an additional factor in play in patients with this lesion. It is likely that abnormal loading of these areas gives rise to the histological changes that are found in these cases that represent a tissue response to excess force in the region. This finding suggests that abnormal structural development is an important component of the disease process.

The Relationship with the Left Atrium and Ventricle

Put most simply, the mitral valve is the door-way from the left atrium to the left ventricle and if the leaflets are the leaves of that door, the annulus is the very flexible door-frame. As such, it bears the origins of the muscle of both the base of the left ventricle and the left atrium. Excessive stretching of these chambers will have a pull on the orifice of the valve, which in turn will disturb the alignment of the leaflets.

Chronic atrial fibrillation causes the atria to stretch and its volume to increase. Blood has significant mass and as the volume increases the mass of blood increases, the weight of which pulls upwards and outwards on the annulus causing malapposition of the leaflets and mitral regurgitation.

A significant number of patients with orifice dilatation are as a result of this mechanism. The use of an appropriately sized annuloplasty ring will restore competence of the valve. Reduction of left atrial mass by excising part of the posterior wall may also contribute to longer term stability.

Patients with dilated cardiomyopathy can also present with orifice dilatation but in these cases as a result of ventricular muscle distortion and distraction of the papillary muscles. This is particularly exaggerated in ischaemic cardiomyopathy. In these patients, the problem will be addressed by rectifying the lesions which may include papillary muscle repositioning and/or annuloplasty ring insertion. These conditions will be considered in more detail later.

Summary

The mitral valve is a complex structure that functions like a machine to both control flow of blood through the heart and to support the left ventricle. The complexity of embryonic formation, much of which is poorly understood, gives room for multiple congenital abnormalities in various combinations and leads to a structure, which is unable to bear the stresses that are loaded on it throughout a normal lifespan. This can lead to the development of a regurgitant valve at almost any time in a person's life dependent upon the severity of the lesions. Recognition of this aetiological pathway can be very helpful in sorting out the appropriate method of reconstruction of the valve to give the best results.

Recommended Reading

Angelini A, Ho SY, Anderson RH, Davies MJ, Becker AE. A histological study of the atrioventricular junction in hearts with normal and prolapsed leaflets of the mitral valve. Br Heart J. 1988;59(6):712–6.

Buckberg G1, Hoffman JI, Mahajan A, Saleh S, Coghlan C. Cardiac mechanics revisited: the relationship of cardiac architecture to ventricular function. Circulation. 2008;118(24):2571–87.

Hinton R, Yutzey E. Heart valve structure and function in development and disease. Annu Rev Physiol. 2011;73:29–46.

Ho SY. Anatomy and myo-architecture of the left ventricular wall in normal and in disease. Eur J Echocardiogr. 2009;10(8):iii3–7.

Levack MM, Jassar AS, Shang EK, Vergnat M, Woo YJ, Acker MA, Jackson BM, Gorman JH 3rd, Gorman RC. Three-dimensional echocardiographic analysis of the mitral annular dynamics. Implications for annuloplasty selection. Circulation. 2012;126(suppl 1):S183–8.

Levine RA, Hagége AA, Judge DP, Padala M, Dal-Bianco JP, Aikawa E, Beaudoin J, Bischoff J, Bouatia-Naji N, Bruneval P, Butcher JT, Carpentier A, Chaput M, Chester AH11, Clusel C, Delling FN, Dietz HC, Dina C, Durst R, Fernandez-Friera L, Handschumacher MD, Jensen MO, Jeunemaitre XP, Le Marec H, Le Tourneau T14, Markwald RR, Mérot J, Messas E, Milan DP, Neri T, Norris RA, Peal D, Perrocheau M, Probst V, Pucéat M, Rosenthal N, Solis J, Schott JJ, Schwammenthal E, Slaugenhaupt SA, Song JK, Yacoub MH. Leducq mitral transatlantic network. Mitral valve disease – morphology and mechanisms. Nat Rev Cardiol. 2015;12(12):689–710.

Lillehei CW, Levy MJ, Bonnabeau RC. Mitral valve replacement with preservation of papillary muscles and chordae tendinae. J Thorac Cardiovasc Surg. 1964;47:532–43.

Ring L, Rana BS, Ho SY, Wells FC. The prevalence and impact of deep clefts in the mitral leaflets in mitral valve prolapse. Eur Heart J Cardiovasc Imaging. 2013;14(6):595–602.

Ring L, Rana BS, Wells FC, Kydd AC, Dutka DP. Atrial function as a guide to timing of intervention in mitral valve prolapse with mitral regurgitation. JACC Cardiovasc Imaging. 2014;7(3):225–32.

Echocardiography of the Mitral and Tricuspid Valves

2

Keywords
Trans-thoracic echocardiography · Trans-oesophageal echocardiography · Doppler · Three-dimensional echocardiography · M-mode echocardiography · Vena contracta · Proximal isovelocity surface area (PISA) · Apical views · Parasternal views · Mid-oesophageal views · Trans-gastric views

Introduction

Normal function of the mitral valve depends on the complex interaction between the leaflets, annulus, subvalvular apparatus (chordae tendineae and papillary muscles) and left ventricle. Echocardiography is the imaging technique of choice to systematically demonstrate anatomical, physiological and pathological aspects of the entire mitral valve complex. It assesses the mitral valve in the beating heart under physiologic loading conditions, as opposed to surgical assessment that is performed on the arrested heart. In addition, quantitative analysis can be performed on frozen frames throughout the cardiac cycle.

Echocardiography is invaluable in the clinical management of mitral valve disease as a non-invasive, readily available investigation that can be used to provide an understanding of the aetiology, lesion and mechanism of valve dysfunction; quantify the severity of valve disease; guide decision-making regarding the timing of intervention; determine the feasibility and give predictors of surgical repair; provide a roadmap for the repair procedure; and assess the completeness of the surgical procedure intra-operatively and post-operatively to determine if any additional intervention is required.

Echocardiography has evolved greatly over the years and has been a major contributor to the technical advances made in mitral valve repair surgery. Most recently, three-dimensional trans-oesophageal echocardiography has been developed, thereby allowing visualisation of the mitral valve from any spatial point of view in real time, especially the left atrial 'en-face' view that replicates the surgical view. Echocardiographical segmental analysis allows the location of mitral valve pathology to be clearly communicated.

The severity of functional MR has been shown to decrease under the effects of general anaesthesia compared with the preoperative state. General anaesthesia alters the haemodynamic loading of the left ventricle by affecting preload, contractility and afterload. In view of this, intra-operative quantification of functional MR should be made with caution and haemodynamic conditions should be optimised with fluid administration and vasoconstrictors to increase the preload and afterload, respectively to replicate the haemodynamic condition of an awake non-anaesthetised patient.

N. Moorjani et al., *Operative Mitral and Tricuspid Valve Surgery*,
https://doi.org/10.1007/978-1-4471-4204-1_2

Echocardiographic Anatomy of the Mitral Valve

Mitral Valve Leaflets

The mitral valve consists of anterior and posterior leaflets, which are normally thin (<5 mm thickness), pliable structures. The thicker, semicircular anterior leaflet covers two-thirds of the height of the mitral valve orifice but is attached anteriorly to only one-third of the mitral valve annulus. Conversely, the crescent-shaped posterior leaflet covers one-third of the height of the mitral valve orifice but is attached posteriorly to two-thirds of the mitral valve annulus.

The leaflets are divided into two zones, including the coaptation zone, which is thicker, rougher and more nodular, and the membranous zone, which is smooth and translucent, and represents the base of the leaflet that can be seen with the en-face view of the valve from the atrium in systole (typically referred to as the surgical view). The total area of the leaflets is approximately twice as large as the valve thereby providing valve competency by allowing the excess leaflet tissue to coapt in the zone of apposition, with the depth of coaptation usually approximately 1 cm. This allows enough leaflet tissue overlap to maintain competency withstanding the chordal tethering forces during systole. Reduction in the zone of apposition increases the likelihood of valve incompetence and progressive regurgitation. The leaflets converge at the anterolateral and posteromedial commissures.

The posterior leaflet is usually divided by indentations into three scallops, whereas the anterior leaflet is usually continuous without scallops. Normally, the indentations do not reach the annulus and are present during diastole but closed in systole. As opposed to indentations, which span <50% of the leaflet height, clefts span >50% of the leaflet height. The lateral P1 scallop is adjacent to the anterolateral commissure and left atrial appendage, the central P2 scallop is the largest segment and the medial P3 scallop is adjacent to the posteromedial commissure. As the P2 scallop is the largest, it is more prone to systolic load bearing and therefore to pathological prolapse or flail. Although the anterior leaflet does not have as clearly identifiable indentations, it is artificially divided into three segments A1, A2 and A3, corresponding to the P1, P2 and P3 scallops, respectively (Fig. 2.1). The A2 and P2 scallop lengths are best measured in the mid-oesophageal long-axis 3-chamber view (135°), whereas the P1 and P3 scallops are best measured in the mid-oesophageal bicommissural or 2-chamber views.

Mitral Annulus

The mitral annulus is a three-dimensional saddle ellipsoid-shaped structure with the highest points formed by the central part of the anterior and posterior annulus and nadirs at the anterolateral and posteromedial commissures. The non-planar

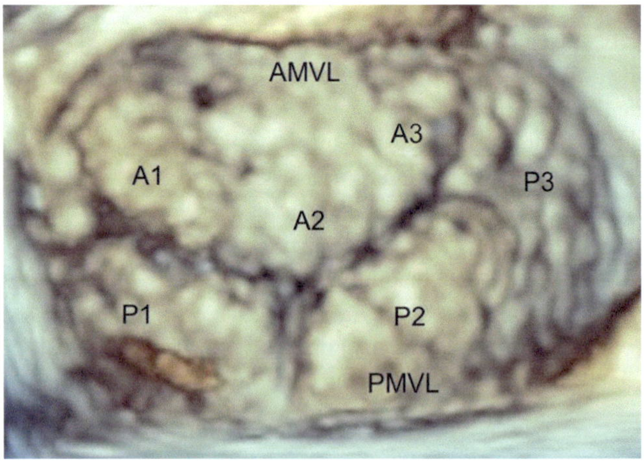

Fig. 2.1 Scallops of the anterior and posterior mitral valve leaflets. AMVL anterior mitral valve leaflet, PMVL posterior mitral valve leaflet

shape of the annulus reduces the mechanical stress on the valve leaflets. The annulus represents the attachment of the mitral valve leaflets at their bases to the atrioventricular junction and fibrous skeleton. The anterior mitral annulus consists mainly of fibrous tissue, is demarcated by the left and right fibrous trigones and is connected to the aortic annulus, at the level of the left and non-coronary sinuses, via the aorto-mitral curtain. Although both the anterior and posterior parts of the annulus can dilate, the posterior annulus is less fibrotic and is more muscular and membranous than the anterior annulus, and hence likely to dilate to a greater extent.

The anteroposterior distance (minor axis) is approximately three-fourth of the inter-commissural distance (major axis). The anteroposterior distance (minor axis) can be measured in the trans-thoracic parasternal long-axis or trans-oesophageal mid-oesophageal long-axis views and the inter-commissural distance (major axis) can be measured directly during in the mid-oesophageal bicommissural view. Annular dilatation is defined as an end-systolic anteroposterior annular diameter >35 mm or an end-diastolic annular to anterior leaflet length ratio >1.3. The annulus undergoes complex conformational changes during the cardiac cycle, secondary to atrial and ventricular contraction and changes in intra-cardiac pressures. This normal motion and contraction of the mitral annulus contributes to valvular competence, with the annular area decreasing by 20–40% in mid- systole.

Chordae Tendineae

The chordae tendineae attach the mitral leaflets to the papillary muscles, creating a dynamic interaction between the mitral valve and the left ventricular wall. They consist of fibrous tissue and provide a suspension system for the mitral valve, determining the tension and position of the leaflets at the end of systole. The chordae are classified according to their site of insertion on the leaflets, with marginal (primary) chordae inserted on the free edge of the leaflets, intermediate (secondary) chordae on the rough zone of the ventricular surface of the leaflets and basal (tertiary) chordae on the base of the posterior leaflet only. There are usually over 100 primary chordae arising from over 25 chordal trunks that act to prevent prolapse of the leaflet margin, thereby maintaining leaflet coaptation. The secondary chordae allow limited bulging of the leaflet body, thereby reducing leaflet tension. The strut chords are thicker secondary chords attached to the body of the anterior leaflet and are part of the ventriculo-valvular fibrous loop, which is important in maintaining the aorto-mitral angle, as well as normal left ventricular geometry and function.

Papillary Muscles

The papillary muscles originate from the left ventricular wall and are divided into two groups. The anterolateral papillary muscle is the largest, arises from a single trabecularised insertion (body) on the apicolateral third of the myocardium and usually has two heads (anterior and posterior), whereas the posteromedial papillary muscle arises from multiple trabecularised insertions (bodies) on the middle third of the inferior wall and has three heads (anterior, intermediate and posterior). Chordae tendineae that originate from the anterolateral papillary muscle attach to the lateral half of the anterior (A1 and part of A2) and posterior (P1 and part of P2) leaflets, whereas the chordae tendineae that originate from the posteromedial papillary muscle attach to the medial half of the anterior (A3 and part of A2) and posterior (P3 and part of P2) leaflets. The commissures receive chordae only from their corresponding papillary muscles located beneath. During ventricular systole, the papillary muscles and adjacent myocardium contract to prevent prolapse of the mitral leaflets by increasing tension on the chordae tendineae.

Functional Mitral Anatomy

In the absence of pathology, the mitral leaflets open during diastole to allow ventricular filling and close during systole to prevent regurgitation.

When the mitral valve is closed, the coaptation line represents the contact between the leaflets on the atrial side of the leaflets (Fig. 2.2a) and the coaptation length represents the overlap between the leaflets from the tips to the coaptation line, with a coaptation length of >8 mm considered ideal for valvular competency (Fig. 2.2b). The coaptation distance or tenting height represents the distance from the coaptation point to mitral annular plane in mid-systole and should be <10 mm (Fig. 2.2c). The tenting area represents the triangular-shaped space between the mitral annular plane, the leaflet surfaces and the coaptation line, and should be <1.0 cm^2 (Fig. 2.2c). The anterior and posterior angles are measured between the mitral annular plane and the anterior and posterior mitral leaflets, respectively, and can be assessed at the level of A1-P1, A2-P2 or A3-P3 (Fig. 2.2d).

Leaflet motion is usually categorised as normal (leaflets reach annular plane), excessive (leaflet displaced beyond annular plane) or restricted (leaflet do not reach annular plane). Excessive leaflet motion can be further sub-classified as billowing, prolapse or flail (Fig. 2.3). Billowing represents systolic bulging of the leaflet body (but not the tip) into the atrium above the annular plane but with preserved coaptation of the leaflet free edge. Prolapse represents displacement of the coaptation point >2 mm above the annular plane into the atrium. On TTE, this should be identified on parasternal long-axis or apical 3-chamber but not the apical 4-chamber view, because the saddle-shape of the annulus may result in a false positive diagnosis. Flail represents displacement of the leaflet edge above the annular plane with systolic reversal of the leaflet tip towards the left atrium (compared to prolapse where the leaflet

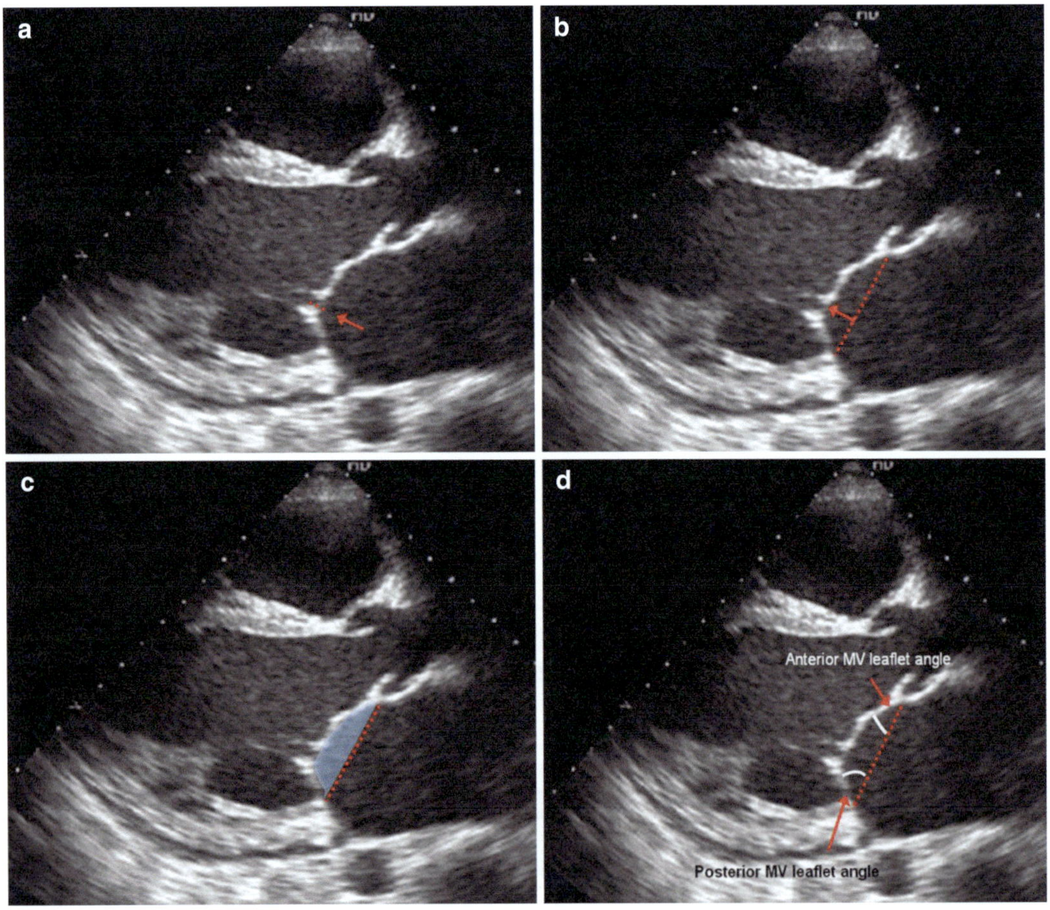

Fig. 2.2 Echocardiographical images demonstrating the (**a**) coaptation length; (**b**) tenting height; (**c**) tenting area; and (**d**) anterior and posterior angles. MV mitral valve

tip points towards the left ventricle), as there is chordal detachment from the ventricular wall. It is usually associated with chordal (or papillary muscle) rupture.

'Restricted' motion represents leaflet tissue that is fixed and does not reach the annular plane during systole.

The different types of mitral regurgitation have been classified according leaflet motion (Fig. 2.4). Type I dysfunction represents a mitral valve with normal leaflet motion but regurgitation caused by annular dilatation (secondary to ventricular or atrial enlargement) or leaflet perforation (secondary to infective endocarditis or trauma), resulting in a

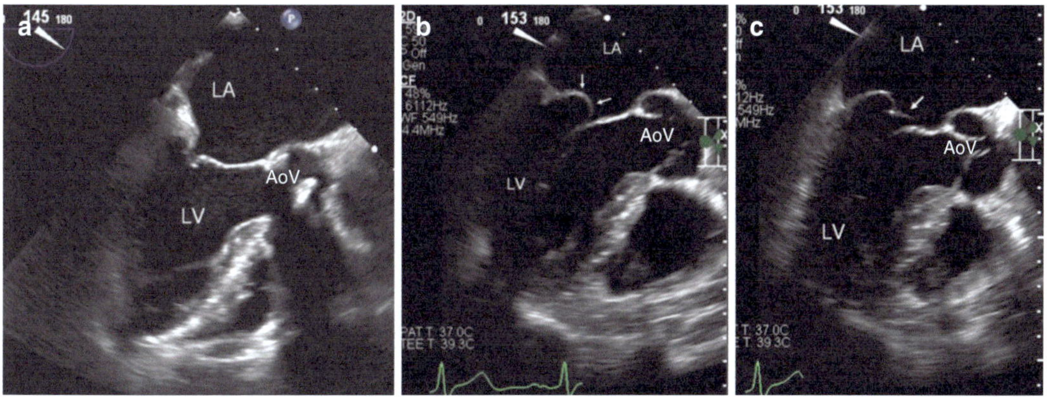

Fig. 2.3 Echocardiographical images demonstrating (**a**) normal leaflet movement; and excessive leaflet motion of the posterior leaflet, sub-classified as (**b**) prolapse and (**c**) flail. LA left atrium, LV left ventricle, AoV aortic valve

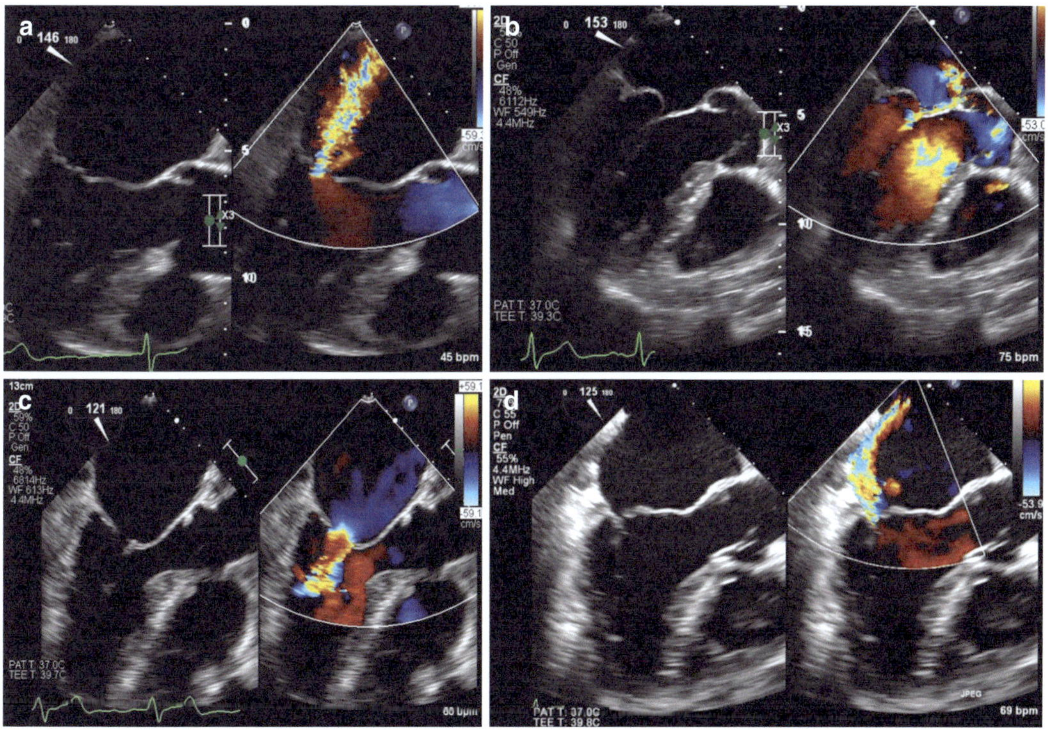

Fig. 2.4 Echocardiographical images demonstrating the functional classification of mitral regurgitation, with (**a**) type I representing normal leaflet motion causing a central regurgitant jet, (**b**) type II representing excessive leaflet motion causing an eccentric regurgitant jet directed away from the lesion, (**c**) type IIIa representing restricted leaflet opening; and (**d**) type IIIb representing restricted leaflet closure causing a central or eccentric jet directed towards the lesion

central regurgitant jet. Type II dysfunction represents a mitral valve with excessive leaflet motion caused by prolapse or a flail leaflet (secondary to chordal elongation or rupture, or papillary muscle rupture), resulting in an eccentric regurgitant jet directed in the opposite direction to the predominant pathology. Type III dysfunction represents a mitral valve with restricted leaflet motion caused by leaflet tethering. Type IIIa is caused by apical displacement of both leaflets (secondary to rheumatic disease or dilated cardiomyopathy) producing restricted leaflet motion in systole and diastole, often resulting in a central regurgitant jet. Type IIIb is caused by lateral displacement of the mitral leaflets (secondary to ischaemic cardiomyopathy) causing restricted leaflet motion in systole, resulting an eccentric regurgitant jet directed in the same direction as the predominant leaflet pathology.

Trans-thoracic Echocardiography

A standard trans-thoracic echocardiographic (TTE) examination of the mitral valve includes an M-mode examination, multiple two-dimensional views and Doppler flow evaluation.

M-Mode Echocardiography

The M-mode assessment is guided from the two-dimensional long- and short-axis views. Normally, the anterior mitral valve leaflet exhibits an M-shaped motion pattern that reflects left ventricular inflow, whilst the posterior mitral valve leaflet exhibits a near mirror image W-shaped motion pattern with a reduced excursion (Fig. 2.5).

The E-point represents the initial opening of the mitral valve at the start of diastole secondary to rapid left ventricular filling. The F-point represents where the mitral valve almost closes during mid-diastole, which reflects the deceleration of ventricular filling secondary to reduction of the pressure gradient between the left ventricle and atrium. The E-F slope hence represents early diastolic closure and usually is >60 mm/s. Despite the fact that the mitral valve is almost closed, there is still passive flow from the pulmonary veins through the left atrium into the ventricle. The A-point represents

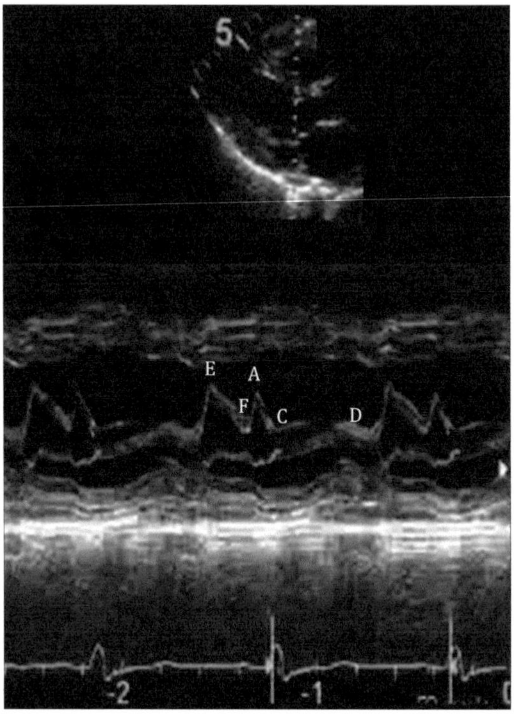

Fig. 2.5 M-mode image of the mitral valve, demonstrating an M-shaped motion pattern of the anterior leaflet and W-shaped motion pattern on the posterior leaflet, with reduced excursion in comparison

the second opening of the mitral valve produced by atrial contraction. The C-point represents final closure of the mitral valve, which occurs secondary to deceleration of atrial inflow and isometric LV contraction. The C-D line represents the leaflet closure line in systole.

In mitral stenosis, the early diastolic closure of the valve (E-F slope) is delayed or abolished, resulting in a slope <10 mm/s (Fig. 2.6). In addition, the motion of the posterior leaflet parallels that of the anterior leaflet, as compared to a normal leaflet where it mirrors the anterior leaflet motion.

Two-Dimensional Trans-thoracic Echocardiographic Views of the Mitral Valve

The mitral valve can be visualised in several different views on 2D trans-thoracic echocardiography, including:

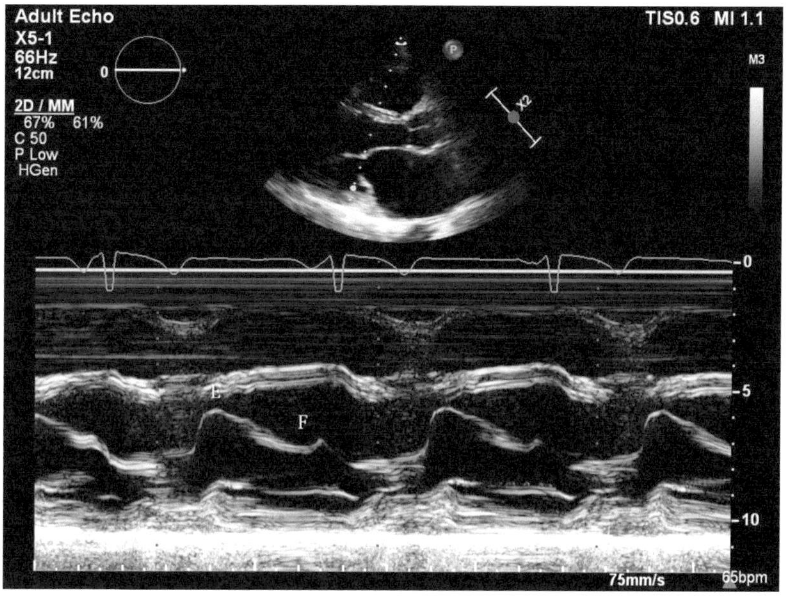

Fig. 2.6 M-mode echocardiography image of mitral stenosis demonstrated by the flat EF slope and paradoxical motion of posterior mitral leaflet

- Parasternal long-axis (PLAX)
- Parasternal short-axis (PSAX)
- Apical 4-chamber (A4C)
- Apical 3-chamber (A3C)
- Apical 2-chamber (A2C)

In order to help appreciate anatomy of the mitral valve relative to surrounding structures, it is important to understand a few constant spatial relations (Fig. 2.7). The aortic valve lies antero-lateral to the mitral valve, with the anterior mitral valve leaflet adjacent to the non-coronary and left coronary cusps of the aortic valve. The left atrial appendage lies superior and lateral to the mitral valve, with A1, P1 and the anterolateral commissure lying in close proximity to the appendage.

Parasternal Long-Axis View (PLAX)

The parasternal long-axis view reveals motion of the mitral valve leaflets in systole and diastole. The thickness and length of the leaflets can be appreciated, with the anterior leaflet longer than the posterior leaflet. Whereas the chordae tendineae can often be seen, the papillary muscles are usually difficult to visualise in this view. In addition, the left atrial diameter and the minor axis (anteroposterior diameter) of the mitral annulus can be measured in this view. Annular dilatation is defined as an annulus diameter >35 mm or when the annulus to anterior leaflet length ratio is >1.3, with both measured in the same image in diastole. In the standard parasternal long-axis view, the A2 and P2 scallops of the mitral valve can be viewed. By tilting the probe superiorly (angulation of the probe towards the aortic valve), the A1 and P1 scallops become visible (Fig. 2.8). Conversely, by tilting the probe inferiorly (angulation of the probe toward the tricuspid valve), the A3 and P3 scallops can be seen.

This view can also be used to measure the leaflet tenting height or coaptation distance (centre of the annular plane to the coaptation point, which is normally ≤10 mm), tenting area (area within the annular plane, coaptation point and leaflets edges), and the anterior and posterior angles (angles between the annulus and the leaflet insertions) (Fig. 2.2).

Parasternal Short-Axis View (PSAX)

The parasternal short-axis view at the level of the mitral valve leaflets demonstrates motion of the anterior and posterior mitral valve leaflets, which resemble an ovoid 'fish-mouth' shape (Fig. 2.9). Planimetry of the mitral valve measured at the level of the leaflet tips in this view is the gold standard for measuring mitral valve area, as it is not as dependent on loading conditions. In diastole, all

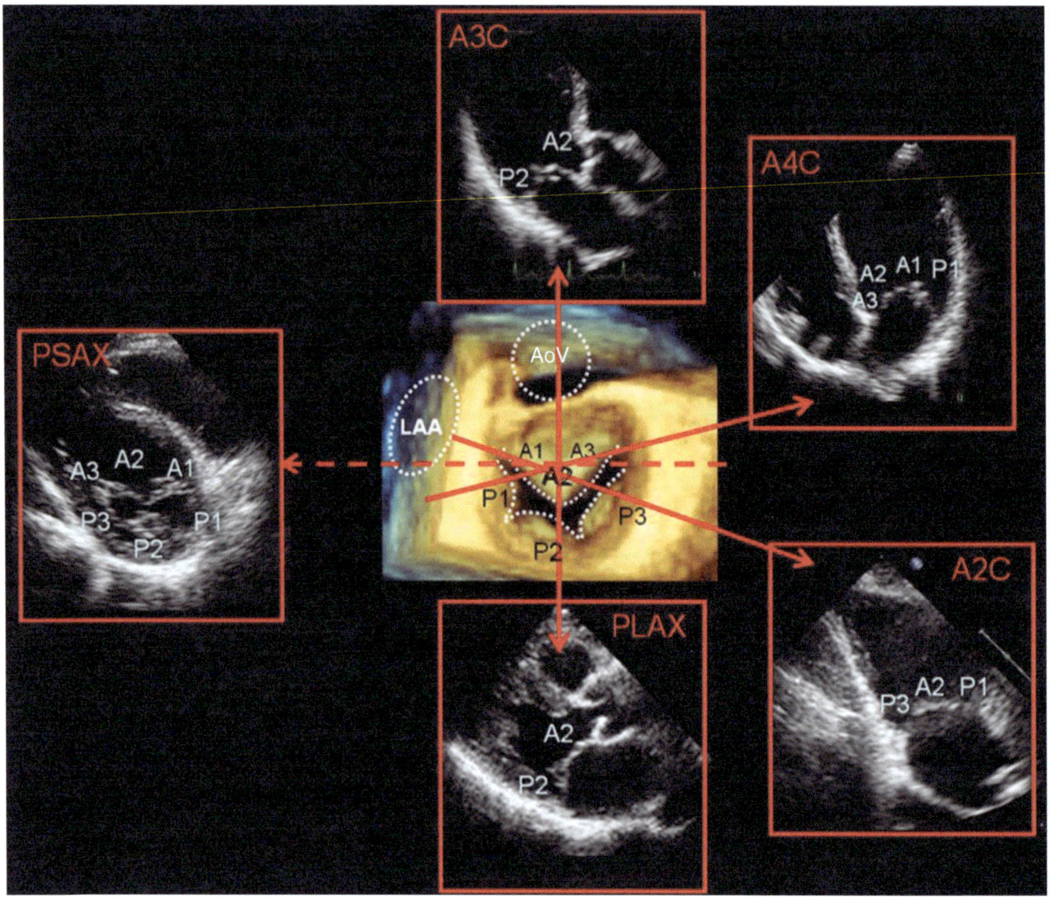

Fig. 2.7 Trans-thoracic echocardiographical views depicting the mitral valve segments. In addition, the spatial anatomical relations of the mitral valve, with the aortic valve (AoV) and left atrial appendage (LAA), can be seen in the central three-dimensional image. A2C apical 2-chamber, A3C apical 3-chamber, A4C apical 4-chamber, PLAX parasternal long-axis, PSAX parasternal short-axis

six scallops can be visualised, as well as separation of the commissures. In systole, any prolapsing or restricted scallop can be identified by analysing the location of the regurgitant jet. As the mitral valve is viewed from the left ventricular aspect, the posteromedial commissure, as well as the P3 and A3 scallops, will be on the left, and the anterolateral commissure, as well as the A1 and P1 scallops, will be on the right. The corresponding trans-gastric short-axis view on trans-oesophageal echocardiography, however, views the mitral valve from the left atrial aspect, and hence the posteromedial commissure, as well as the P3 and A3 scallops, will be on the right, with the anterolateral commissure, as well as the A1 and P1 scallops, on the left.

The parasternal short-axis mid-ventricular view allows the anterolateral and posteromedial papillary muscles to be seen at 4 o'clock and 8 o'clock, respectively (Fig. 2.10). In this view, the interpapillary muscle distance can be measured as the distance between the heads of the papillary muscles in systole.

Apical 4-Chamber View (A4C)

The apical 4-chamber view usually demonstrates the A3, A2 and A1 scallops medially, with the P1 scallop laterally (Fig. 2.11). Although leaflet motion and coaptation can also be identified in this view, allowing leaflet prolapse or restriction to be visualised, the non-planar saddle

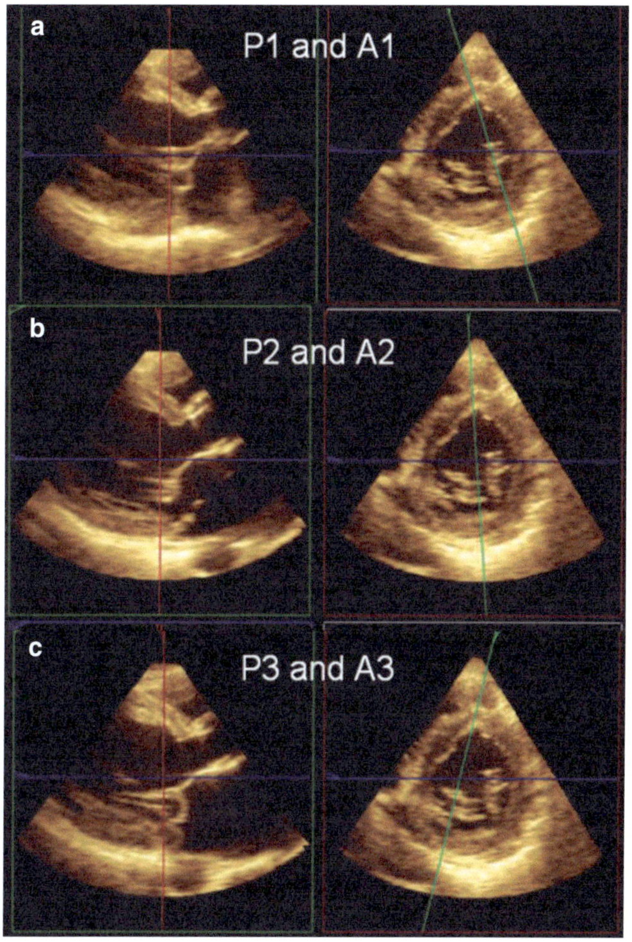

Fig. 2.8 Segmental analysis of the mitral valve on trans-thoracic 3D dataset parasternal long- and short-axis views demonstrating; (**a**) A1 and P1; (**b**) A2 and P2; (**c**) A3 and P3

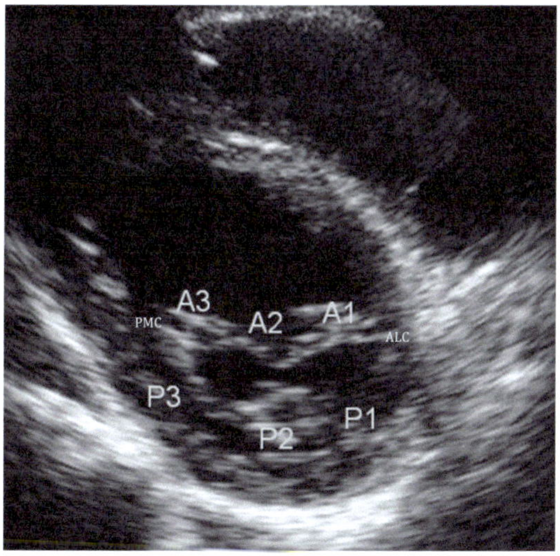

Fig. 2.9 Parasternal short-axis view at the level of the mitral valve, where all six scallops of the anterior (A1, A2 and A3) and posterior (P1, P2 and P3) leaflets can be identified, as well as the anterolateral (ALC) and posteromedial (PMC) commissures

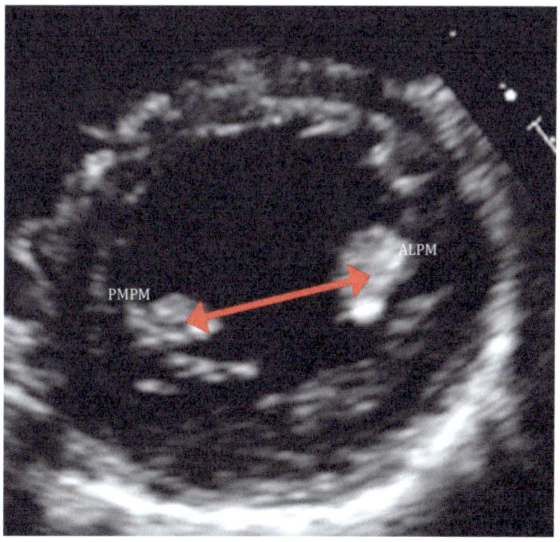

Fig. 2.10 Parasternal short-axis view at the mid-ventricular level, where the anterolateral (ALPM) and posteromedial (PMPM) papillary muscles can be visualised, and the interpapillary muscle distance (red arrow) can be measured

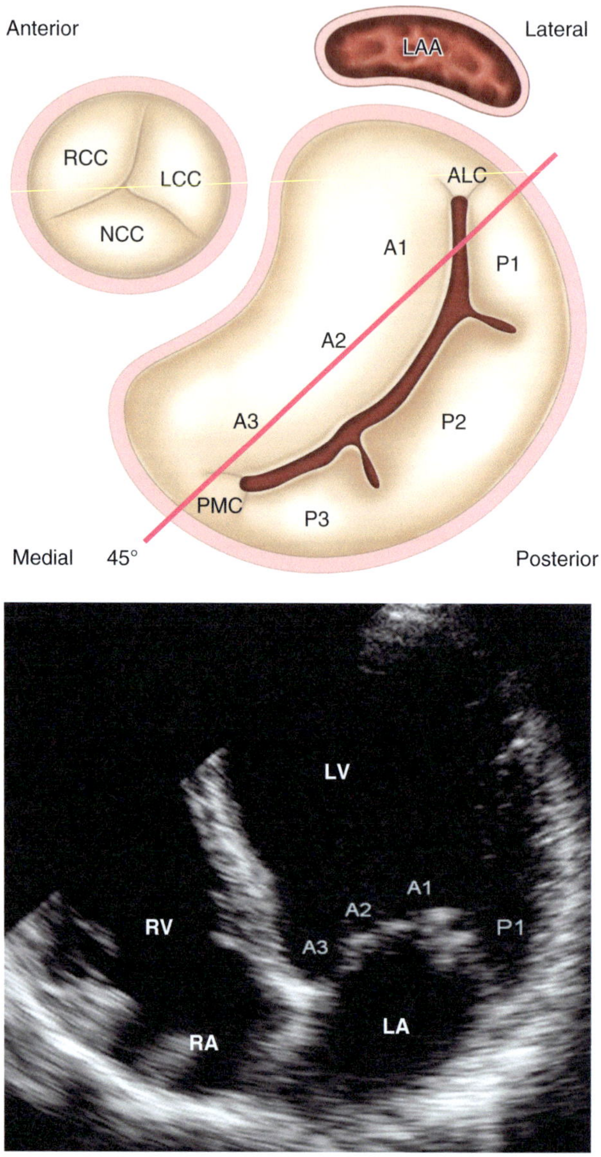

Fig. 2.11 Apical 4-chamber view demonstrating the A3, A2 and A1 scallops of the mitral valve medially, with the P1 scallop laterally. NCC non-coronary cusp of the aortic valve, LCC left coronary cusp of the aortic valve, RCC right coronary cusp of the aortic valve, ALC anterolateral commissure, PMC posteromedial commissure, LAA left atrial appendage, RV right ventricle, RA right atrium, LV left ventricle, LA left atrium

shape of the annulus may lead to a false positive diagnosis of prolapse in this view. The presence of annular calcification can also be determined in this view.

Apical Long-Axis View (3-Chamber View, A3C)

The apical 3-chamber view demonstrates the A2 and P2 scallops of the mitral valve (Fig. 2.12). It also allows the anteroposterior diameter (minor axis) of the mitral annulus to be measured.

Apical Commissural View (Apical 2-Chamber, A2C)

The apical 2-chamber view allows the P3, A2 and P1 scallops, and both commissures of the mitral valve to be identified (Fig. 2.13). The inter-commissural diameter (major axis) can be measured at the end of systole (Fig. 2.14). Both papillary muscles and chordae tendineae can also be seen on this view, allowing the inter-papillary muscle distance and the annulo-papillary muscle distance to be measured. The annulo-papillary muscle distance allows the measurement of the neo-chords length used to maintain annulo-ventricular continuity in patients undergoing mitral valve replacement, where the neo-chords are attached to the annulus rather than the leaflets.

Three-Dimensional Trans-thoracic Echocardiography

Three-dimensional TTE images can be acquired from parasternal and apical views enabling the dataset to be rotated, allowing the valve to viewed from the left ventricle or the surgeon's 'en-face' view from the left atrium (Fig. 2.15a, b). Three-dimensional echocardiography has revolutionised understanding of the surgical perspective of the underlying pathology and provides a road map to guide operative strategy. Improved understanding of the mitral valve complex, including the chordae tendineae and papillary muscles, can also be obtained using 3D imaging (Fig. 2.15c).

Trans-oesophageal Echocardiography

Trans-oesophageal echocardiography (TOE) has revolutionised imaging of the mitral valve and considerably helped to advance surgical repair techniques of the mitral valve. Due to its proximity to the left atrium, TOE is able to obtain more detailed images of mitral valve anatomy than a TTE and hence plays an important role in decision-making regarding the feasibility of mitral valve repair, as well as the technique to be used. Multi-plane imaging allows detailed segmental analysis of the entire mitral valve complex to be constructed and analysed (Fig. 2.16). Key landmarks help orientate the section of valve in view, where left atrial appendage is located adjacent to the lateral portion of the valve (A1, P1 and anterolateral commissure) and the aortic valve is located adjacent to the anterior leaflet.

A standard detailed trans-oesophageal examination of the mitral valve involves obtaining several different mid-oesophageal and trans-gastric views. As the probe is inserted and advanced into the oesophagus, the initial (approximately 30 cm from incisors) 5-chamber view is usually seen at 0°. The lateral portion of the mitral valve is first viewed (A1, P1 and anterolateral commissure), the scan plane being an oblique view through the mitral valve leaflets (Fig. 2.17). In addition, the aortic valve and outflow tract are visualised.

With further probe advancement (30–35 cm from the incisors), the mid-oesophageal 4-chamber view is obtained. This view is an oblique slice through the middle portion (usually A2 and P2) of the mitral valve (Fig. 2.18).

If the probe is advanced (moved inferiorly) from the 4-chamber view (with or without retroflexion of the tip of the probe), the medial portion (A3, P3 and posteromedial commissure) of the mitral valve become visible (Fig. 2.19).

The transducer is then rotated to approximately 60° to obtain a mid-oesophageal bicommissural view, where a combination of both the anterior and posterior leaflets (P3, A2 and P1 scallops) can be seen (Fig. 2.20). Clockwise and anticlockwise rotation of the probe will demonstrate the posteromedial and anterolateral

Fig. 2.12 Apical 3-chamber view demonstrating the P2 and A2 scallops of the mitral valve. NCC non-coronary cusp of the aortic valve, LCC left coronary cusp of the aortic valve, RCC right coronary cusp of the aortic valve, ALC anterolateral commissure, PMC posteromedial commissure, LAA left atrial appendage, LV left ventricle, LA left atrium, Ao aorta

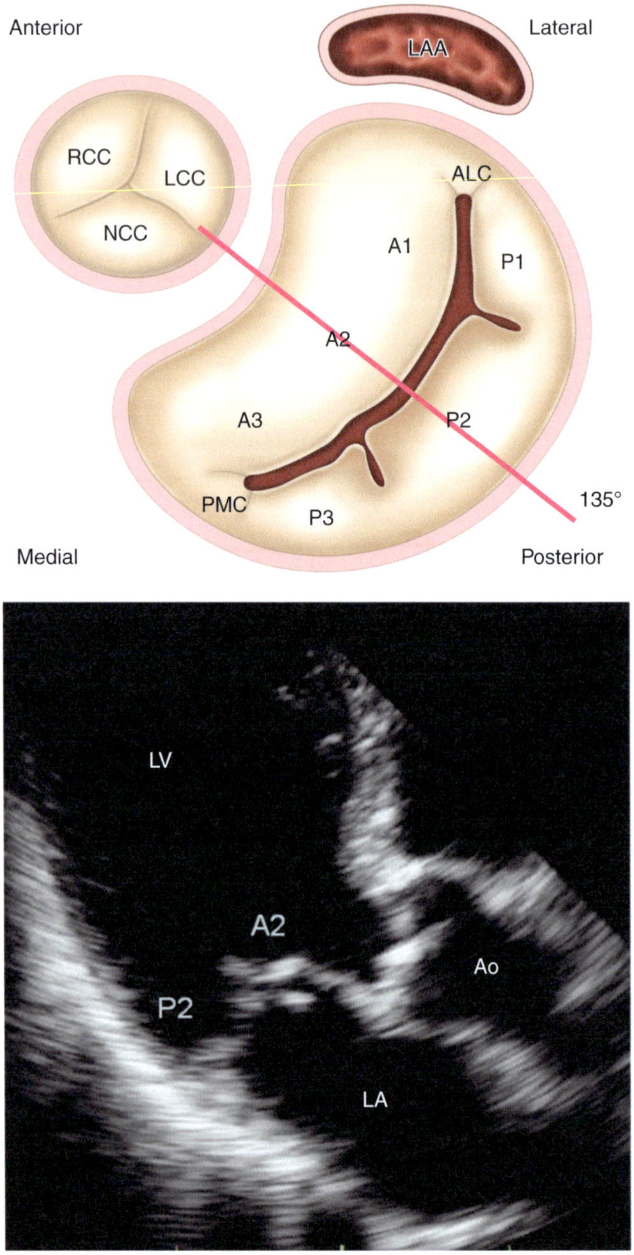

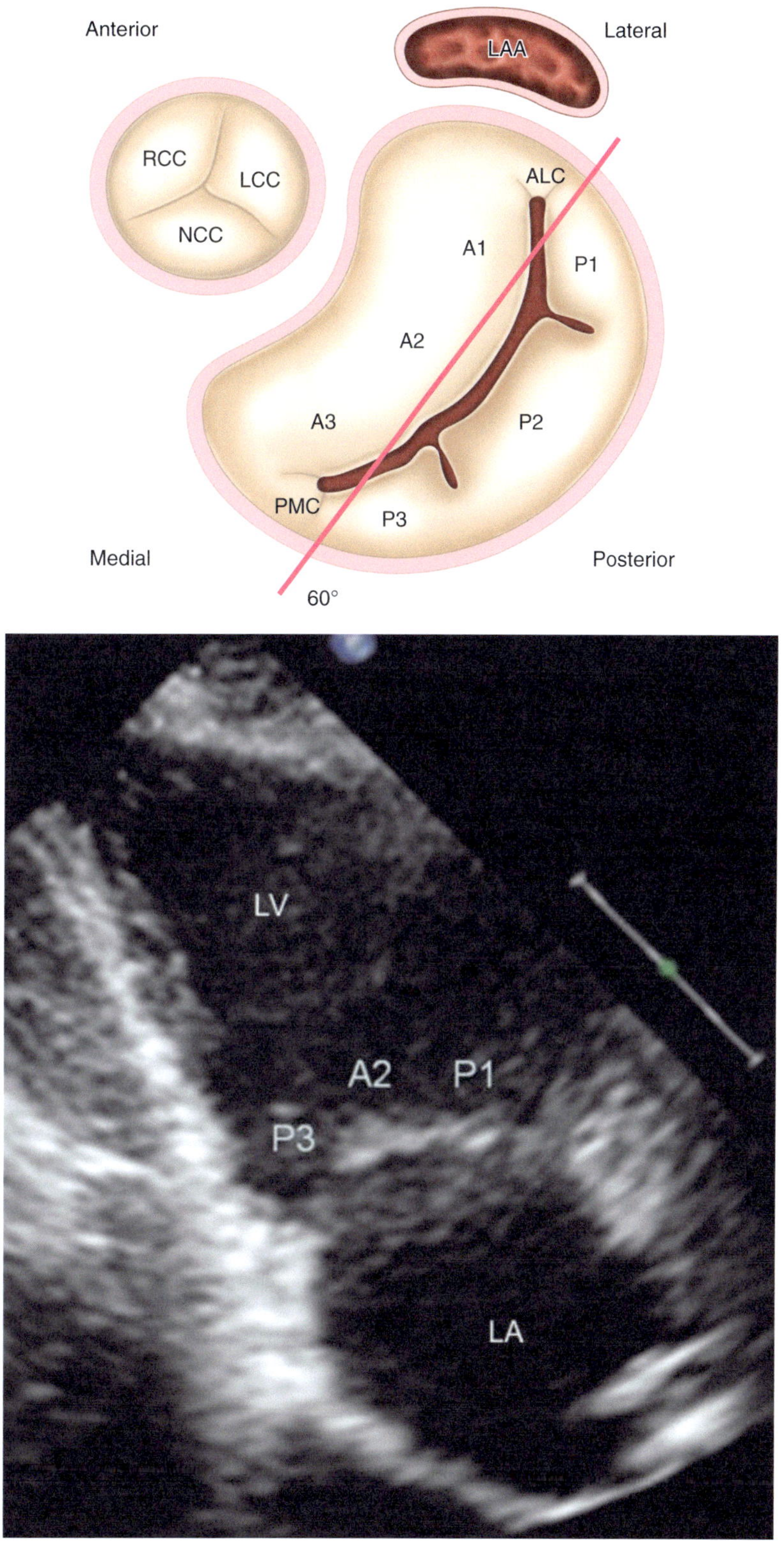

Fig. 2.13 Apical 2-chamber bicommissural view, demonstrating the P3, A2 and P1 scallops of the mitral valve. NCC non-coronary cusp of the aortic valve, LCC left coronary cusp of the aortic valve, RCC right coronary cusp of the aortic valve, ALC anterolateral commissure, PMC posteromedial commissure, LAA left atrial appendage, LV left ventricle, LA left atrium

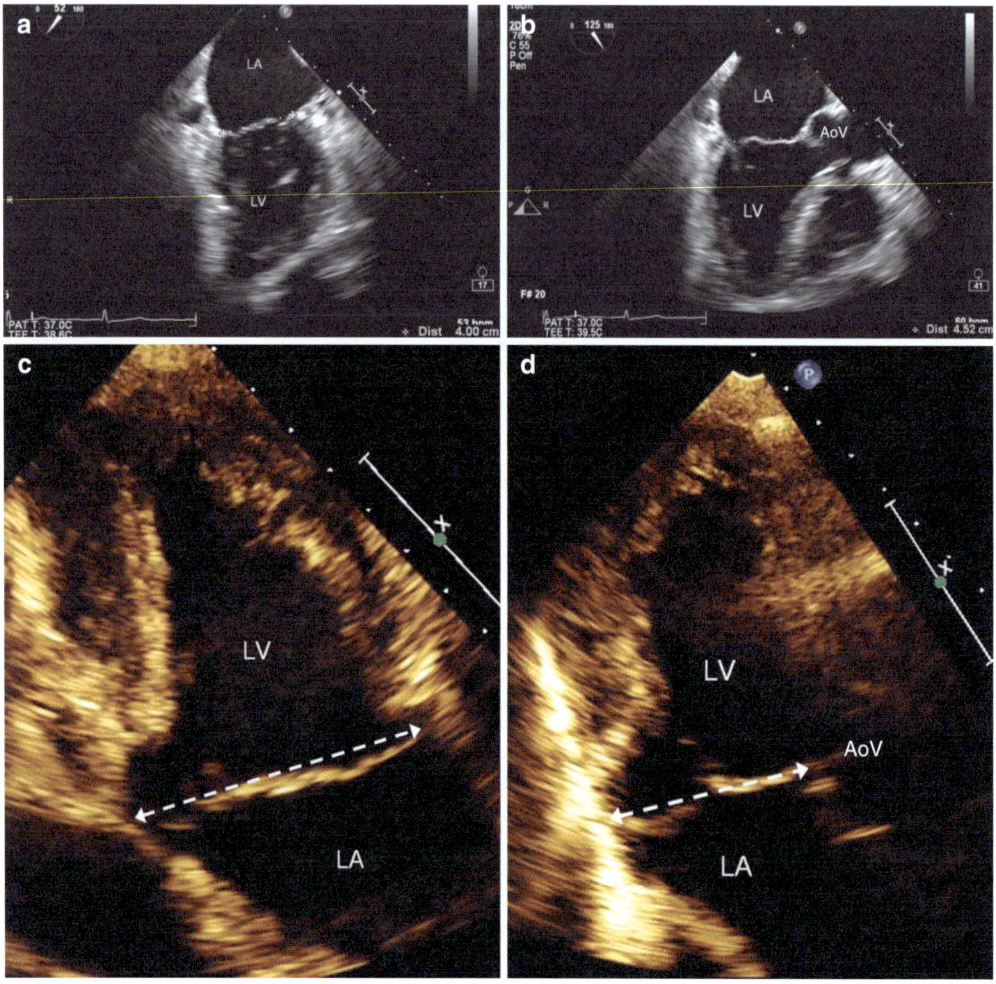

Fig. 2.14 Mitral valve major and minor axis measurement in TOE mid-oesophageal and TTE apical views; (**a**) major axis on TOE bicommissural view at 60°, (**b**) minor axis on TOE long-axis view at 135°, (**c**) major axis on TTE apical 2-chamber view and (**d**) minor axis on TTE apical 3-chamber view. LV left ventricle, LA left atrium, AoV aortic valve

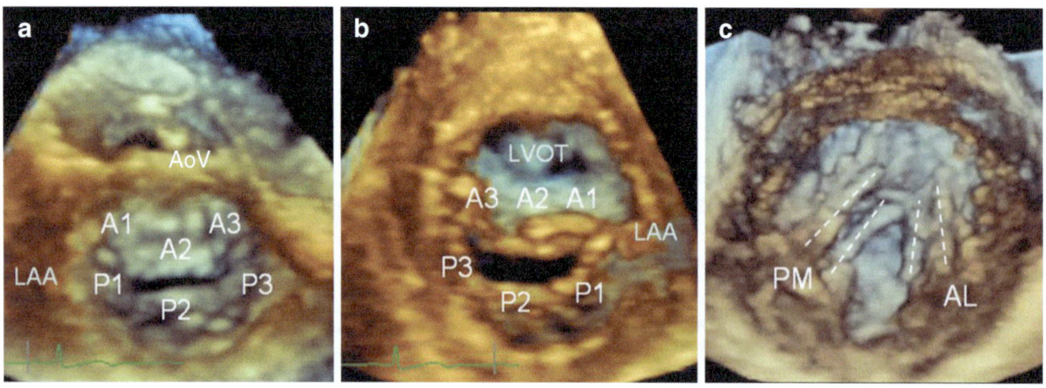

Fig. 2.15 Three-dimensional trans-thoracic echo images, with (**a**) left atrial view of the mitral valve (surgeon's view), (**b**) left ventricular view of the mitral valve, which replicates the 2D parasternal short-axis view, and (**c**) left ventricular view of the anterolateral (AL) and posteromedial (PM) papillary muscles and chordae tendineae (dashed white lines). LAA left atrial appendage, LVOT left ventricular outflow tract, AoV aortic valve

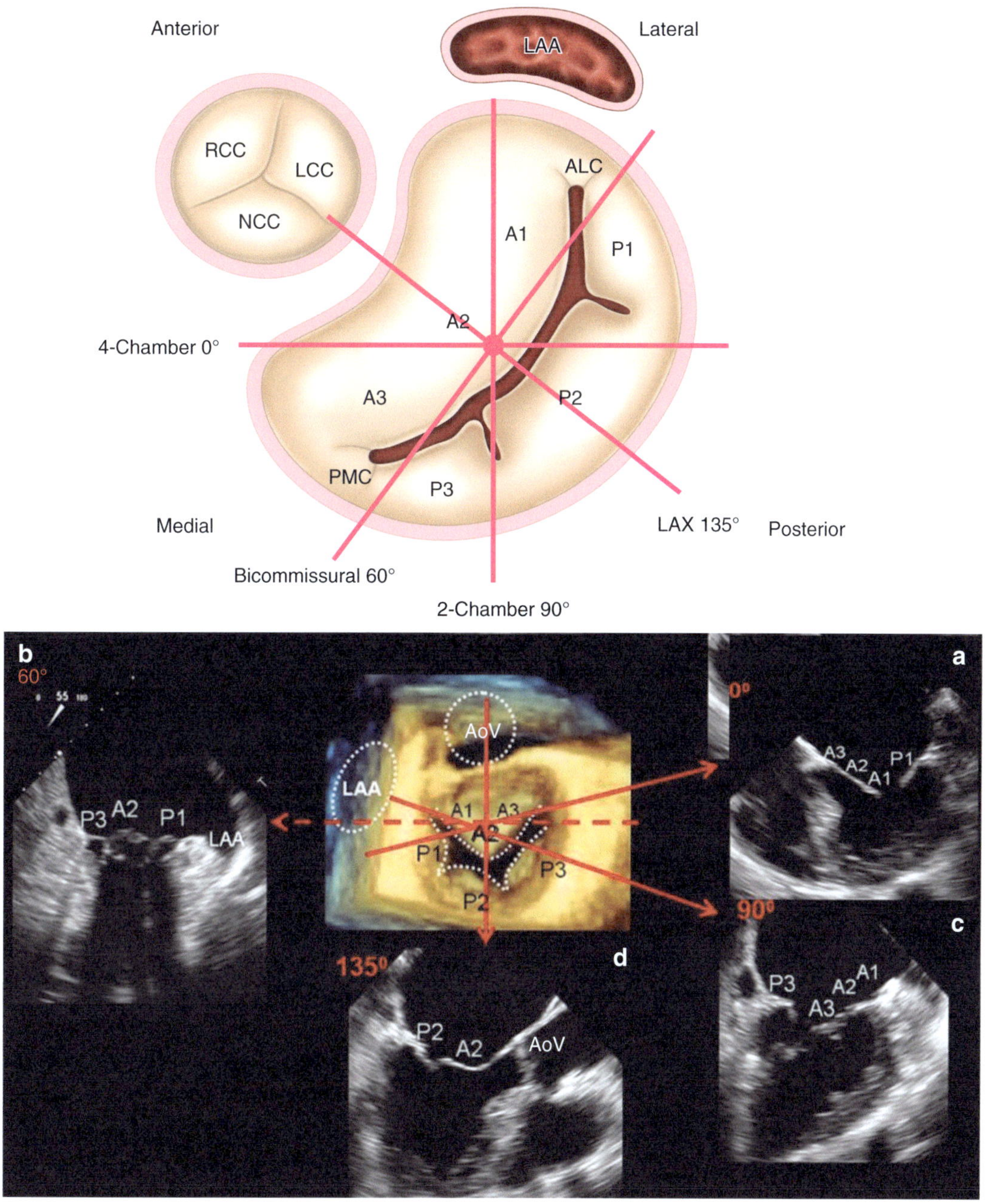

Fig. 2.16 Trans-oesophageal echocardiography mid-oesophageal views; (**a**) 0° 4-chamber view, (**b**) 60° bicommissural view, (**c**) 90° 2-chamber view and (**d**) 135° long-axis view (LAX). NCC non-coronary cusp of the aortic valve, LCC left coronary cusp of the aortic valve, RCC right coronary cusp of the aortic valve, ALC anterolateral commissure, PMC posteromedial commissure, LAA left atrial appendage. AoV aortic valve

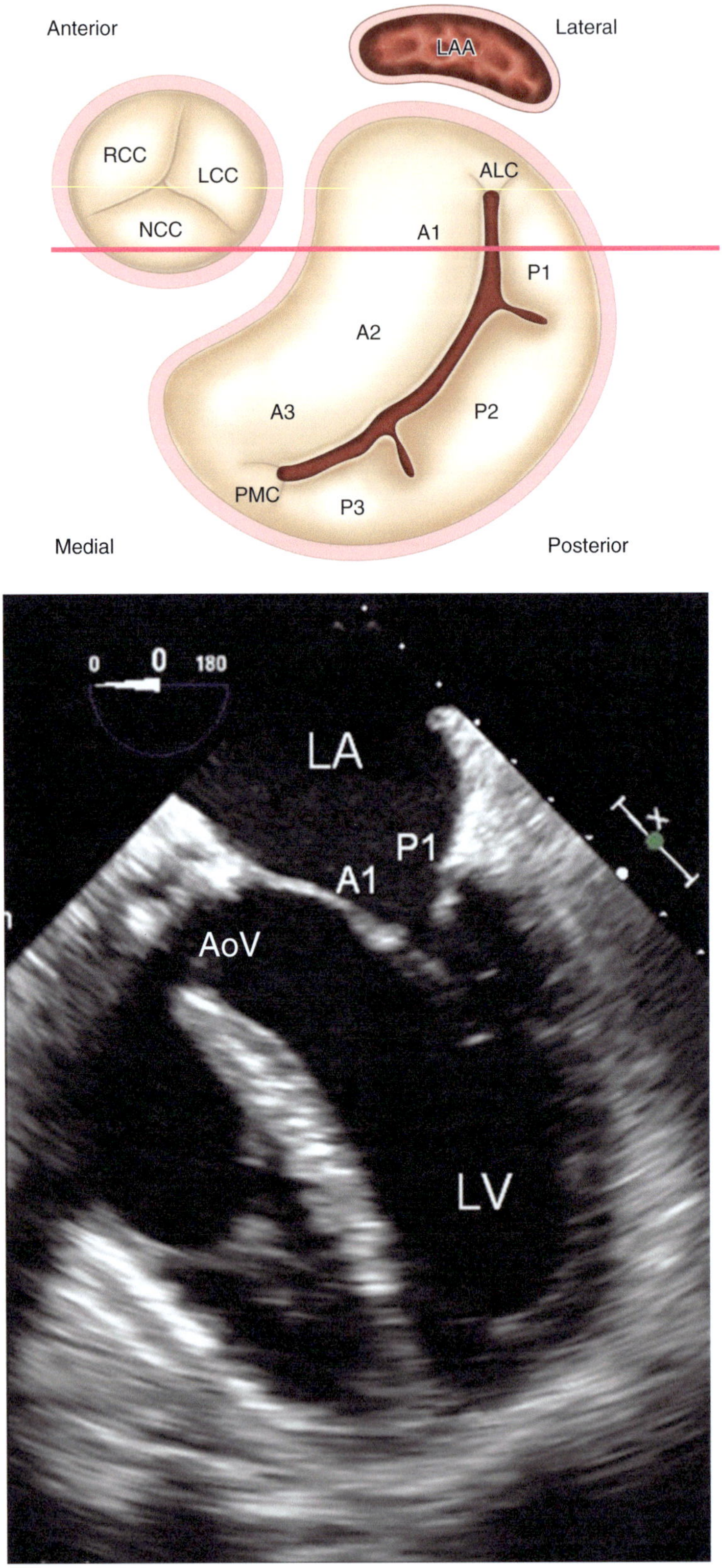

Fig. 2.17 Mid-oesophageal 5-chamber view (0°) at the level of the A1 and P1 scallops, with the aorta visible. NCC non-coronary cusp of the aortic valve, LCC left coronary cusp of the aortic valve, RCC right coronary cusp of the aortic valve, ALC anterolateral commissure, PMC posteromedial commissure, LAA left atrial appendage, AoV aortic valve, LV left ventricle, LA left atrium

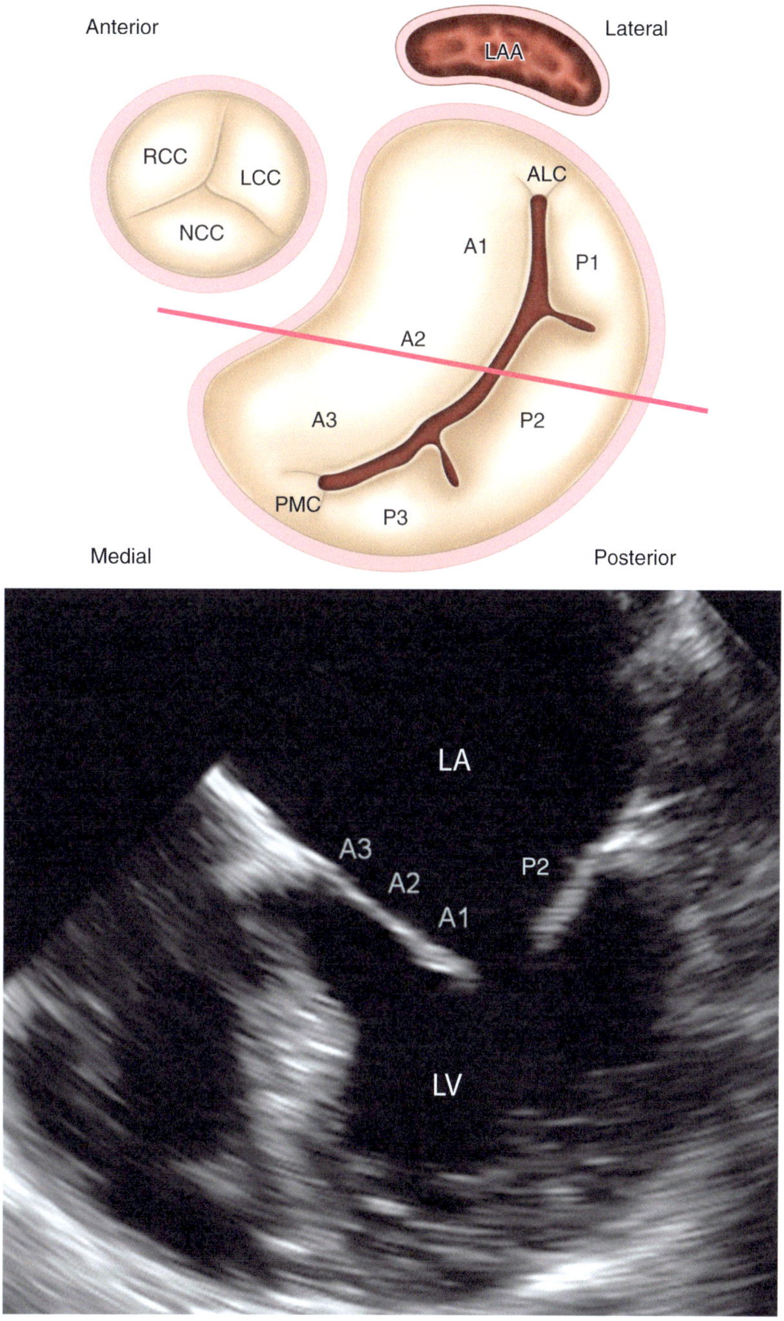

Fig. 2.18 Mid-oesophageal 4-chamber view (0°) at the level of the A2-P2 scallops, with the left ventricular outflow tract visible. NCC non-coronary cusp of the aortic valve, LCC left coronary cusp of the aortic valve, RCC right coronary cusp of the aortic valve, ALC anterolateral commissure, PMC posteromedial commissure, LAA left atrial appendage, LV left ventricle, LA left atrium

commissures, respectively. The intercommissural distance (major axis), leaflet height of the P1 and P3 scallops, distance from the papillary muscle heads to the annulus and respective angles can be measured in the bicommissural view. The left atrial appendage may or may not be seen adjacent to the P1 scallop of the mitral valve in this view.

The transducer is then further rotated to approximately 90° to obtain a mid-oesophageal 2-chamber (2C) view, where the P3 scallop of the posterior leaflet and the entire anterior leaflet (A3, A2 and A1) are visible (Fig. 2.21). The left atrial appendage is usually seen adjacent to the A1 scallop of the mitral valve in this view.

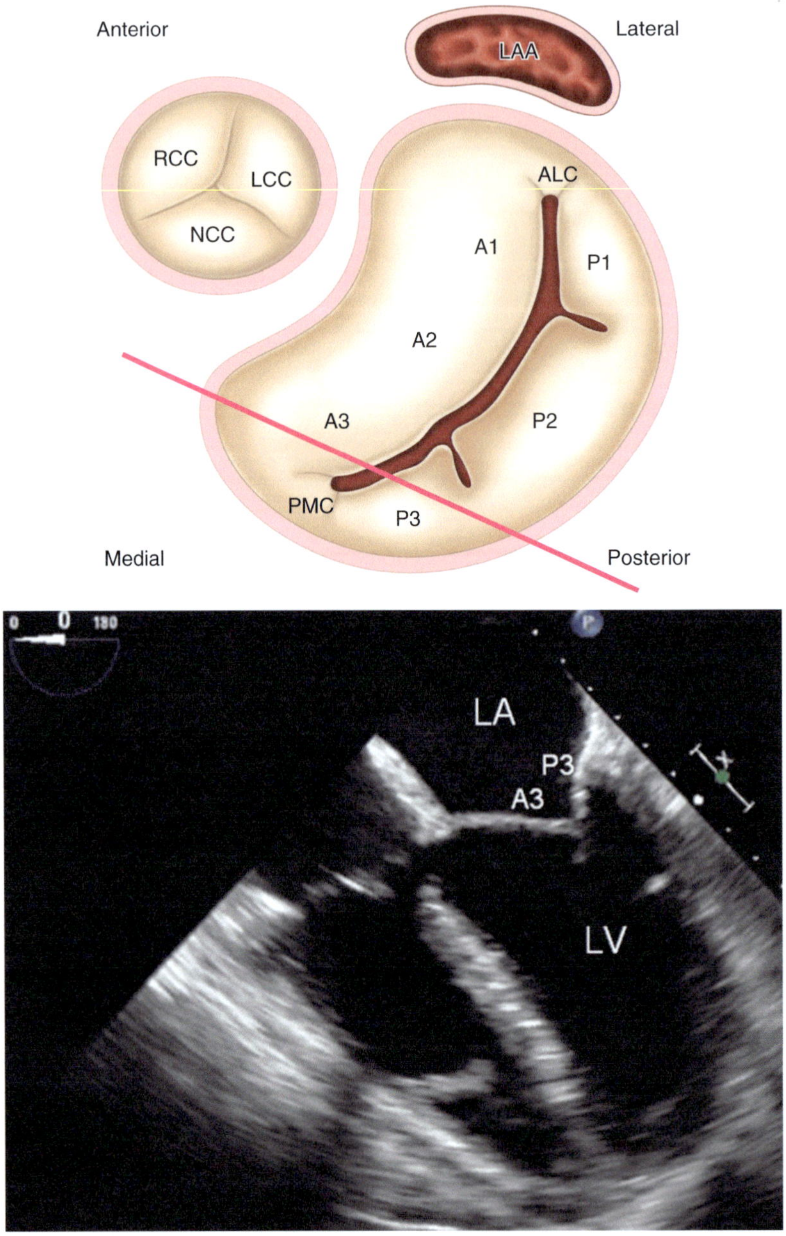

Fig. 2.19 Mid-oesophageal 4-chamber view (0°) at the level of the A3–P3 scallops, with neither the aorta nor the left ventricular outflow tract visible. NCC non-coronary cusp of the aortic valve, LCC left coronary cusp of the aortic valve, RCC right coronary cusp of the aortic valve, ALC anterolateral commissure, PMC posteromedial commissure, LAA left atrial appendage, LA left atrium, LV left ventricle

Clockwise rotation of the probe in this view enables analysis of the posteromedial aspect of the coaptation line (at A3-P3) and posteromedial commissure, whereas counter clockwise rotation of the probe in this view enables analysis of the anterolateral aspect of the coaptation line (at A1-P1) and anterolateral commissure.

Finally, the transducer is rotated to approximately 135° to obtain a mid-oesophageal long-axis view, with the LVOT, aortic valve, and aortic root visible, at which level the A2 and P2 scallops can be seen (Fig. 2.22). Similar to the mid-oesophageal 4-chamber view, the probe can be slightly withdrawn or advanced to allow the A1-P1 or A3-P3 scallops to be visualised, respectively.

The leaflet lengths of P2 and A2 can also be measured in this view (or on the 5-chamber view). In the determination of the risk of SAM, these measurements are made in systole during

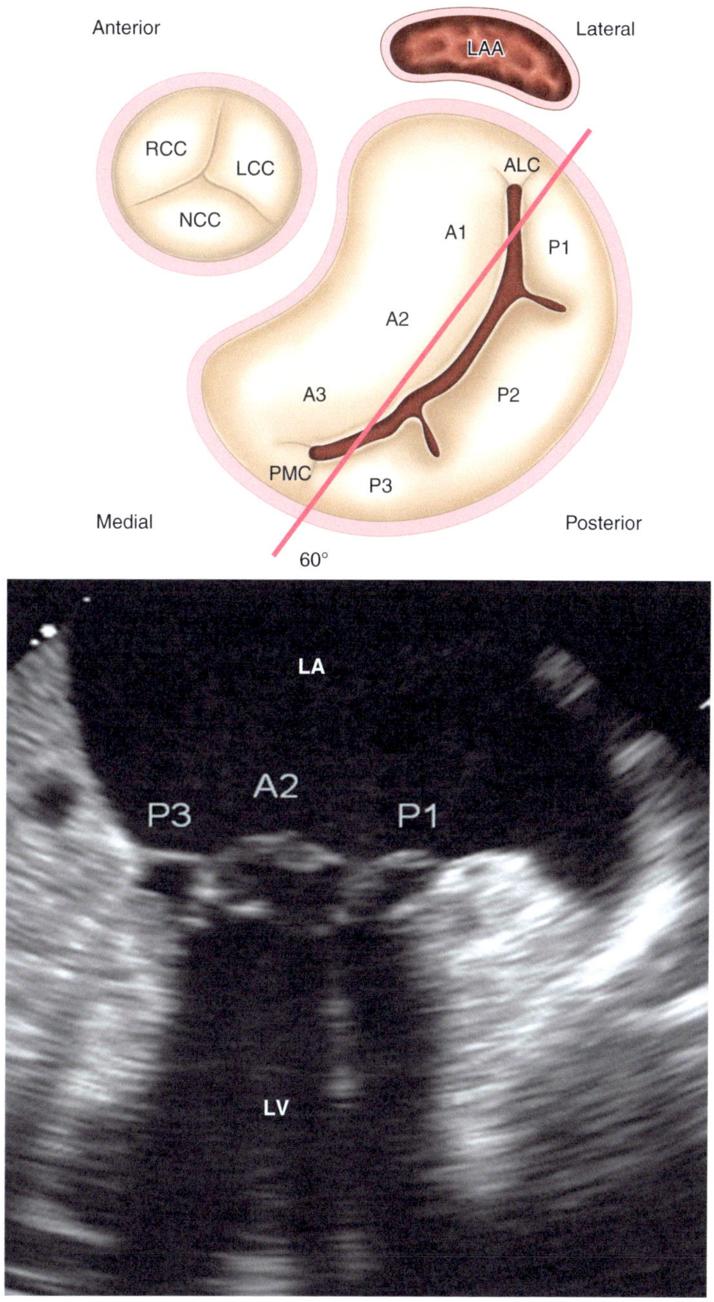

Fig. 2.20 Mid-oesophageal bicommissural view (60°), demonstrating the P3, A2 and P1 scallops of the mitral valve. NCC non-coronary cusp of the aortic valve, LCC left coronary cusp of the aortic valve, RCC right coronary cusp of the aortic valve, ALC anterolateral commissure, PMC posteromedial commissure, LAA left atrial appendage, LA left atrium, LV left ventricle

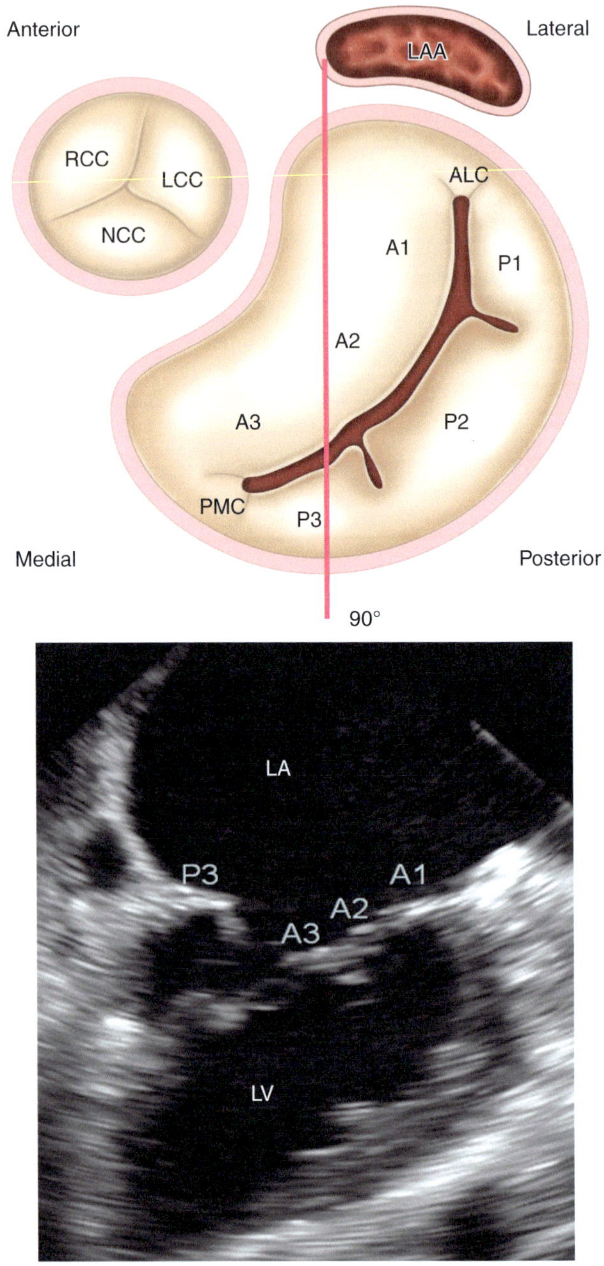

Fig. 2.21 Mid-oesophageal 2-chamber view (90°), demonstrating the P3 scallop and entire anterior leaflet (A3, A2 and A1 scallops) of the mitral valve. NCC non-coronary cusp of the aortic valve, LCC left coronary cusp of the aortic valve, RCC right coronary cusp of the aortic valve, ALC anterolateral commissure, PMC posteromedial commissure, LAA left atrial appendage. LA left atrium, LV left ventricle

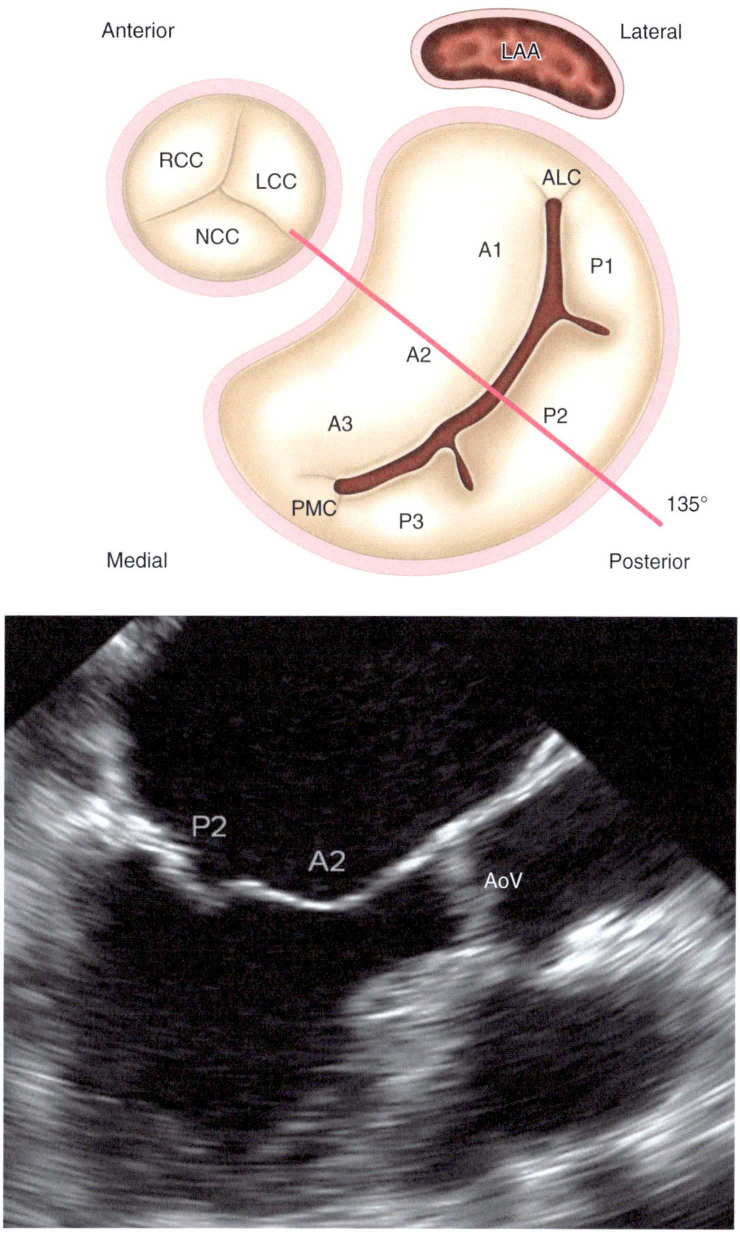

Fig. 2.22 Mid-oesophageal long-axis view (135°), demonstrating the A2 and P2 scallops of the mitral valve. NCC non-coronary cusp of the aortic valve, LCC left coronary cusp of the aortic valve, RCC right coronary cusp of the aortic valve, ALC anterolateral commissure, PMC posteromedial commissure, LAA left atrial appendage, LA left atrium, LV left ventricle, AoV aortic valve

leaflet coaptation, rather than in diastole when the leaflets are straightened. The anteroposterior diameter (minor axis) of the mitral annulus can be measured in this view. Annular dilatation is defined as an annulus diameter >35 mm or when the annulus to anterior leaflet length ratio is >1.3, with both measured in the same image in diastole.

The mid-oesophageal long-axis view can also be used to measure the leaflet tenting height or coaptation distance (centre of the annular plane to the coaptation point, which is normally ≤10 mm), tenting area (area within the annular plane, coaptation point and leaflets edges), and the anterior and posterior angles (angles between the annulus and leaflet insertions).

After completion of imaging at the mid-oesophageal level, the probe is advanced below the diaphragm into the stomach to obtain the trans-gastric views of the mitral valve. Initially at 0°, a basal short-axis view of the mitral valve can be obtained, which gives an 'en-face' view of the mitral valve when the image is rotated (Fig. 2.23). In this view, all the anterior and posterior leaflet scallops and both commissures can be seen, with the A3-P3 scallops closest to the probe. Planimetry of the mitral valve measured at the level of the leaflet tips in this view was the gold standard for measuring mitral valve area, as it is not as dependent on loading conditions. This requires carefully optimised on-axis views of the mitral valve orifice to avoid over estimation of the valve area. The use of three-dimensional imaging is now the preferred method, requiring less operator experience and has been shown to correlate with surgical findings.

A trans-gastric mid short-axis view (0°) can be used to assess any regional wall abnormalities at the time of surgery (Fig. 2.24). In addition, the inter-papillary muscle distance can be measured in this view between the bases or the heads of the papillary muscles in systole.

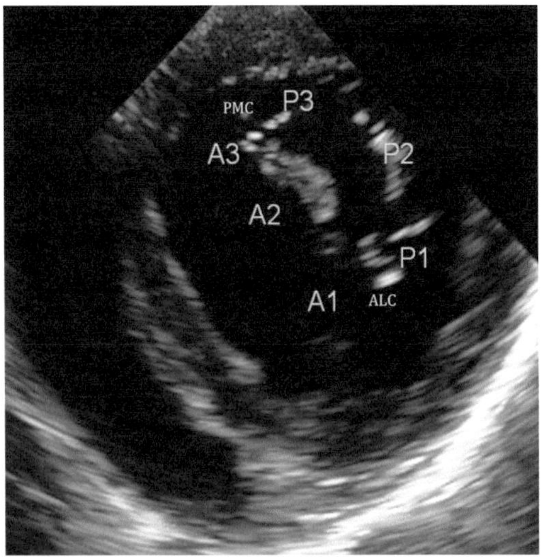

Fig. 2.23 Trans-gastric basal short-axis view (0°) demonstrating all six scallops (A1, A2, A3, P1, P2 and P3) and both commissures (anterolateral, ALC, and posteromedial, PMC) of the mitral valve

The transducer is then rotated to 90–120° to obtain the left ventricular long-axis view, which as well as assessing the mitral valve leaflets, can give a detailed view of the sub-valvular apparatus, including the chordae tendineae and papillary muscles (Fig. 2.25). The chordal lengths and distance between the heads of the papillary muscle and the leaflet free edge can also be measured.

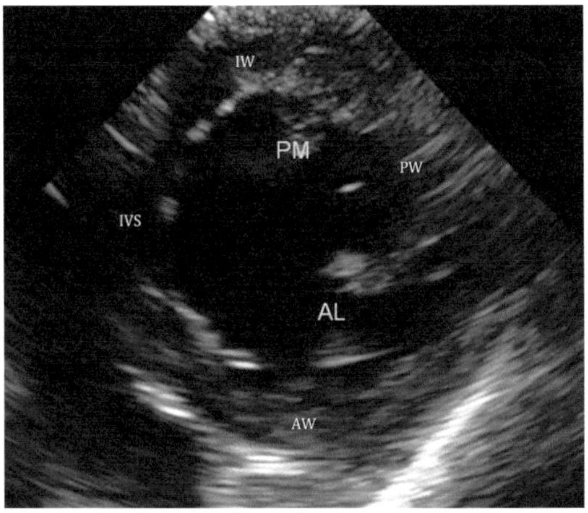

Fig. 2.24 Trans-gastric mid short-axis view (0°) demonstrating the regional walls of the left ventricle and the papillary muscles. PM posteromedial papillary muscle, AL anterolateral papillary muscle, IW inferior wall, PW posterior wall, AW anterior wall and IVS interventricular septum

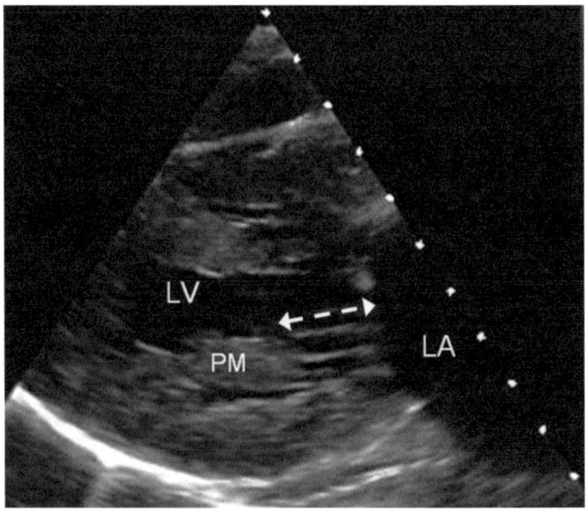

Fig. 2.25 Trans-gastric LV long-axis view (90–120°) demonstrating measurement of the chordal length from the head of the papillary muscle to the leaflet free edge. PM papillary muscle, LA left atrium, LV left ventricle

Three-Dimensional Trans-oesophageal Echocardiography of the Mitral Valve

Real-time three-dimensional echocardiography has revolutionised segmental analysis of the mitral valve. The 'en-face' view allows easy identification of all the scallops and both commissures of the mitral valve from the atrial perspective, similar to the surgeon's view during mitral valve surgery. Three-dimensional trans-oesophageal echocardiography provides better spatial resolution than 3D trans-thoracic images with more anatomical detail visible (Fig. 2.26).

In addition, geometric analysis of the mitral valve is possible, enabling leaflet areas, leaflet angles and tenting volumes to be determined (Fig. 2.27). The leaflets can also be visualised as

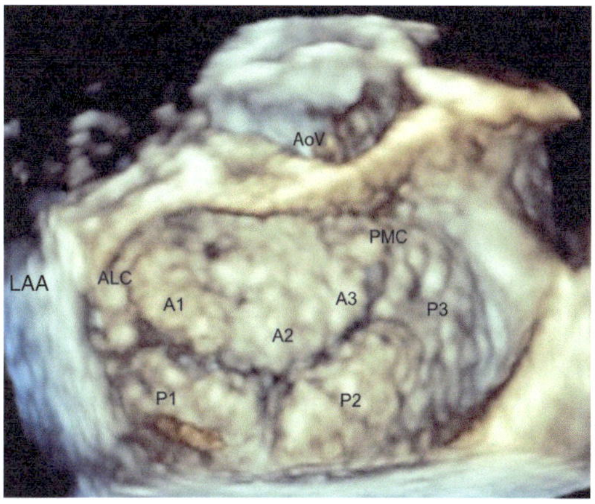

Fig. 2.26 Three-dimensional trans-oesophageal echocardiographical image demonstrating all six scallops and both commissures in the surgical 'en-face' view of the mitral valve viewed from the left atrium. AoV aortic valve, LAA left atrial appendage, ALC anterolateral commissure, PMC posteromedial commissure

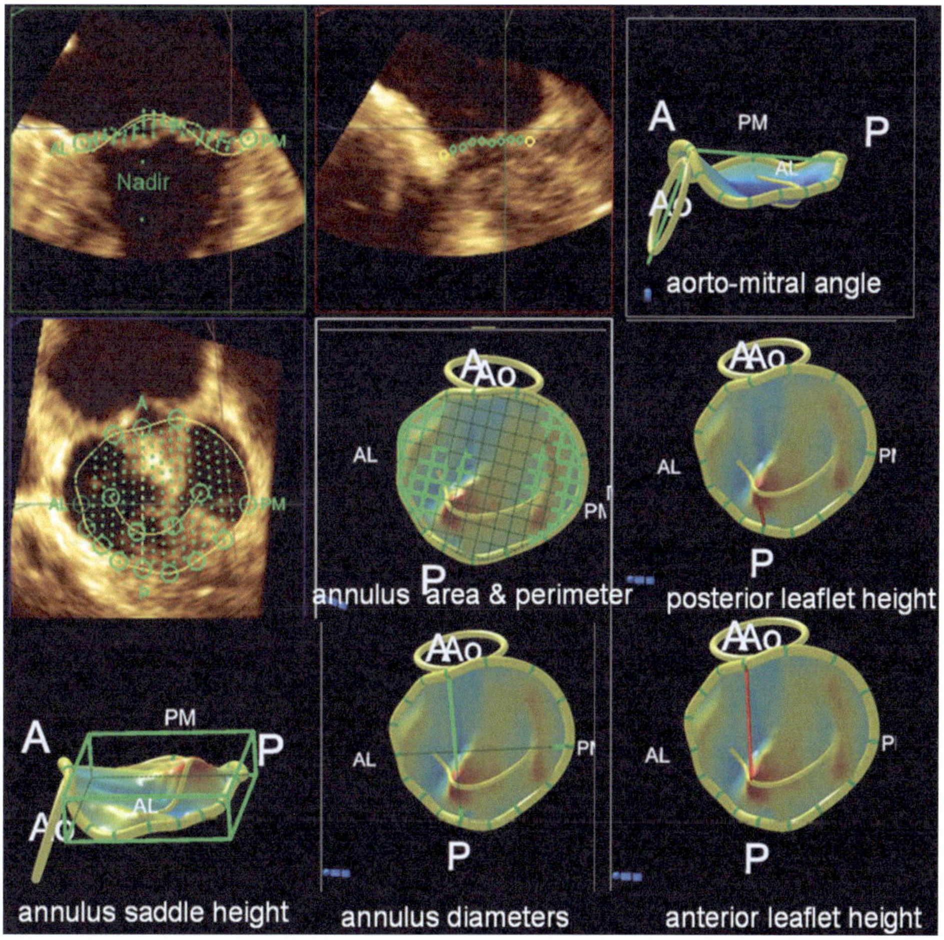

Fig. 2.27 Three-dimensional trans-oesophageal analysis of the mitral valve geometric indices. A anterior, P posterior, Ao aorta, AL anterolateral papillary muscle, PM posteromedial papillary muscle

protruding or restricted as compared to the annular plane, to further delineate the exact location of the mitral valve pathology.

Doppler Echocardiography

Doppler echocardiography allows assessment of the velocity pattern of blood flow during diastole and systole across the mitral valve. In the absence of pathology, the velocity flow pattern across the mitral valve resembles the M-shaped pattern of M-mode echocardiography, with blood flow most rapid during the early (E) phase of left ventricular filling and then falling to low levels during mid-diastole, before accelerating again during atrial (A) contraction (Fig. 2.28a). The peak velocity is measured using pulsed wave Doppler and velocity time integral (area under the mitral inflow pattern) is measured using continuous wave Doppler. Normal peak flow velocity across the mitral valve is usually just under 1 m/s. Using the modified Bernoulli equation $p = 4\ v^2$, where p = pressure (in mmHg) and v = velocity (in m/s), the peak and mean pressure gradient across the valve can be calculated from the peak velocity and velocity time integral, respectively. A mean pressure gradient >10 mmHg is suggestive of severe mitral stenosis (Fig. 2.28b).

Doppler flows across the mitral valve can also be used to assess the pressure half-time, which represents the time required for the pressure gradient between the left atrium and left ventricle to reduce by 50% (Fig. 2.29a). The mitral valve area can then be calculated using the formula MVA = 220/PHT, where MVA = mitral valve area (in cm^2) and PHT = pressure half-time (in ms). A pressure half-time >220 ms is suggestive of severe mitral stenosis, as it will result in a valve area <1 cm^2 (Fig. 2.29b). Assessment of the mitral valve area using the pressure half-time method may be inaccurate in patients where the pressure gradient between the left atrium and left ventricle is altered by other factors, such as severe aortic regurgitation. As well as mitral valve assessment, the trans-mitral waveform (pulsed wave Doppler) can be used to assess diastolic function of the left ventricle with measurement of the E:A ratio, isovolumetric relaxation time and deceleration time.

Colour Flow Doppler

Colour flow Doppler can be used to determine the severity of mitral regurgitation. The colour scale and gain should be optimised, and assessment should integrate multiple echo views, including all apical and parasternal views. Colour flow Doppler allows determination of all three components of the regurgitant jet from which the severity of mitral regurgitation can be assessed;

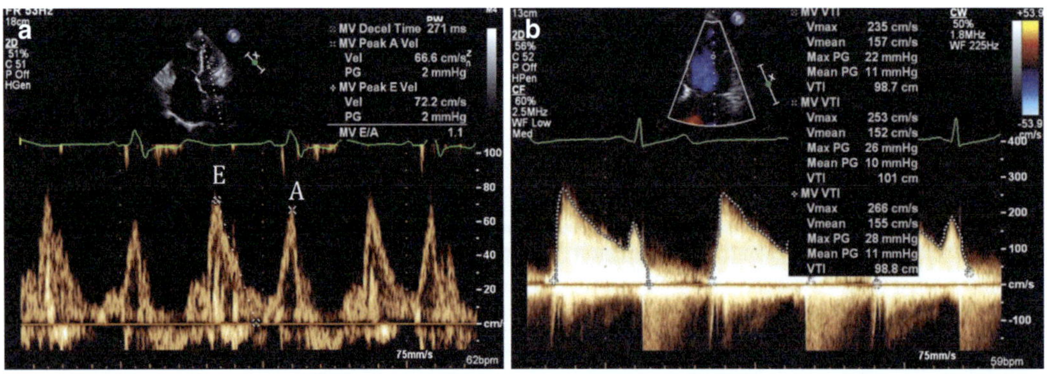

Fig. 2.28 (**a**) Pulsed wave Doppler assessment of blood flow with the sampling volume placed across the mitral wave from an apical 4-chamber view, demonstrating rapid early (E) filling of the left ventricle and late filling following atrial (A) contraction in a patient with a normal mitral valve. Left ventricular diastolic function and mitral valve area can also be calculated from these waveforms by measuring E:A ratio and deceleration time. (**b**) Continuous wave Doppler echocardiography across the mitral valve, in a patient with severe mitral stenosis, where the mean pressure gradient is calculated from the velocity time integral using the modified Bernoulli equation

the regurgitant jet area, vena contracta and flow convergence (PISA radius).

Regurgitant Jet Area

This is a qualitative method to assess the severity of mitral regurgitation that is based on the principle that the severity of MR is proportional to the size of the regurgitant jet into the left atrium. On trans-thoracic echocardiography, it is typically visualised in the apical 4-chamber view. The colour flow Doppler scale is adjusted to a Nyquist limit of 50–60 cm/s. A small jet occupying <20% of the left atrial cavity area and typically where a flow convergence is not visible is classified as mild, whilst a jet occupying >40% of the left atrial area with a large flow convergence region is classified as severe (Fig. 2.30). Although jet size is a useful qualitative method used to assess MR severity, it is dependent on loading conditions, such as a high blood pressure, where the jet size is increased in response to increased left ventricular pressures; or a high left atrial pressure or low blood pressure, both of which reduced the jet size. Therefore, quantitative methods are required, including the vena contracta and flow convergence (PISA) methods. Where an eccentric regurgitant jet is directed towards and sweeps along the left atrial wall, it cannot entrain blood on all sides and appears smaller than a central jet into the left atrial cavity, known as the Coanda effect.

Vena Contracta

The vena contracta is defined as the width of the narrowest part of the mitral regurgitation jet immediately distal to the regurgitant orifice (on the left atrial side). It therefore can be used as a surrogate to represent the regurgitant orifice and is used as a semi-quantitative method of assessing the severity of mitral regurgitation. Accurate assessment requires visualisation of all three jet components (flow convergence, vena contracta and jet expansion into the left atrium). Optimal views include the parasternal long-axis or the apical 4-chamber views on trans-thoracic echocardiography, and mid-oesophageal long-axis or 4-chamber views on trans-oesophageal echocardiography. The probe is carefully angled to optimize the regurgitant jet profile and zoom views help to identify the neck of the jet, while the Doppler colour sector is made as narrow as possible to improve resolution (image frame rates) and accuracy of measurement (Fig. 2.31). Mild mitral regurgitation is usually associated with a vena contracta <3 mm, whereas ≥7 mm is suggestive of severe MR. Intermediate values are not accurate at distinguishing moderate from mild or severe MR, as there is a large overlap.

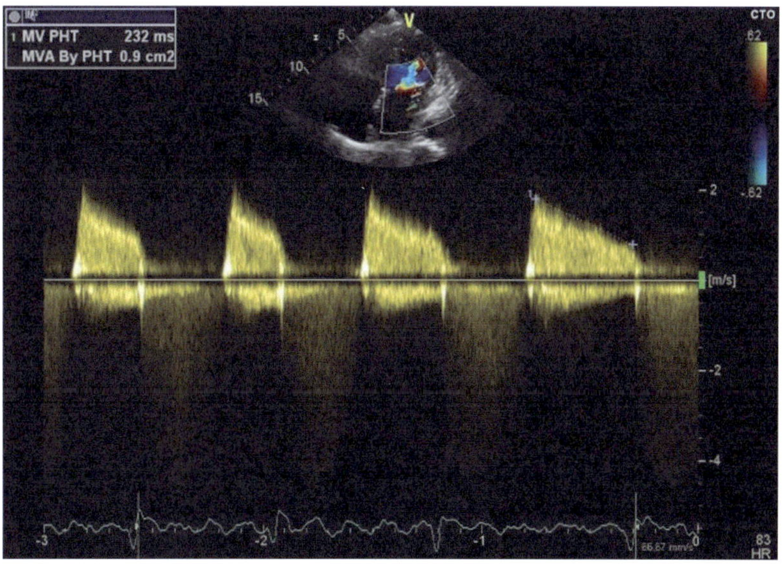

Fig. 2.29 Continuous wave Doppler echocardiography across the mitral valve, in a patient with severe mitral stenosis, where the pressure half-time (PHT) is measured, allowing the mitral valve area (MVA) to be calculated, MVA (cm^2) = 220/PHT (ms)

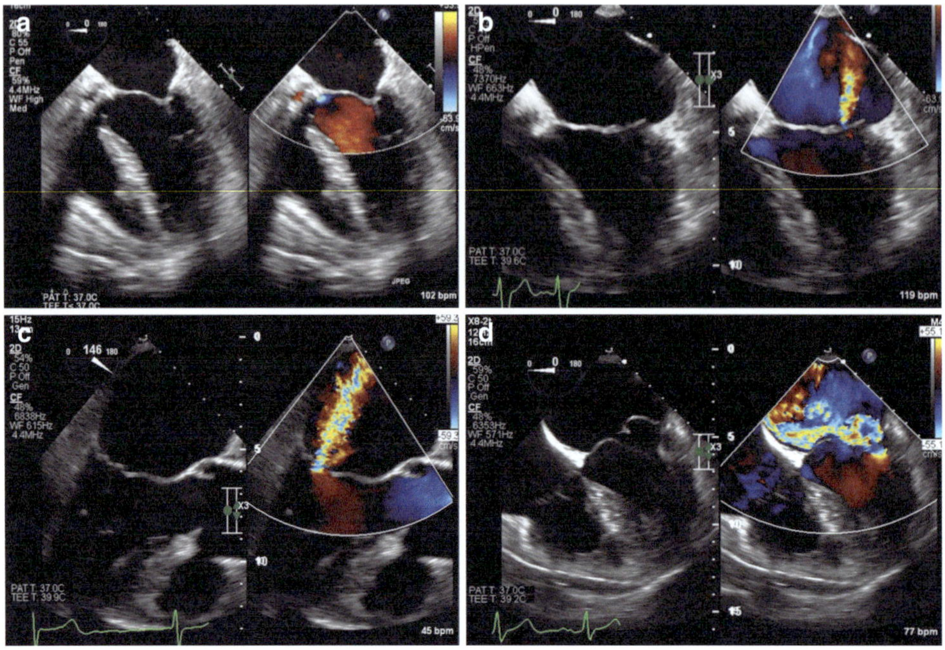

Fig. 2.30 TOE mid-oesophageal views with 2D and colour flow Doppler images across the mitral valve, demonstrating (**a**) no mitral regurgitation, (**b**) mild mitral regurgitation, (**c**) moderate mitral regurgitation and (**d**) severe eccentric regurgitant jet with a 'wall-hugging' jet and Coanda effect that causes the jet size to appear smaller

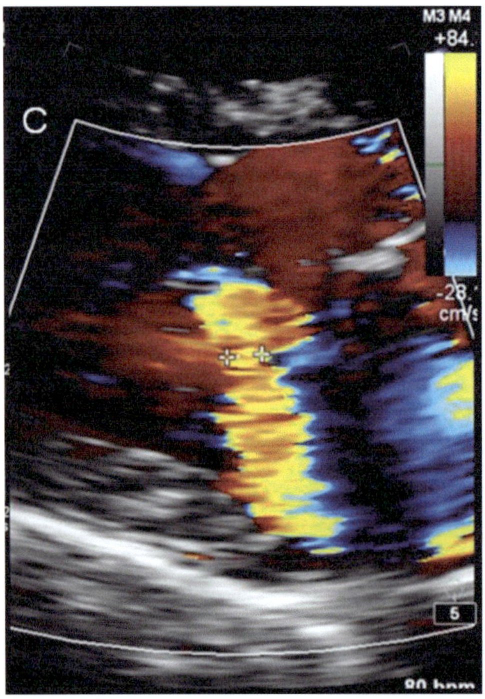

Fig. 2.31 Vena contracta assessment in the TTE parasternal long-axis view, obtained by measuring the width of the narrowest part of the mitral regurgitation jet as it leaves the regurgitant orifice

The principle of vena contracta is based on the assumption that the regurgitant orifice is almost circular, typically seen in mitral valve prolapse. This method is reliable in central and eccentric jets. It is, however, dependant on orifice geometry and may underestimate severity in the presence of multiple jets. In the case of functional MR, where the orifice is elliptical, two orthogonal planes transecting the regurgitant jet may be utilised to measure the vena contracta and the average of the two measurements is a useful guide to severity. More recently, the evolution of three-dimensional echo has allowed visualisation of the entire vena contracta area at the level of the regurgitant orifice allowing direct planimetry.

Proximal Isovelocity Surface Area (PISA)

Quantitative assessment of mitral regurgitation is usually performed using the proximal isovelocity surface area (PISA) or flow convergence method on the apical 4-chamber view (on TTE) or mid-oesophageal 4-chamber view (on TOE). As blood accelerates towards the regurgitant orifice the flow organises into isovelocity hemispheres of decreasing surface area but increasing velocities. Using colour flow Doppler, flow converging towards the regurgitant orifice can be identified as a hemispherical shell with its surface velocity equal to the chosen aliasing velocity. To optimise the analysis, the image of the regurgitant mitral valve is enlarged by reducing the image depth and then zoom mode followed by reducing the Nyquist limit. The PISA radius (r) is measured in mid-systole using the first aliasing threshold (where the displayed colour changes from red or blue to yellow) (Fig. 2.32). The identified PISA radius is measured from the surface of the hemisphere to the level of the orifice, allowing the surface area of the hemisphere of flow convergence to be calculated ($2\pi r^2$), and by multiplying it with the aliasing velocity of the flow convergence, the regurgitant flow can be calculated. The peak velocity and velocity time integral (VTI) of the regurgitant jet are measured using continuous wave Doppler. The continuity equation is then used to calculate the effective regurgitant orifice area (EROA) by dividing the regurgitant flow by the peak velocity of the regurgitant jet. The regurgitant volume (RV) can be calculated by multiplying the EROA by the velocity time integral of

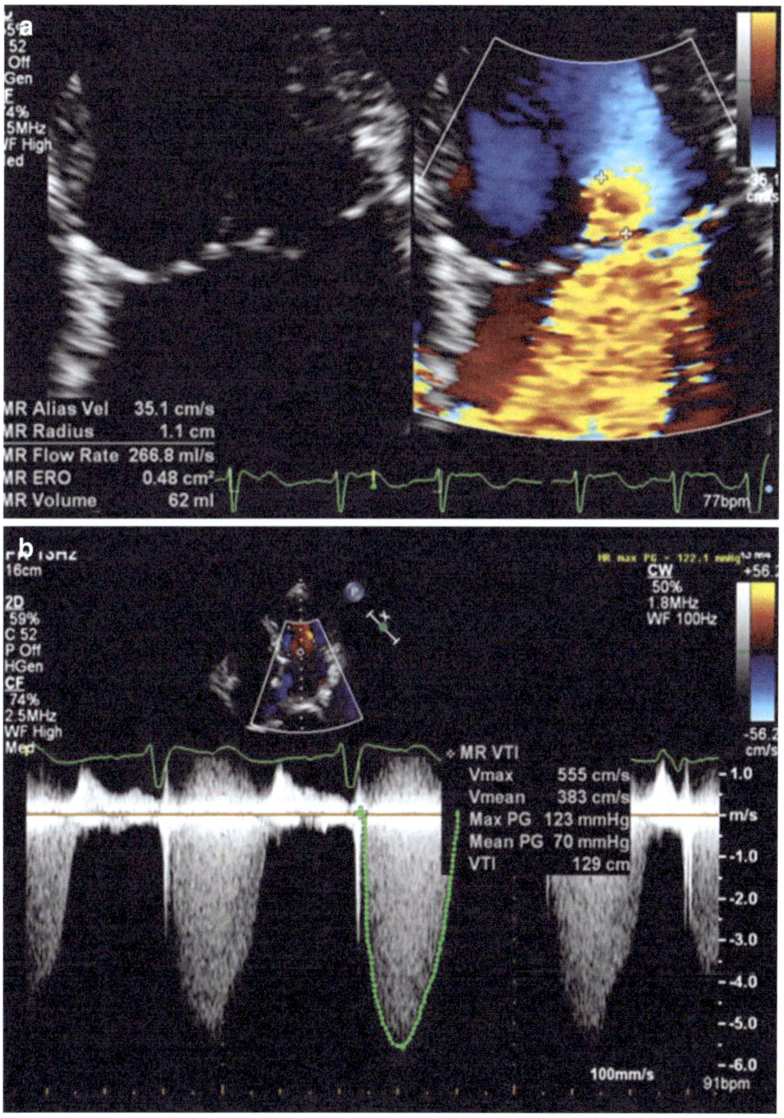

Fig. 2.32 Quantitative assessment of the severity of mitral regurgitation (MR) using the flow convergence method. (**a**) The radius of the hemispheric proximal isovelocity surface area (PISA) is measured using the first aliasing threshold with colour flow Doppler across the mitral valve in a zoomed apical 4-chamber view. (**b**) The velocity time integral (VTI) of the MR jet is measured using continuous wave Doppler

the regurgitant jet. Finally, the regurgitant fraction (RF) can be calculated by dividing the regurgitant volume by the mitral inflow volume and multiplying by 100.

$$\text{Regurgitant flow} = 2\pi r^2 \times \text{aliasing velocity}$$

$$\text{EROA} = \text{Regurgitant flow} / \text{peak velocity of regurgitant jet}$$

$$\text{RV} = \text{EROA} \times \text{VTI of the regurgitant jet}$$

$$\text{RF} = \left(\text{RV} / \text{mitral inflow volume}\right) \times 100$$

Mitral regurgitation can then be classified as mild, moderate or severe (see Table 2.1).

The PISA method is based on the assumption that the mitral regurgitation jet shell is a complete symmetrical hemisphere. The shape of the PISA hemisphere reflects the regurgitant orifice morphology and is hemispherical and roughly circular in mitral valve prolapse or flail, but is hemi-elliptical in functional mitral regurgitation, and risks underestimation of severity. Other limitations include the duration of regurgitation, dynamic jets (where the regurgitation is worse in early and late systole reducing in mid systole) and alteration in the shape of the PISA from adjacent structures (such as leaflet tenting with constraint of the hemisphere from a non-planar orifice). There is also inter-observer variability, especially as any errors in PISA radius are squared in the calculation of flow. A simplified method assumes mitral regurgitant peak velocity measured with continuous wave Doppler falls between 4 and 6 m/s (true for the majority of cases) where a PISA radius of 1 cm equates to roughly 0.4 cm^2. Regurgitation is classified as mild if the PISA radius is <0.4 cm and severe if the PISA radius is >1 cm. The most recent AHA guidelines have reclassified the recommended definition of severe secondary MR as the same values as primary MR (effective regurgitant orifice ≥0.4 cm^2 and regurgitant volume ≥60 mL).

Pulmonary Vein Flow

Pulsed wave Doppler flow, measured by placing the sample volume within the pulmonary veins as they enter the left atrium, can give additional information regarding the severity of mitral regurgitation. Although sampling of pulmonary flow from the left and right superior pulmonary vein can be performed with trans-thoracic echocardiography (apical 4-chamber view), sampling of all four pulmonary veins is recommended, as an eccentric MR jet can cause flow reversal in only one or two pulmonary veins, and this is best performed by trans-oesophageal echocardiography. In patients without diastolic dysfunction or mitral regurgitation, where left atrial pressure is normal, flow from the pulmonary veins into the left atrium is continuous during ventricular systole and diastole, except in late diastole where flow is momentarily reversed due to atrial contraction (when in sinus rhythm). Hence, the normal pulmonary venous trace includes a positive larger systolic (S) wave followed by a smaller diastolic (D) wave and a small reversed atrial contraction wave (Fig. 2.33). In patients with increasing mitral regurgitation, the size of the S wave progressively reduces, until flow reversal into the pulmonary veins is seen in severe mitral regurgitation, with systolic flow reversal of the S wave. Blunting of systolic pulmonary vein flow, however, is not specific for mitral regurgitation as it reflects increasing left atrial pressure from any aetiology including atrial fibrillation or left ventricular dysfunction.

Table 2.1 Classification of mitral regurgitation according to effective orifice area, regurgitant volume and regurgitant fraction

	Mild	Moderate	Severe	Severe IMR
Regurgitant volume (mL)	<30	30–59	>60	>60
Regurgitant fraction (%)	<30	30–49	>50	>50
Effective regurgitant orifice area (mm^2)	<20	20–39	>40	>40

IMR ischaemic mitral regurgitation

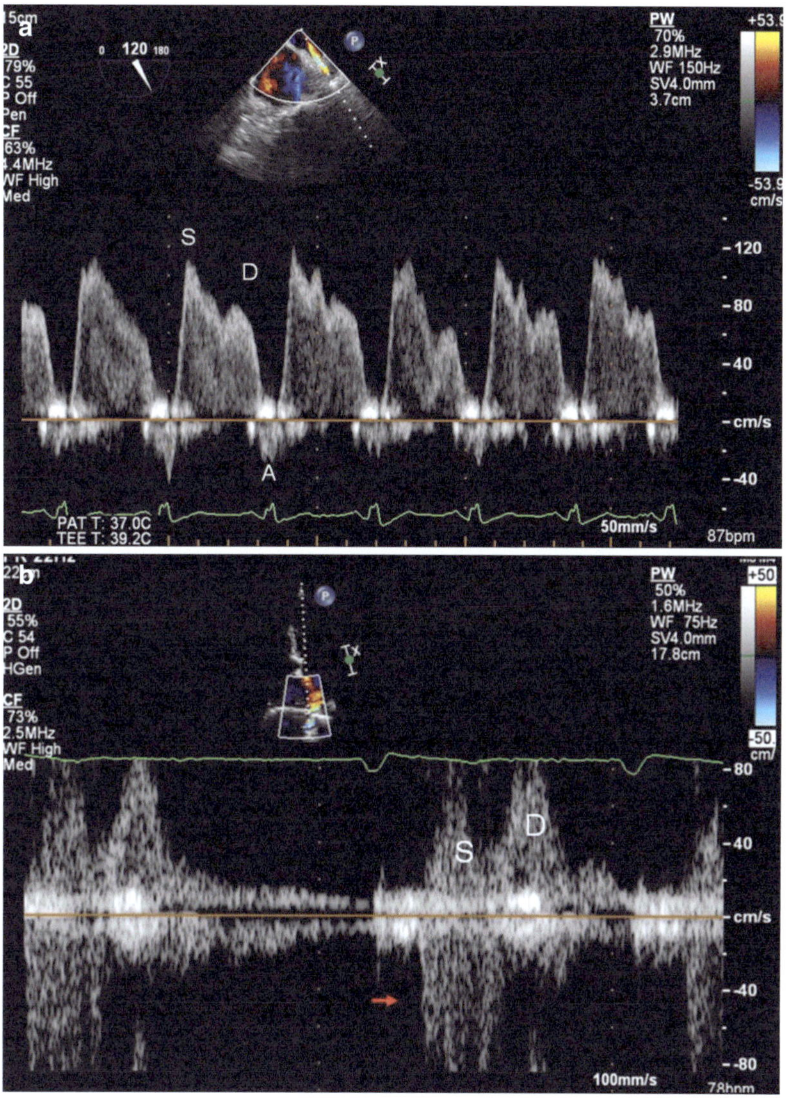

Fig. 2.33 Pulsed wave Doppler flow patterns across the pulmonary veins, demonstrating (**a**) normal flow pattern, and (**b**) pulmonary vein systolic flow reversal (below the line, red arrow) in a patient with severe MR. S systolic wave, D diastolic wave

Left Ventricular Size and Function

Changes in left ventricular size and function secondary to volume overload from the mitral regurgitation can be measured by assessing left ventricular dimensions and ejection fraction. The standardised method for left ventricular internal diameter measurements are performed at end-diastole and end-systole in the parasternal long-axis view at the level of the tips of the mitral valve. For ejection fraction, the biplane Simpson's method is applied to the apical 2- and 4-chamber orthogonal views on transthoracic echocardiography. An end-systolic diameter of >45 mm (European guidelines) or >40 mm (or >22 mm/m^2, American guidelines) and an ejection fraction of <60% are Class I indications for surgery in patients with severe mitral regurgitation. Three-dimensional echocardiography correlates closely with cardiac magnetic resonance imaging (MRI) and is increasingly used in clinical practice. More recently, myocardial contractility has been defined by myocardial tissue speckle tracking methods. Abnormal global longitudinal strain has been shown to identify individuals who go on to develop post-operative left ventricular dysfunction despite normal chamber size and ejection fraction.

Left Atrial Size and Pulmonary Pressures

Changes in left atrial size has been shown to be an importance prognostic marker in many disease states, including systemic hypertension and left ventricular dysfunction. Volume overload with mitral regurgitation or pressure overload with mitral stenosis will result in progressive left atrial dilatation. Similar to left ventricular volume, quantification using two orthogonal planes apical 4-chamber and apical 2-chamber views on trans-thoracic echocardiography are traced in (ventricular) end-systole (Fig. 2.34). If significant mitral pathology is present, the left atrium is usually enlarged, except in the acute setting. Reverse remodelling of the left atrium may also occur following mitral valve surgery. Left atrial linear dimension can be measured in the parasternal long-axis view and area in the apical 4-chamber view. Normal left atrial size parameters are diameter <4 cm, area <20 cm^2 and indexed volume <34 mL/m^2. Significant left atrial dilatation is defined as diameter >5 cm, area >40 cm^2 and indexed volume >50 mL/m^2.

In addition, the presence of mitral valve disease may result in raised pulmonary artery systolic pressures. This can be calculated, if any tricuspid regurgitation is present, using continuous wave Doppler of the tricuspid valve flow in the apical 4-chamber view. The velocity of the tricuspid regurgitation jet is used to calculate the right ventricular systolic pressure (RVSP) using the modified Bernouli equation, $RVSP = 4\ v^2 + RA$ (where RA = right atrial pressure). The pulmonary artery systolic pressure is assumed to equate the RVSP in the absence of pulmonary stenosis or RV outflow tract obstruction. In a patient with severe mitral regurgitation, the presence of pulmonary hypertension (pulmonary artery systolic pressure >50 mmHg at rest) may also be an indication for mitral valve surgery.

Post-cardiopulmonary Bypass Echocardiography

Following separation from cardiopulmonary bypass, there are a number of factors that need to be assessed following mitral valve repair surgery, including:

1. Competency of the mitral valve – with no more than trace regurgitation. Following a long, complex repair, with poor underlying tissue, mild regurgitation (vena contracta <3 mm) may be acceptable. The risk of a further spell on cardiopulmonary bypass is balanced against the risk of leaving residual mild regurgitation. Severity of mitral regurgi-

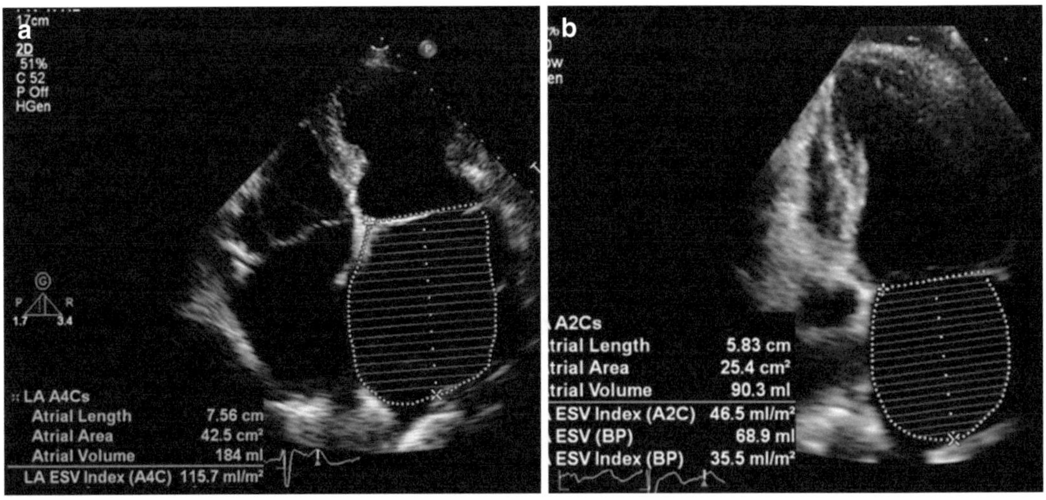

Fig. 2.34 Trans-thoracic echocardiographical left atrial size measurement on (**a**) apical 4-chamber and (**b**) apical 2-chamber views

tation greater than mild warrants further repair to the valve or replacement, as once the normal haemodynamic state is established postoperatively, its severity is invariably worse.
2. Bileaflet function with a good surface area of coaptation – mobility of both leaflets and a depth of coaptation >8 mm is usually associated with a good long term outcome and durability of repair.
3. Absence of systolic anterior motion (SAM) of the mitral valve. If present, this can often be treated with conservative measures, such as increased preload (fluid administration), reduced tachycardia (to allow ventricular filling), avoidance of inotropic agents (such as adrenaline or phosphodiesterase inhibitors) and increased afterload (such as with noradrenaline vasoconstriction). If these fail, the patient will need to be placed back on cardiopulmonary bypass to reduce the height of the posterior leaflet by resection or neo-chordae implantation to displace the coaptation line posteriorly away from the left ventricular outflow tract, implant a larger annuloplasty ring or perform a mitral valve replacement.
4. Absence of mitral stenosis (valve area >1.8 cm^2 and mean gradient <6 mmHg). In patients who have undergone complex repair, including leaflet resection and implantation of a small annuloplasty ring (<32 mm in size), there is a risk of obstruction to mitral inflow.
5. Ventricular contractility – both left and right ventricular contractility need to be assessed following mitral valve surgery. In particular, it is important to exclude the presence of left ventricular regional wall motion abnormalities involving the lateral wall, as this may highlight injury to the circumflex coronary artery, which lies in close proximity to the posterior annulus adjacent to P1 and P2.

Exercise Stress Echocardiography

Exercise stress echocardiography is used in risk stratification where MR is severe in the absence of symptoms, presence of equivocal symptoms or borderline left ventricular changes (EF 60–65%, LVESD 40–45 mm), to determine whether surgical intervention is warranted. A positive exercise stress echocardiography test is suggested by the unmasking of symptoms, worsening of MR severity, increase in pulmonary artery systolic pressure >60 mmHg or worsening (or absence of contractile reserve) left ventricular function.

Echocardiography of the Tricuspid Valve

As with the mitral valve, competency of the tricuspid valve depends on the complex interaction of the valve leaflets, annulus, chordae tendineae, papillary muscles and right ventricle. The valve consists of the anterior (largest), septal and posterior (smallest) leaflets. It is the most apically located valve and has the largest orifice of the cardiac valves, thereby maintaining a low forward velocity and pressure gradient across the ventricular inflow. The tricuspid annulus is an elliptical saddle-shaped structure, with the highest points in an anterior-posterior orientation and the lowest points in a medial-lateral orientation. The tricuspid annulus lies more apically and is slightly larger than the mitral valve annulus. In the apical 4-chamber view, the normal tricuspid valve annulus diameter is 28 ± 5 mm, with >40 mm representing annular dilatation. During the cardiac cycle, contraction of the tricuspid annulus contributes to valvular competency, with a 25% decrease in annular size in systole. The anterior, posterior and septal papillary muscles give rise to chordae tendineae attaching to the leaflets and are positioned beneath the commissures. The anterior papillary muscle is the largest and is attached to the moderator band. The septal papillary muscle is the smallest and may sometimes be absent.

Trans-thoracic echocardiography is usually the investigation of choice to image the tricuspid valve, since the right heart sits anteriorly in the chest. Where views may be suboptimal, however, TOE can be useful. The tricuspid valve can be seen on the parasternal right ventricular inflow view, parasternal short-axis view (at the level of the aortic valve), apical 4-chamber view and subcostal 4-chamber view (Fig. 2.35). The parasternal long-axis view of the right ventricular inflow can be obtained by tilting the probe inferomedially and rotating it clockwise from the parasternal long-axis view of the left ventricle, allowing the anterior leaflet (adjacent to the aortic valve) and posterior leaflet to be visualised. The septal and anterior (or posterior leaflet if the liver, and hence the inferior wall, is adjacent to the right ventricle) leaflets can be seen in the parasternal short-axis, apical 4-chamber and subcostal views.

On trans-oesophageal echocardiography, the tricuspid valve can be visualised on the basal oesophageal 4-chamber view (0°), RV inflow-outflow and bicaval views, and the trans-gastric RV basal short-axis and RV inflow views (Fig. 2.36). It is rare to visualise all three leaflets in the same 2D image but is possible on real-time 3D echocardiography.

It is important to appreciate that in a fasted patient under general anaesthesia, the sever-

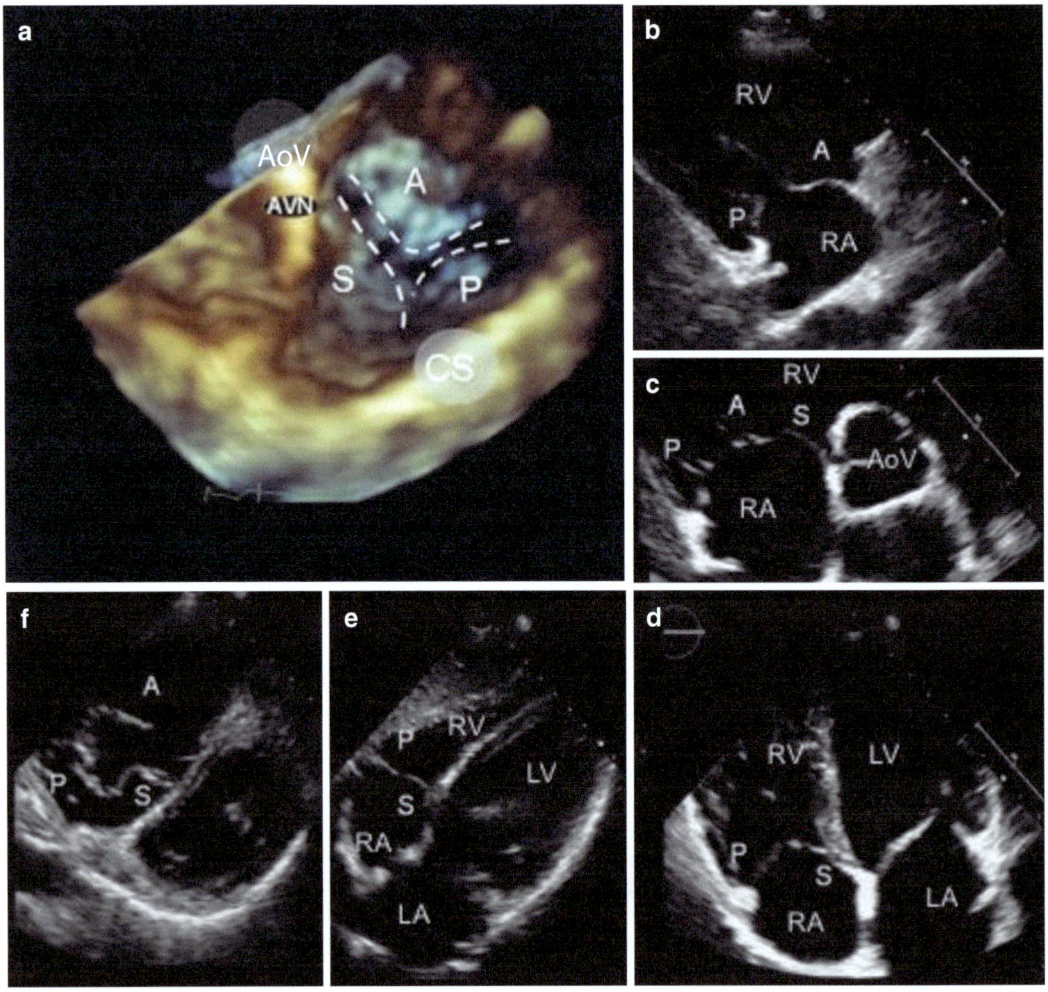

Fig. 2.35 Trans-thoracic echocardiographical images of the tricuspid valve. (**a**) 3D view from the right atrium, (**b**) parasternal long-axis view of the right ventricular inflow, (**c**) parasternal short-axis view (at the level of the aortic valve), (**d**) apical 4-chamber view, (**e**) subcostal 4-chamber view and (**f**) subcostal short-axis view. A anterior leaflet, P posterior leaflet, S septal leaflet, AVN atrioventricular node, AoV aortic valve, CS coronary sinus, RV right ventricle, RA right atrium, LV left ventricle, LA left atrium

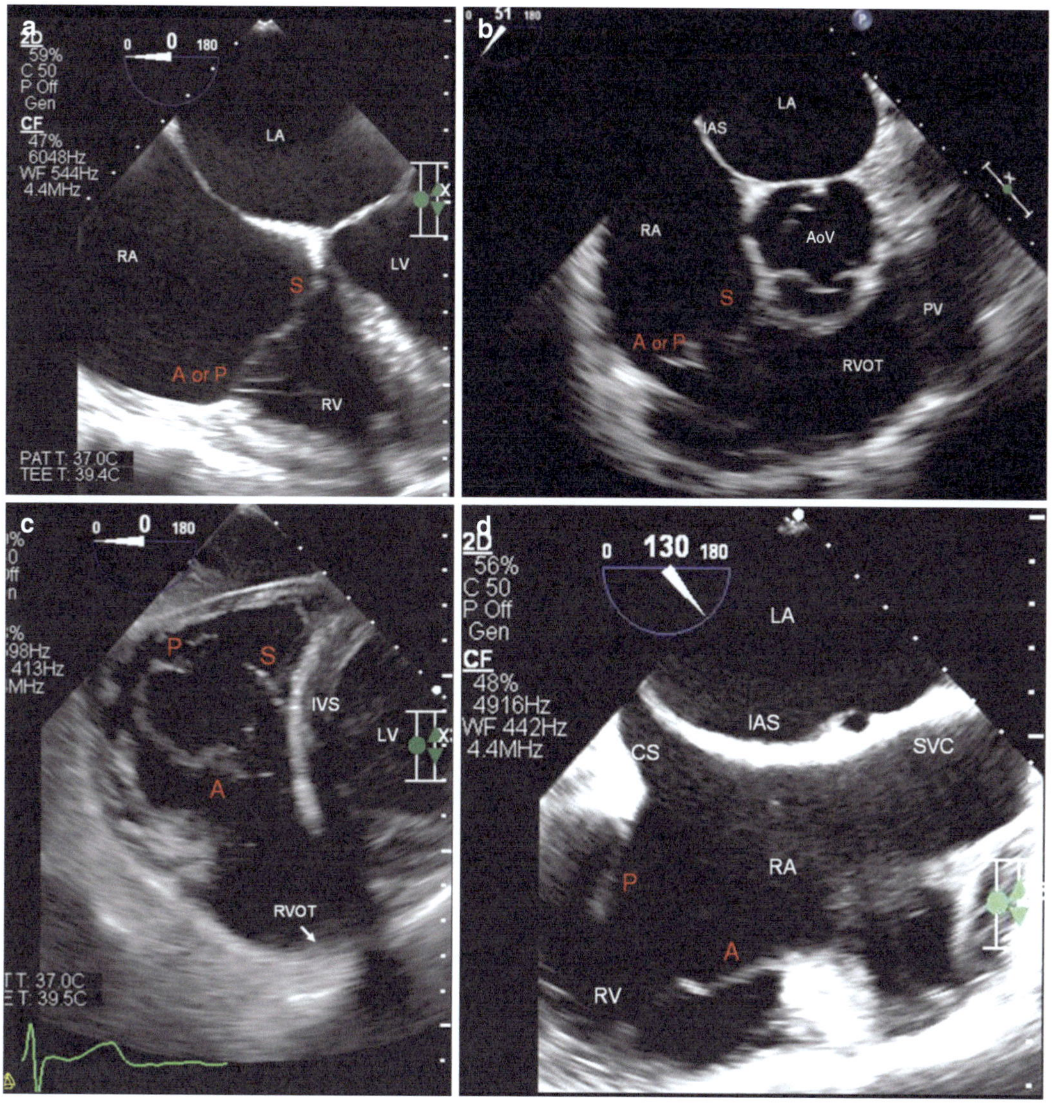

Fig. 2.36 Trans-oesophageal echocardiographic images of the tricuspid valve, (**a**) mid-oesophageal 4-chamber view (0°); (**b**) mid-oesophageal RV inflow-outflow view; (**c**) trans-gastric RV basal short-axis view; and (**d**) trans-gastric RV inflow view. A anterior tricuspid valve leaflet, P posterior tricuspid valve leaflet, S septal tricuspid valve leaflet, RA right atrium, RV right ventricle, LA left atrium, LV left ventricle, IAS inter-atrial septum, RVOT right ventricular outflow tract, AoV aortic valve, PV pulmonary valve, IVS inter-ventricular septum, CS coronary sinus, SVC superior vena cava

ity of tricuspid regurgitation measured is usually attenuated due to reduced preload, afterload and right ventricular function. It should therefore be interpreted with caution and other measures of tricuspid valve dysfunction be assessed, such as the dimensions of the tricuspid annulus, which should be measured on the trans-thoracic apical or trans-oesophageal mid-oesophageal 4-chamber view, with >4.0 cm considered to be dilated.

Regurgitant Jet Area

Colour flow Doppler assessment of regurgitant jet area is a useful qualitative marker for the severity of TR (Fig. 2.37). The measurement should be made in multiple views, including the parasternal inflow and short-axis, apical 4-chamber and subcostal views. As described for mitral regurgitation, however, loading conditions can impact on

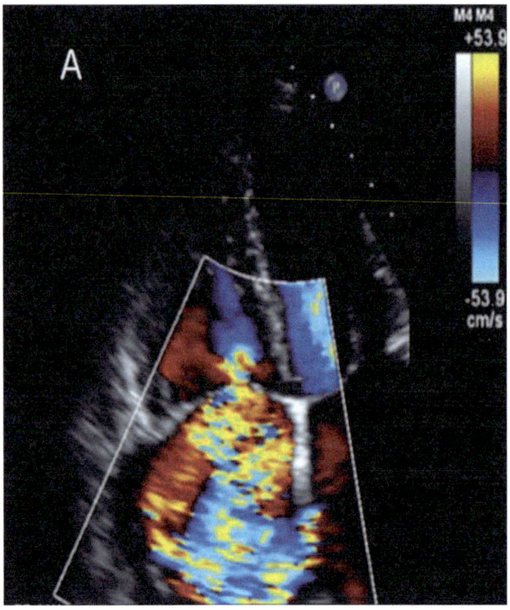

Fig. 2.37 Qualitative assessment of tricuspid regurgitation severity using colour flow Doppler measurement of the regurgitant jet area

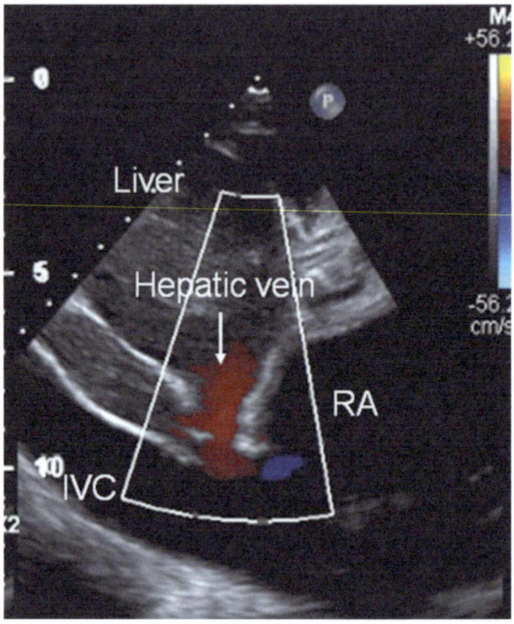

Fig. 2.38 Pulsed wave Doppler analysis on a transthoracic echocardiography subcostal view demonstrating systolic hepatic flow reversal

jet size, as well as eccentric wall-hugging jets in a large right atrium may appear less pronounced than a central regurgitant jet of equal severity.

Vena Contracta

The width of the vena contracta of the tricuspid regurgitant jet can be measured in an apical 4-chamber view using the same Nyquist limit scale as for MR, with >7 mm suggestive of severe TR. Lower values are unreliable in differentiating mild from moderate TR due to similar limitations already described for mitral regurgitation, including regurgitant jet orifice morphology.

PISA Analysis

The PISA radius and derived regurgitant volume (RV), regurgitant fraction (RF) and effective regurgitant orifice area (EROA) can be quantified using a similar methodology to MR PISA analysis, from the apical 4-chamber and the parasternal RV inflow and short-axis views. A PISA radius >9 mm, EROA >40 mm^2 or a RV >45 mL are suggestive of severe TR. A PISA radius 1–4 mm represents mild TR and 5–8 mm moderate TR.

Hepatic Vein Flow

Using pulsed wave Doppler, hepatic vein systolic flow reversal may indicate the presence of severe TR (Fig. 2.38). Although blunting or decrease of hepatic vein systolic flow occurs with increasing degrees of TR, it is less specific than flow reversal, as it can occur with atrial fibrillation or other causes of raised right atrial pressure.

Recommended Reading

Bhave NM, Ward RP. Echocardiographic assessment and clinical management of tricuspid regurgitation. Curr Cardiol Rep. 2011;13(3):258–64.

Hahn RT, Abraham T, Adams MS, Bruce CJ, Glas KE, Lang RM, Reeves ST, Shanewise JS, Siu SC, Stewart W, Picard MH. Guidelines for performing a comprehensive transesophageal echocardiographic examination: recommendations from the American Society of Echocardiography and the Society of Cardiovascular Anesthesiologists. J Am Soc Echocardiogr. 2013;26(9):921–64.

Lancellotti P, Moura L, Pierard LA, Agricola E, Popescu BA, Tribouilloy C, Hagendorff A, Monin JL, Badano L, Zamorano JL. European Association of Echocardiography recommendations for the assessment of valvular regurgitation. Part 2: mitral and tricuspid regurgitation (native valve disease). Eur J Echocardiogr. 2010;11:307–32.

Lancellotti P, Tribouilloy C, Hagendorff A, Popescu BA, Edvardsen T, Pierard LA, Badano L, Zamorano JL. Scientific Document Committee of the European Association of Cardiovascular Imaging. Recommendations for the echocardiographic assessment of native valvular regurgitation: an executive summary from the European Association of Cardiovascular Imaging. Eur Heart J Cardiovasc Imaging. 2013;14(7):611–44.

Lang RM, Badano LP, Mor-Avi V, Afilalo J, Armstrong A, Ernande L, Flachskampf FA, Foster E, Goldstein SA, Kuznetsova T, Lancellotti P, Muraru D, Picard MH, Rietzschel ER, Rudski L, Spencer KT, Tsang W, Voigt JU. Recommendations for cardiac chamber quantification by echocardiography in adults: an update from the American society of Echocardiography and the European Association of Cardiovascular Imaging. J Am Soc Echocardiogr. 2015;28:1–39.

Mahmood F, Matyal R. A quantitative approach to the intraoperative echocardiographic assessment of the mitral valve for repair. Anesth Analg. 2015;121(1): 34–58.

Poelaert JI, Bouchez S. Perioperative echocardiographic assessment of mitral valve regurgitation: a comprehensive review. Eur J Cardiothorac Surg. 2016;50: 801–12.

Zoghbi WA, Adams D, Bonow RO, Enriquez-Sarano M, Foster E, Grayburn PA, Hahn RT, Han Y, Hung J, Lang RM, Little SH, Shah DJ, Shernan S, Thavendiranathan P, Thomas JD, Weissman NJ. Recommendations for noninvasive evaluation of native valvular regurgitation: a report from the American Society of Echocardiography developed in collaboration with the Society for Cardiovascular Magnetic Resonance. J Am Soc Echocardiogr. 2017;30(4):303–71.

Indications for Surgery on the Mitral and Tricuspid Valves

3

Keywords
Mitral regurgitation · Mitral stenosis · Tricuspid regurgitation · Tricuspid stenosis · Infective endocarditis · Atrial fibrillation · American College of Cardiology/American Heart Association guidelines · European Society for Cardiology guidelines · Class of recommendation (COR) · Level of evidence (LOE)

Introduction

The indications for surgery on the mitral and tricuspid valves and rationale for intervention have been very clearly described in the most recent international guidelines from the American College of Cardiology/American Heart Association and European Society for Cardiology. This chapter summarises the recommendations from these guidelines, which are categorized into a number of classes of recommendations based on three different levels of evidence. The Class of Recommendation (COR) represents an estimate of the size of the treatment effect, with consideration given to the risks versus benefits, as well as the evidence and agreement that a given treatment or procedure is or is not useful or effective, or in some situations may cause harm. The Level of Evidence (LOE) represents an estimate of the certainty or precision of the treatment effect.

A class I recommendation is for a procedure or treatment that is useful or effective and should be performed or administered. A class IIa recommendation is in favour of a treatment or procedure being useful or effective, where it is reasonable for it to be performed or administered. A class IIb recommendation is where the usefulness or efficacy is less well established and the procedure or treatment may be considered. A class III recommendation is for a procedure or treatment that is not useful or effective and may be harmful, and therefore should not be performed or administered.

The strength of evidence that exists to support these recommendations has been also been described. Level A evidence represents data derived from multiple randomized clinical trials or meta-analyses, where multiple populations have been evaluated. Level B evidence represents data derived from a single randomized clinical trial or non-randomised studies, where limited populations have been evaluated. Level C evidence represents only consensus opinion of experts, case studies or standard of care, where very limited populations have been evaluated.

Mitral Regurgitation

Mitral valve surgery is recommended for symptomatic patients with chronic severe primary mitral regurgitation (MR) and a left ventricular

N. Moorjani et al., *Operative Mitral and Tricuspid Valve Surgery*,
https://doi.org/10.1007/978-1-4471-4204-1_3

ejection fraction >30%. As the presence of even mild symptoms in patients with severe MR is associated with an adverse effect on long-term patient outcomes, even in the absence of left ventricular changes, the onset of symptoms should initiate a prompt referral for surgery.

Mitral valve surgery is recommended for asymptomatic patients with chronic severe primary MR and the presence of left ventricular dysfunction, evidenced by an ejection fraction (EF) of 30–60% and/or left ventricular end-systolic diameter (LVESD) ≥40 mm. As the onset of LV systolic dysfunction is associated with a worse prognosis, mitral valve surgery ideally should be performed on patients before the deterioration of EF below 60% or dilatation of the left ventricle (LVESD ≥40 mm). Imaging surveillance is important as LV changes may occur before the onset of symptoms. If operated on early enough, reverse remodelling of impaired ventricles may occur following mitral surgery, thereby allowing for recovery of left ventricular function. An ejection fraction of 60% is used as a cut-off in the presence of mitral regurgitation, as the left ventricle ejects blood into the left atrium as well as the aorta, and impaired contractility may be present with a 'normal' EF of 50%. Among asymptomatic patients with severe primary MR with preserved LV systolic function (LV EF >60%, LVESD <40 mm), mitral valve surgery is reasonable in the setting of serial imaging studies that reveal a progressive increase in LV size or decrease in LVEF.

Mitral valve repair is recommended in preference to replacement when surgical treatment is indicated for patients with chronic severe primary MR limited to the posterior leaflet. Although there are no prospective randomised controlled trials, mitral valve repair is associated with lower operative mortality, better preservation of LV function (due to better preservation of the mitral valve apparatus), and a lower incidence of complications associated with prosthetic heart valves (such as thromboembolism, anticoagulation-related events or structural valve deterioration), when compared to mitral valve replacement. As mitral valve repair is the standard of care for isolated degenerative posterior mitral valve prolapse, it should be performed in a high volume centre with surgical expertise achieving a repair rate >90%, operative mortality <1%, long-term survival similar to that of an age-matched general population, 95% freedom from reoperation and >80% freedom from recurrent moderate + MR at 15–20 years. If there is any doubt regarding the durability of the repair, replacement is preferable.

Mitral valve repair is recommended in preference to replacement when surgical treatment is indicated for patients with chronic severe primary MR involving the anterior leaflet or both leaflets when a successful and durable repair can be accomplished. These patients require a more complex and extensive repair and have an inferior durability compared to isolated posterior leaflet prolapse, with a freedom from reoperation of 80% and freedom from moderate + MR 60% at 15–20 years. Despite this, the outcomes are still superior to replacement; therefore, repair should be attempted in these patients but in the hands of an experienced mitral valve surgeon. In young patients where very complex repair of the mitral valve is required, mechanical mitral valve replacement may be able to provide comparable results.

Concomitant mitral valve repair or replacement is indicated in patients with chronic severe primary MR undergoing cardiac surgery for other indications, such as coronary revascularization and other valvular surgery.

Mitral valve repair is reasonable in asymptomatic patients with chronic severe primary MR with preserved LV function (LVEF >60% and LVESD <40 mm) in whom the likelihood of a successful and durable repair without residual MR is greater than 95%, with an expected mortality rate of less than 1%, when performed at a heart valve centre of excellence. As the onset of symptoms, LV dysfunction or pulmonary hypertension is associated with a worse prognosis, performing early surgery in these patients is an attractive option. This option necessitates the requirement of an experienced mitral valve surgeon to perform a successful repair procedure in order to avoid exposing the patient to the risks associated with valve replacement, or repair failure and reoperation.

Mitral valve repair is reasonable for asymptomatic patients with chronic severe nonrheumatic primary MR and preserved LV function (LVEF >60% and LVESD <40 mm) in whom there is a high likelihood of a successful and durable repair, with new onset of atrial fibrillation (AF) or resting pulmonary hypertension (pulmonary artery systolic pressure >50 mm Hg). The presence of AF or pulmonary hypertension due to MR is associated with poorer surgical outcome. Restoration of valvular competency and subsequent reverse remodelling may help to restore sinus rhythm, although the addition of a concomitant ablation procedure may be required. In rheumatic MR, the presence of atrial inflammation and valve scarring may make restoration of sinus rhythm and a successful repair less likely.

Concomitant mitral valve repair is reasonable in patients with chronic moderate primary MR when undergoing cardiac surgery for other indications. The added risk of mitral valve surgery, however, must be weighed against the potential for progression of MR.

Mitral valve surgery may be considered in symptomatic patients with chronic severe primary MR and LVEF ≤30%. Although most patients with decompensated MR and poor left ventricular function have secondary MR, there are a small number of patients with advanced LV dysfunction that may still benefit from surgery. The effect of mitral surgery on the long-term outcome of these patients, however, is unclear.

Mitral valve repair may be considered in patients with rheumatic mitral valve disease when surgical treatment is indicated if a durable and successful repair is likely or when the reliability of long-term anticoagulation management is questionable. Rheumatic mitral valve disease is characterised by extensive calcification and thickening of the entire mitral valve apparatus and hence less amenable to a successful repair procedure. Repair of a rheumatic valve should therefore only be considered if a durable repair is likely or in patients where anticoagulation management is a concern.

Mitral valve replacement should not be performed for the treatment of isolated severe primary MR limited to less than one half of the posterior leaflet unless mitral valve repair has been attempted and was unsuccessful, due to the excellent long-term outcomes of repair when operated on by an experienced mitral valve surgeon.

Acute mitral regurgitation due to rupture of the papillary muscle should be treated by immediate surgery and revascularization, after stabilization of the haemodynamic status, using an intra-aortic balloon pump, positive inotropic agents and vasodilators. Most patients require valve replacement.

Mitral valve surgery is reasonable for patients with chronic severe secondary MR who are undergoing CABG or AVR. The benefit of mitral valve repair in these patients is unclear and replacement may provide a greater freedom from recurrent mitral regurgitation.

Mitral valve surgery may be considered for severely symptomatic patients (New York Heart Association, NYHA, class III–IV) with chronic severe secondary MR who have persistent symptoms despite optimal medical therapy for heart failure. It is reasonable to choose chordal-sparing mitral valve replacement over reduction annuloplasty mitral valve repair for these patients. Although volume overload caused by chronic secondary mitral regurgitation is associated with a worse prognosis, there is minimal evidence that correcting the severe MR improves symptoms long-term or prolongs life.

In patients with chronic, moderate, ischaemic MR (stage B) undergoing CABG, the usefulness of mitral valve repair is uncertain.

Mitral Stenosis

Mitral valve surgery (repair, commissurotomy or valve replacement) is indicated in severely symptomatic patients (NYHA, class III–IV) with significant mitral stenosis (MS, mitral valve area ≤1.5 cm^2) who are not high risk for surgery and who are not candidates for or who have failed previous percutaneous mitral balloon commissurotomy. Replacement is usually preferred due to the presence of severe thickening and calcification of the entire mitral valve complex. As MS is a slowly progressive disease, surgery should only be performed once the patient has severe symptoms (NYHA class III–IV).

Concomitant mitral valve surgery is indicated for patients with significant MS (mitral valve area ≤1.5 cm^2) undergoing cardiac surgery for other indications.

Concomitant mitral valve surgery may be considered for patients with a mitral valve area 1.6–2.0 cm^2 undergoing cardiac surgery for other indications.

Mitral valve surgery and excision of the left atrial appendage may be considered for patients with significant MS (mitral valve area ≤1.5 cm^2) who have had recurrent embolic events while receiving adequate anticoagulation. MS is a risk factor for recurrent embolism among patients with prior embolic events irrespective of the presence or absence of AF. The appendage should be excised and not just excluded from the circulation, due to the risk of residual communication with the appendage.

Tricuspid Regurgitation

Tricuspid valve (TV) surgery is recommended for patients with severe tricuspid regurgitation (TR) undergoing left-sided valve surgery, as the TR will not improve following reduction of right ventricular (RV) afterload following the left-sided surgery. Furthermore, reoperation for severe, isolated TR following previous left-sided valve surgery is associated with an operative mortality rate of 10–25%, whereas the addition of tricuspid valve repair at the time of the left-sided valve surgery does not appreciably increase the operative risks. Tricuspid valve repair is preferable to replacement. If replacement is required, the standard criteria should be used when determining whether to implant a mechanical or tissue valve, as there is no difference in survival between the two.

Tricuspid valve repair can be beneficial for patients with mild, moderate or greater functional TR at the time of left-sided valve surgery with either tricuspid annular dilation or prior evidence of right-sided heart failure. Approximately 25% of patients with mild or moderate functional TR uncorrected at the time of left-sided surgery progress, which is associated with reduced long-term functional outcome and survival. The risk factors for progression of TR include TV annular dilation (>40 mm or 21 mm/m^2 on preoperative trans-thoracic echocardiogram (TTE); >70 mm diameter on direct intraoperative measurement); RV dysfunction or dilatation; leaflet tethering; pulmonary artery hypertension; AF; non-myxomatous aetiology of MR; and intra-annular RV pacemaker leads. Surgery should be carried out early enough to avoid the risks of developing irreversible RV dysfunction.

Tricuspid valve surgery can be beneficial for patients with symptoms due to severe primary TR that are unresponsive to medical therapy. Patients with symptomatic severe primary TR without left-sided valve disease should undergo surgical intervention before the onset of significant RV dysfunction. TV replacement may be required because of the extent and severity of the underlying pathology, such as in patients with carcinoid, radiation-induced disease or Ebstein's anomaly. In the presence of severe RV systolic dysfunction or irreversible pulmonary hypertension, the operative risks should be carefully considered, due to the possibility of RV failure after the operation.

Tricuspid valve repair may be considered for patients with moderate functional TR and pulmonary artery hypertension at the time of left-sided valve surgery. It was previously thought that pulmonary hypertension caused by left-sided valve disease usually decreased following successful left-sided valve surgery, with improvement of mild to moderate functional TR, but this may not always be the case. In these patients, addition of TV repair at the time of left-sided valve surgery should be made on an individual case basis.

Tricuspid valve surgery may be considered for asymptomatic or minimally symptomatic patients with severe primary TR, associated with moderate or greater RV dilation or systolic dysfunction.

Reoperation for isolated tricuspid valve repair or replacement may be considered for persistent symptoms due to severe TR in patients who have undergone previous left-sided valve surgery and who do not have severe pulmonary hypertension or significant RV systolic dysfunction. The presence of either severe irreversible pulmonary hypertension or significant RV dysfunction constitutes a relative contraindication to reoperation, due to the high associated risks.

Tricuspid Stenosis

Tricuspid valve surgery is recommended for patients with severe tricuspid stenosis (TS) at the time of operation for left-sided valve disease. If repair is not feasible due to valve destruction, replacement may be required and the choice of prosthesis should be made on an individual case basis.

Tricuspid valve surgery is recommended for patients with isolated, symptomatic severe TS. In the presence of TR, tricuspid valve surgery is preferred over percutaneous balloon tricuspid commissurotomy for the treatment of symptomatic severe TS.

Infective Endocarditis

Early surgery (during initial hospitalization before completion of a full therapeutic course of antibiotics) is indicated in patients with infective endocarditis (IE) who present with valve dysfunction resulting in symptoms of heart failure (HF). Repair of the mitral valve following infective endocarditis is not always possible but may be feasible when leaflet perforation occurs without extensive leaflet destruction or annular involvement.

Emergency surgery is indicated for patients with mitral native or prosthetic valve endocarditis with severe acute regurgitation, obstruction or fistula causing refractory pulmonary oedema or cardiogenic shock.

Early surgery (during initial hospitalization before completion of a full therapeutic course of antibiotics) is indicated in patients with left-sided IE caused by *Staphylococcus aureus*, fungal or other highly resistant organisms. Infection from these organisms is difficult to cure with medical therapy alone and they are associated with local tissue destruction, including abscess and fistula formation.

Early surgery (during initial hospitalization before completion of a full therapeutic course of antibiotics) is indicated in patients with IE complicated by heart block, annular or aortic abscess, or destructive penetrating lesions. Abscess formation involving the native valves or paravalvular structures, with or without extension to the cardiac conduction system is a life-threatening complication that cannot be cured with antibiotic therapy alone and urgent surgical intervention is required.

Early surgery (during initial hospitalization before completion of a full therapeutic course of antibiotics) for IE is indicated in patients with evidence of persistent infection as manifested by persistent bacteraemia or fevers lasting longer than 5–7 days after the onset of appropriate antimicrobial therapy. Blood cultures usually become negative after 48 h of appropriate antimicrobial therapy (or within 7 days for methicillin-resistant *staphylococcus aureus*, MRSA, and other resistant organisms). Ongoing infection despite antibiotic therapy may suggest abscess formation or the presence of a large vegetation. It is also important to consider causes of infection other than the valve in patients who develop recurrent fever after an initially successful response to antibiotics.

Operation without delay may be considered in patients with IE and an indication for surgery who have suffered a stroke, but have no evidence of intracranial haemorrhage or extensive neurological damage. If hemodynamically stable, delaying valve surgery for ≥4 weeks may be considered among patients with IE and major ischemic stroke or intracranial haemorrhage.

Surgery is recommended for patients with prosthetic valve endocarditis (PVE) and relapsing infection (defined as recurrence of bacteraemia after a complete course of appropriate antibiotics and subsequently negative blood cultures) without other identifiable source for portal of infection.

Early surgery (during initial hospitalization before completion of a full therapeutic course of antibiotics) is reasonable in patients with IE who present with recurrent emboli and persistent vegetations despite appropriate antibiotic therapy.

The risk of embolism is highest during the 1st few days after initiation of antibiotic treatment and decreases after 2 weeks to 9–21%. Risk factors associated with a new embolic event include vegetation >10 mm diameter and marked vegetation mobility (especially on the anterior leaflet of the mitral valve).

Early surgery (during initial hospitalization before completion of a full therapeutic course of antibiotics) may be considered in patients with native valve endocarditis (NVE) who exhibit a mobile vegetation >10 mm diameter (with or without clinical evidence of embolic phenomenon). In patients with a vegetation >10 mm, with or without embolic events, there is no mortality benefit between early surgery versus conventional surgery, but there is a significant reduction in the number of embolic events in the early surgery group.

Atrial Fibrillation

A concomitant maze procedure is reasonable at the time of mitral valve repair or replacement for the treatment of chronic, persistent AF. This is made on the basis that persistent AF is an independent risk factor for stroke and mortality following surgery for mitral valve disease and that mitral surgery alone is unlikely to restore stable sinus rhythm to a patient if AF has been present for >1 year. Combining the maze procedure does not significantly increase the risk of surgery and is associated with significantly increased freedom from AF at 1 year (75–95%), as compared to mitral surgery alone (10–40%). The addition of a maze procedure, however, does not seem to improve long-term survival or freedom from stroke. Although left atrial appendage excision is commonly performed in patients with AF, there are no randomised controlled trials to have shown a beneficial impact.

A full bi-atrial maze procedure, when technically feasible, is reasonable at the time of mitral valve surgery, compared with a lesser ablation procedure, in patients with chronic, persistent AF. Lesser procedures, such as pulmonary vein isolation or left-sided maze, are associated with a reduced freedom from AF, although may be advocated in paroxysmal AF. The full bi-atrial maze is, however, associated with an increased incidence of permanent pacemaker requirement.

A concomitant maze procedure or pulmonary vein isolation may be considered at the time of mitral valve repair or replacement in patients with paroxysmal AF that is symptomatic or associated with a history of embolism on anticoagulation.

Concomitant maze procedure or pulmonary vein isolation may be considered at the time of cardiac surgical procedures other than mitral valve surgery in patients with paroxysmal or persistent AF that is symptomatic or associated with a history of emboli on anticoagulation.

Exclusion/excision of the left atrial appendage may be considered in patients undergoing cardiac surgery with AF, although there is insufficient evidence to prove that LAA exclusion has a benefit in terms of stroke reduction or mortality.

Recommended Reading

Baumgartner H, Falk V, Bax JJ, De Bonis M, Hamm C, Holm PJ, Iung B, Lancellotti P, Lansac E, Rodriguez Muñoz D, Rosenhek R, Sjögren J, Tornos Mas P, Vahanian A, Walther T, Wendler O, Windecker S, Zamorano JL; ESC Scientific Document Group. 2017 ESC/EACTS Guidelines for the management of valvular heart disease. Eur Heart J. 2017;38(36):2739–791.

January CT, Wann LS, Alpert JS, Calkins H, Cigarroa JE, Cleveland JC Jr, Conti JB, Ellinor PT, Ezekowitz MD, Field ME, Murray KT, Sacco RL, Stevenson WG, Tchou PJ, Tracy CM, Yancy CW, ACC/AHA Task Force Members. 2014 AHA/ACC/HRS guideline for the management of patients with atrial fibrillation: a report of the American College of Cardiology/American Heart Association task force on practice guidelines and the Heart Rhythm Society. Circulation. 2014;130(23):e199–267.

Kirchhof P, Benussi S, Kotecha D, Ahlsson A, Atar D, Casadei B, Castella M, Diener HC, Heidbuchel H, Hendriks J, Hindricks G, Manolis AS, Oldgren J, Popescu BA, Schotten U, Van Putte B, Vardas P, Agewall S, Camm J, Baron Esquivias G, Budts W, Carerj S, Casselman F, Coca A, De Caterina R, Deftereos S, Dobrev D, Ferro JM, Filippatos G, Fitzsimons D, Gorenek B, Guenoun M, Hohnloser SH, Kolh P, Lip GY, Manolis A, McMurray J, Ponikowski P, Rosenhek R, Ruschitzka F, Savelieva I, Sharma S, Suwalski P, Tamargo JL, Taylor CJ, Van Gelder IC, Voors AA, Windecker S, Zamorano JL, Zeppenfeld K. 2016 ESC guidelines for the management of atrial fibrillation developed in collaboration with EACTS. Eur J Cardiothorac Surg. 2016;50(5):e1–e88.

Nishimura RA, Otto CM, Bonow RO, Carabello BA, Erwin JP 3rd, Guyton RA, O'Gara PT, Ruiz CE, Skubas NJ, Sorajja P, Sundt TM 3rd, Thomas JD, Anderson JL, Halperin JL, Albert NM, Bozkurt B, Brindis RG, Creager MA, Curtis LH, DeMets D, Guyton RA, Hochman JS, Kovacs RJ, Ohman EM, Pressler SJ, Sellke FW, Shen WK, Stevenson WG, Yancy CW, American College of Cardiology, American College of Cardiology/American Heart Association, American Heart Association. 2014 AHA/ACC guideline for the management of patients with valvular heart disease. J Thorac Cardiovasc Surg. 2014;148(1):e1–e132.

Nishimura RA, Otto CM, Bonow RO, Carabello BA, Erwin JP 3rd, Fleisher LA, Jneid H, Mack MJ, McLeod CJ, O'Gara PT, Rigolin VH, Sundt TM 3rd, Thompson A. 2017 AHA/ACC focused update of the 2014 AHA/ACC guideline for the management of patients with valvular heart disease: a report of the American College of Cardiology/American Heart Association task force on clinical practice guidelines. Circulation. 2017;135(25):e1159–95.

Operative Set Up, Exposure and Analysis of the Mitral and Tricuspid Valves

4

Keywords
Patient positioning · Surgical incision · Minimally invasive surgery · Robotic surgery · Exposure of the valve · Standard left atriotomy · Vertical trans-septal bi-atrial incision · Superior left atrial roof incision · Horizontal trans-septal bi-atrial incision · Right atriotomy

Introduction

Reproducible and safe surgery requires both visibility and vision. The first comes through the correct positioning of the patient on the operating table and the maximal utilization of the surgical incision. The second is harder won and comes with increasing experience and an ever open and questioning mind. Both require a close involvement by the surgeon responsible for the case at all times.

There is much contemporary debate about the pros and cons of minimal access or open surgery to reach the mitral valve. This chapter does not set out to explore this conundrum but to give clear guide lines on how to reliably expose the valve through a midline sternotomy, as all surgeons of the mitral valve need to be able to achieve this safely and reproducibly.

Positioning of the Patient on the Operating Table

This is the responsibility of the surgeon in charge of the case and should not be left to the anaesthetic and operating department staff. It is not other's fault if poor positioning of the patient restricts surgical access.

The patient is positioned on the operating table in the supine position. The head should be a comfortable distance from the upper end of the operating table to give good clearance between the anaesthetist's territory and that of the surgeon. Clashing hands and elbows through the surgical drapes is unnecessary but it is surprising how often it is encountered. If the patient is tall then it is important to make sure that the feet are properly supported, so as not to allow for the potential of foot drop through over extension of the common peroneal nerve, as it passes around the lateral head of the fibula. Properly designed silicone gel rests should be placed under the dorsal aspect of each lower leg to prevent stasis in the deep soleal plexus of veins.

N. Moorjani et al., *Operative Mitral and Tricuspid Valve Surgery*,
https://doi.org/10.1007/978-1-4471-4204-1_4

A similar silicone gel roll is also placed horizontally beneath the patient's shoulders to push the upper chest forwards. This brings the thorax into a horizontal plane to the operating table. In some patients, especially deep chested men, the diameter of the thorax at the level of the 10th thoracic vertebra is much larger than that at the thoracic inlet. Without this support, the sternum slopes downwards, sometimes at a steep angle and once inside the thorax, the heart tends to fall towards the superior mediastinum. If the intercaval distance is short this will worsen the access to the left atrium. This simple manoeuvre improves this access.

The patient's arms are comfortably secured to the patient's side. The essential final check of patient identity and procedure, along with the presence of cross-matched blood and sterile instruments, as laid out in the WHO guidelines, is completed. The patient is then ready for full and careful skin preparation with the chosen antiseptic solution and surgical draping. The surgical team should be present for all of this process.

Surgical Incision

The skin incision must be central allowing access to the sternal notch superiorly and the xiphisternum inferiorly. The length can vary from the middle two-thirds to the full length of the sternum depending upon the experience of the surgeon. Before the sternum is divided, the suprasternal space is developed and a finger used to free the upper mediastinal space. Similarly, the sub-xiphisternal space is developed with a finger and the xiphisternum divided with heavy scissors. Separation of the sub-sternal tissues for as far as possible, along with interrupting ventilation and disconnecting the endotracheal tube for a moment, will allow the lungs to fall away from the anterior mediastinum, thereby reducing the chance of opening either of the pleural spaces when using the sternal saw.

The sternal saw should be allowed to pass through the bone without excessive pressure and following the anterior convexity of the sternum. Once divided, the edges of the sternum are sealed with softened bone wax and the periosteal vessels sealed with diathermy. The sternal retractor can then be inserted over drapes to ease the pressure on the edge of the bone.

The fat in the anterior mediastinal space is then separated in the mid-line. The thymic remnant, which is mainly fat in the adult, is separated and any vessels cauterised. Often, however, there are significant vessels within it crossing the midline. These vessels can be clamped on each side, divided and then the tissue within the clamps can be ligated. This will ensure haemostasis. The left innominate vein is identified and the thymic vein, which drains into it, identified and clipped, as it is often of significant size. It is important to ensure that the there is no bleeding prior to the institution of cardiopulmonary bypass. During this process, the appropriate dose of heparin is given in preparation for cannulation of the heart for the establishment of cardiopulmonary bypass. The pericardium is then opened along a vertical line two-thirds of the way towards the left side of the visible pericardium. This allows for the pericardium on the right side to be more easily slung under the retractor blades, thus elevating the heart in the pericardial cavity and rotating the left atrium towards the surgeon thereby improving access. The visceral pericardial reflection between the pulmonary artery and the aorta is then divided, separating these vessels to allow easy application of the aortic cross-clamp.

Two aortic purse string sutures are then placed concentrically, just at the beginning of the arch of the aorta, using a braided polyester suture. The cardiopulmonary bypass tubing is then clamped and divided at an appropriate place so as to allow the tubing to lie comfortably on either side of the sternotomy. The aortic cannula is inserted into the aorta in the centre of the purse string sutures, which are snugged down to secure the cannula in place. The snugger tubing is then secured to the cannula with a heavy gauge tie to prevent any outward migration of the aortic cannula during the procedure. It is then further secured with a heavy-duty suture to the wound edge, so as to secure the aortic pipe in a gentle curve.

Next the venae cavae are cannulated. One purse-string suture is placed around the right atrial appendage and a second just above the inferior cavo-atrial junction. Venous cannulae are chosen depending upon the surface area of the patient. For superior caval cannulation, a gently curved vascular clamp is applied across the base of the atrial appendage. The first assistant then steadies this and the tip of the atrial appendage is amputated. As the clamp is removed, the venous pipe is slid into the atrium. The retaining suture is gently pulled downwards towards the feet of the patient. This allows easy passage of the venous pipe up into the superior vena cava. Its tip should rest close to the confluence of the innominate vein and the superior vena cava. The snugger is then secured and tied to the pipe with a heavy gauge tie. For inferior caval cannulation, the atrial wall is incised in the centre of the purse-string suture with a pointed blade and then gently dilated with the tip of a Robert's clamp to allow easy passage of the cannula into the atrium. A finger is placed over the hole until the pipe is ready to be inserted. Once the cannula is within the atrium, the first assistant gently retracts the purse-string suture towards the head of the patient and the tube will then pass easily into the inferior cava as the cranial tension causes the caval valve to flatten against the atrial wall. It is essential that if resistance is encountered, as a result of the venous valve, that undue force is not used, as that can result in a tear to the posterolateral wall of the inferior cavo-atrial junction. Once again, the venous pipe is secured to the snugger with a heavy tie (Fig. 4.1).

Cardiopulmonary bypass can then be commenced once the pipes are connected to the circuit. A left ventricular vent is then inserted, via the right superior pulmonary vein or left ventricular apex. The apical approach keeps the operative field free of blood on the ventricular side. A purse-string is then placed in the ascending aorta for the insertion of the cardioplegia line, which again is secured in place using a strong tie. Systemic cooling is then commenced, usually at a systemic temperature of 32 °C.

The aortic cross-clamp is then applied with reduced pump flow to minimise the potential for trauma to the aorta. One litre of antegrade cold blood cardioplegia is then administered. The heart is bathed in cold saline at 4 °C. Using this technique, the heart will arrest rapidly and the ventricle cannot distend, as there is a left ventricular vent in place. Once the heart has been arrested, the superior and inferior vena cavae are mobilised and tapes are passed around each of the cavae. It is done at this stage, as it is very easily done in the arrested heart with no risk of damage to the pulmonary artery superiorly or the back of the inferior vena cava inferiorly.

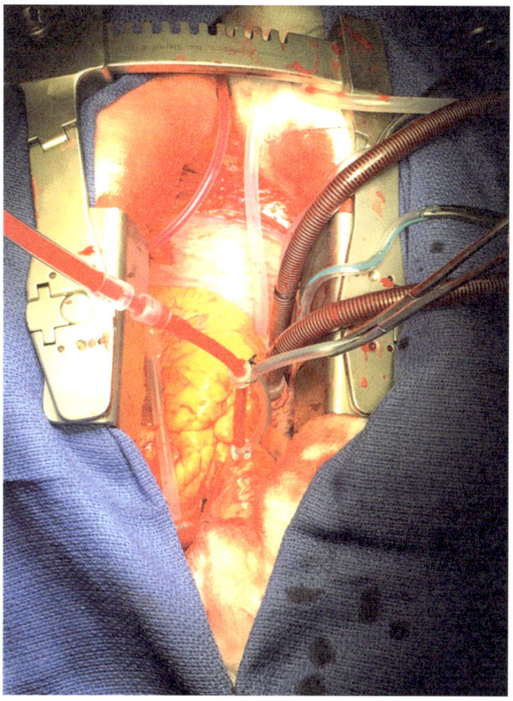

Fig. 4.1 Operative image illustrating the set-up for cardiopulmonary bypass prior to performing mitral valve surgery

Exposure of the Mitral Valve

Standard Left Atriotomy

The standard left atriotomy approach requires mobilisation of Sondergaard's inter-atrial groove to reach the intra-atrial septum (Fig. 4.2).

Following snaring of the cavae, the caval snares are elevated under some tension bringing

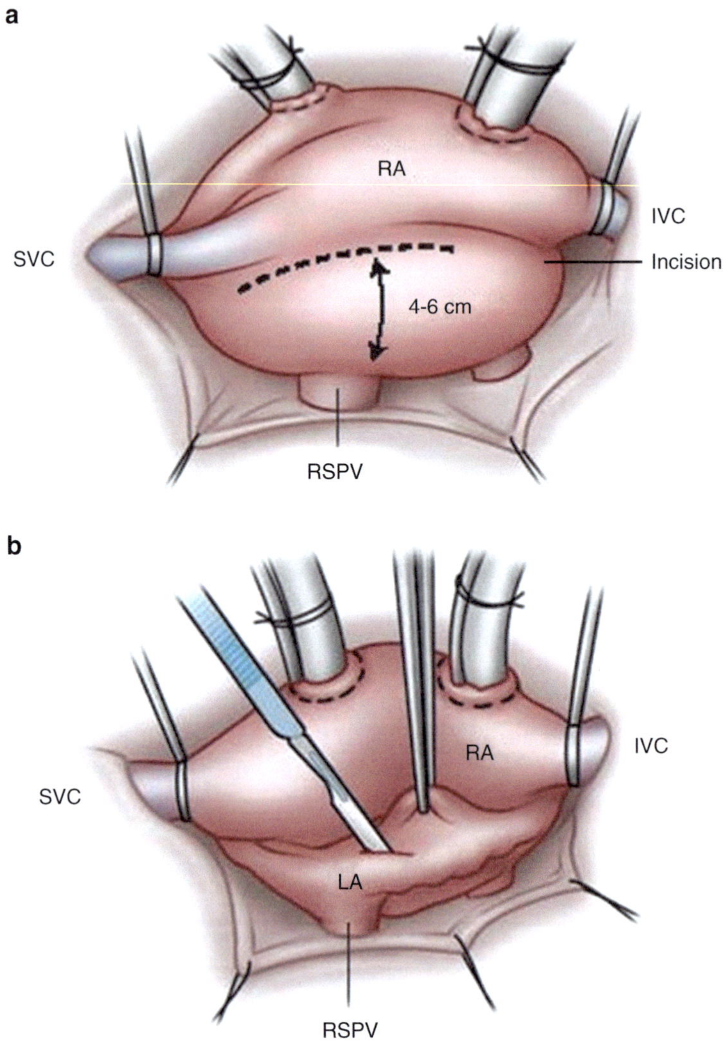

Fig. 4.2 Standard left atriotomy approach to the mitral valve with (**a**) an incision made just inferior to Sondergaard's inter-atrial groove; (**b**) the incision is then extended cranially beneath the superior vena cava just onto the roof of the left atrium and caudally beneath the right atrium. RA right atrium, SVC superior vena cava, IVC inferior vena cava, RSPV right superior pulmonary vein, LA left atrium

the heart a little further anteriorly in the pericardial space. This also places a little tension on Sondergaard's inter-atrial groove at the superior margin of the right superior pulmonary vein. A line of tension will appear as the atrium is retracted upwards and if the incision is begun here then the groove opens with ease. This makes it easier to find the correct place to begin the separation of the right and left atria. All of these small manoeuvres give improved access to the interior of the left atrium (Fig. 4.3).

Sondergaard's inter-atrial groove is then mobilised to reach the level of the fossa ovalis and an incision is made in the left atrium. The incision is extended cranially beneath the superior vena cava just onto the roof of the left atrium and caudally beneath the right atrium, taking care not to circumcise the inferior pulmonary vein (Fig. 4.4). Care should also be taken not to open the right atrium, which can overhang the left atrium as it approaches the inferior vena caval origin.

A further pump sucker is then placed into the left atrium and secured in place with two polypropylene sutures passed through the opened free edge of the left atrium and the parietal pericardium, taking great care not to injure the phrenic nerve by placing them quite high on the

Fig. 4.3 Operative images demonstrating (**a**) mobilisation of the superior vena cava and (**b**) tension placed on the caval snuggers to raise a line of tension at the superior margin of the right superior pulmonary vein

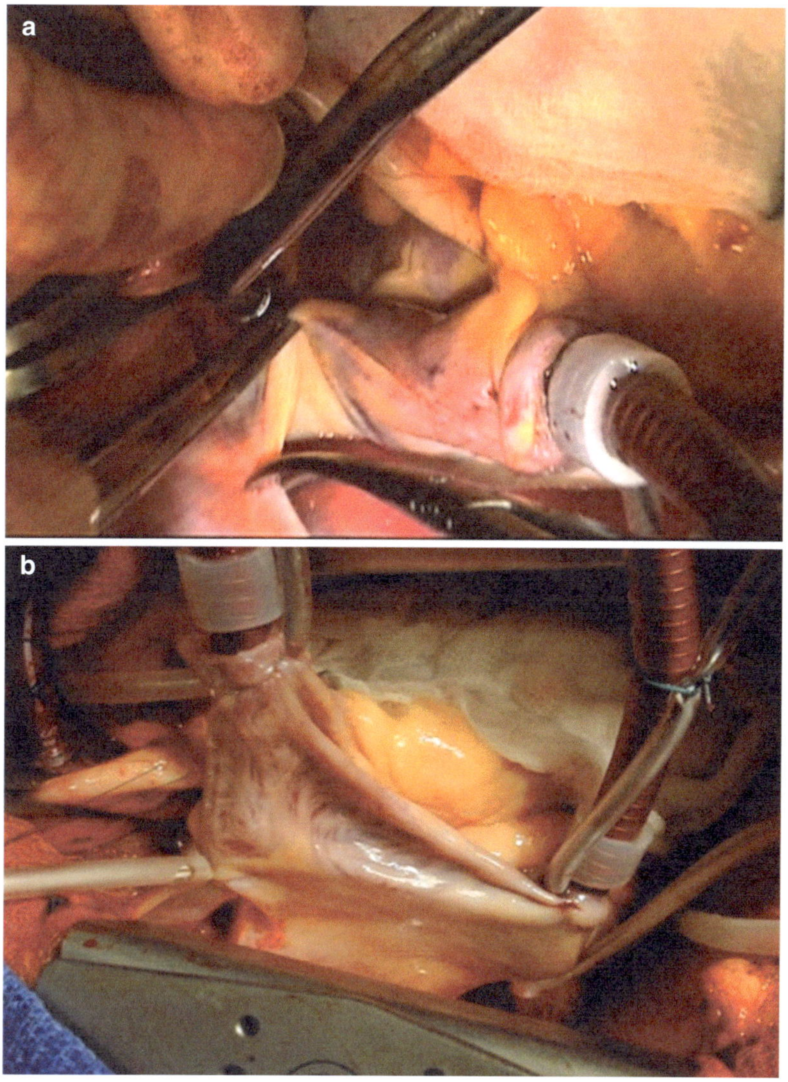

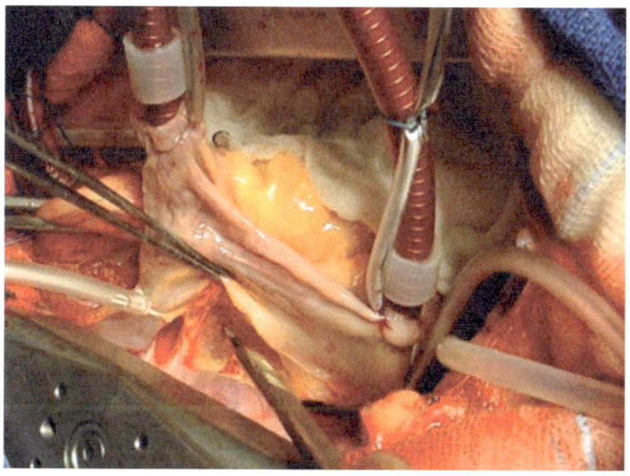

Fig. 4.4 Operative image demonstrating mobilisation of Sondergaard's inter-atrial groove and incision into the left atrium

pericardium. Self-retaining retractor blades can then be inserted into the left atrium to give a very good view of the mitral valve (Fig. 4.5).

In addition, placement of annuloplasty sutures prior to any mitral valve repair brings the leaflets closer to the operating surgeon. Through these simple manoeuvres, a satisfactory operative view of almost all mitral valves will be obtained (Fig. 4.6).

The left atriotomy is usually closed with a single layer continuous 3/0 prolene suture, started at either end of the incision and tied in the middle.

In some patients, access to the mitral valve through a standard left atriotomy may be limited, such as in a patient with dense adhesions

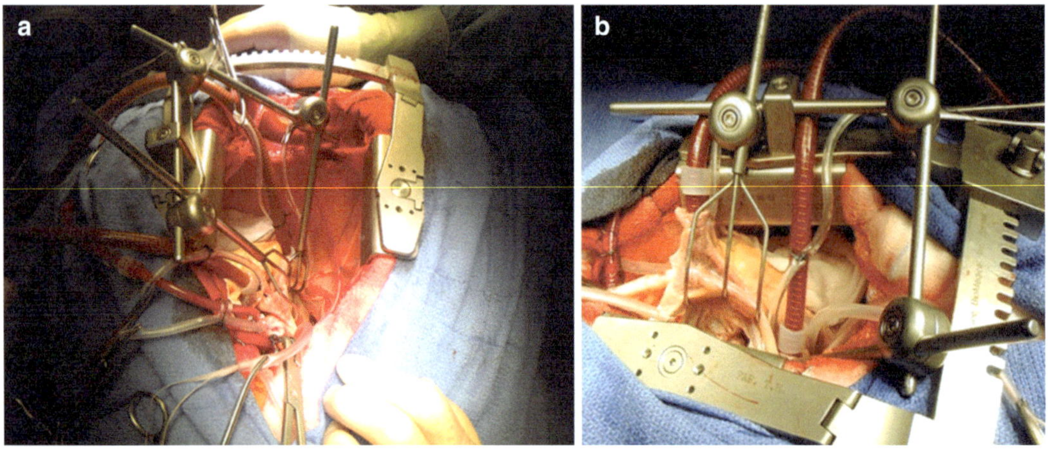

Fig. 4.5 Operative images demonstrating the self-retaining mitral valve retractor blades in situ from the (**a**) superior aspect of the operating table and (**b**) right side of the operating table

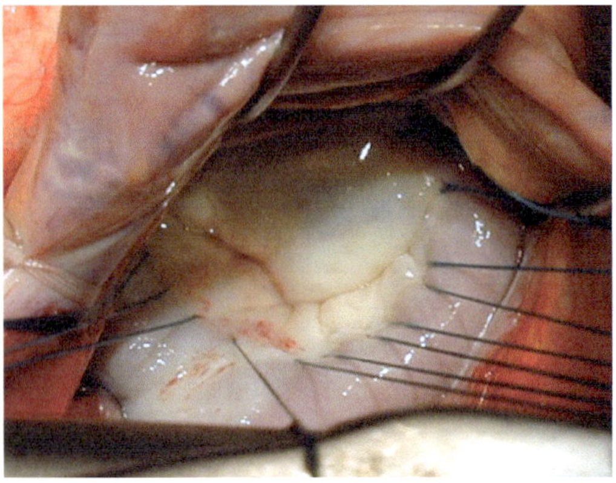

Fig. 4.6 Operative image demonstrating surgical view of the mitral valve following insertion of self-retaining retractor blades and annuloplasty sutures

following previous mitral valve surgery or in patients with a small left atrium. In these patients, alternative approaches need to be considered to access the mitral valve, including a vertical trans-septal bi-atrial incision, superior left atrial roof incision or horizontal trans-septal bi-atrial incision. For some surgeons, these approaches may be the preferred access to the mitral valve.

Vertical Trans-septal Bi-atrial Approach

An oblique incision is made from the right atrial free wall through the right atrial appendage and down to the left atrial roof (Fig. 4.7a). This is joined by a second incision through the fossa ovalis, medial to the crista terminalis, from the Eustachian valve to the edge of the superior limbus (Fig. 4.7b). Although this incision affords excellent exposure to the mitral and tricuspid valves (Fig. 4.7c), it may require considerable time to close the incision. In addition, the sino-atrial nodal artery is at risk during this incision.

Superior Left Atrial Roof Approach

An incision is made across the right atrial free wall and continued between the superior vena cava and the right atrial appendage (Fig. 4.8a). From there, it is extended across the interatrial septum and the roof of the left atrium passing behind the aortic root towards the commissure between the left coronary cusp and the non-coronary cusp (Fig. 4.8b). Although this incision gives good access to the mitral valve (Fig. 4.8c), the roof is the weakest part of the left atrium and this tissue can be relatively friable when closing the incision. In addition, the sino-atrial node artery, left main coronary artery, non-coronary sinus of aorta and superior vena cava are at risk due to their proximity to the incision.

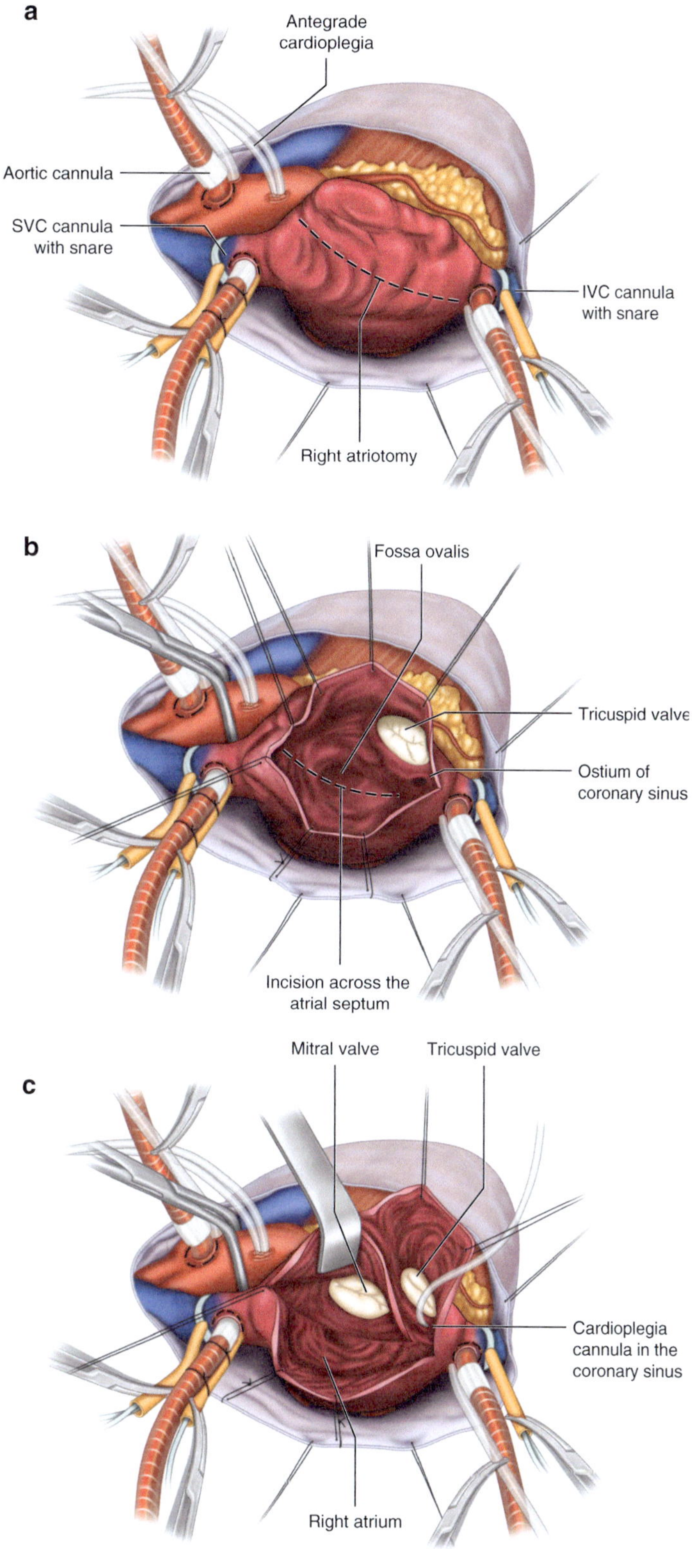

Fig. 4.7 Vertical trans-septal bi-atrial approach to the mitral valve, with (**a**) an incision made across the right atrial free wall through the right atrial appendage and down to the left atrial roof; (**b**) the incision extended across the interatrial septum through the fossa ovalis; and (**c**) giving excellent access to the mitral and tricuspid valves. SVC superior vena cava, IVC inferior vena cava

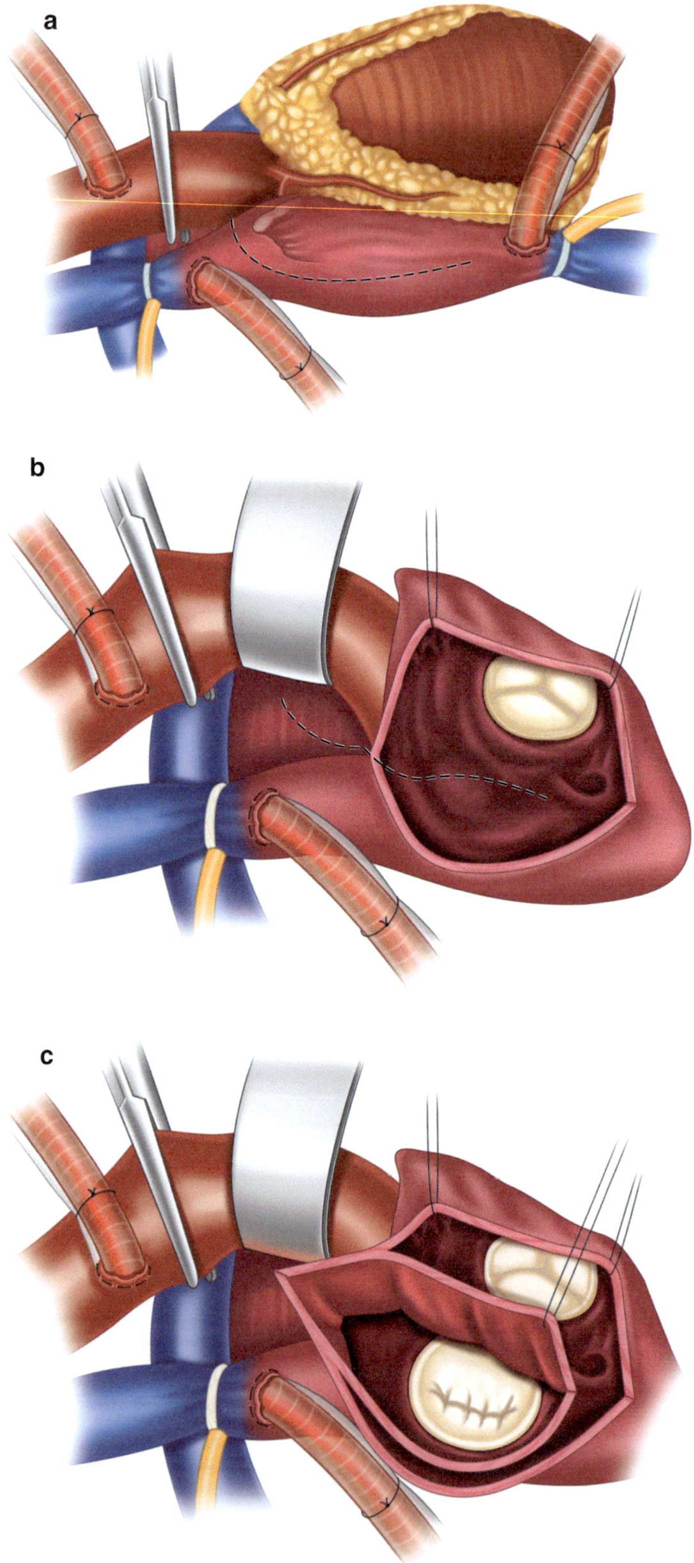

Fig. 4.8 Superior left atrial roof approach to the mitral valve, with (**a**) an incision made across the right atrial free wall and continued between the superior vena cava and the right atrial appendage; (**b**) the incision extended across the interatrial septum and the roof of the left atrium passing behind the aortic root; and (**c**) giving excellent access to the mitral and tricuspid valves. Caution must be excercised here as the roof of the left atrium is one of the weakest parts of the heart and excessive traction can cause a tear to extend beneath the aorta into a relatively inaccessible part or the heart

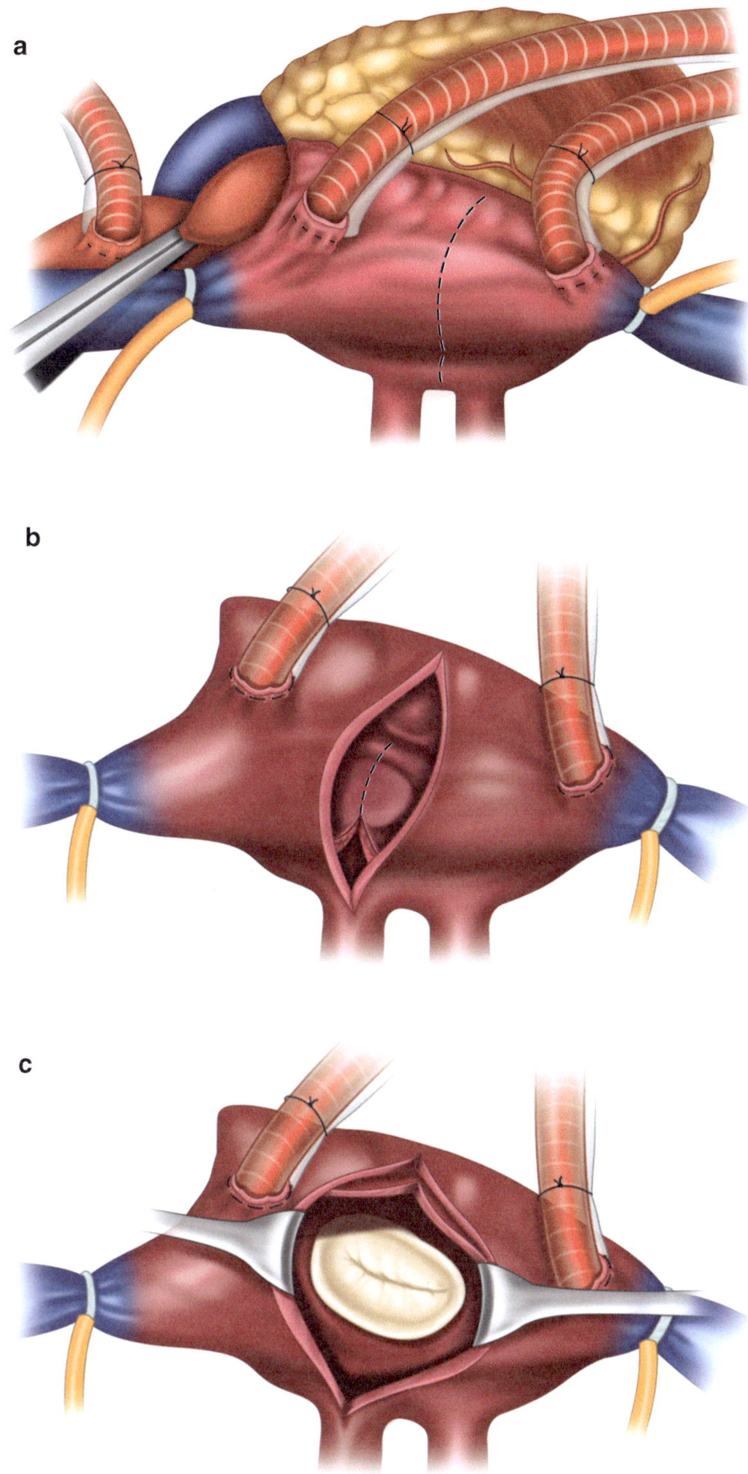

Fig. 4.9 Horizontal trans-septal bi-atrial approach to the mitral valve, with (**a**) an incision made between the right superior and inferior pulmonary veins across the right atrium; (**b**) the incision extended across the interatrial septum through the fossa ovalis; and (**c**) giving excellent access to the mitral and tricuspid valves

Horizontal Trans-septal Bi-atrial Approach

A horizontal incision is made between the right superior and inferior pulmonary veins across the free wall of the right atrium (Fig. 4.9a). The incision is then continued across the inter-atrial septum through the fossa ovalis and the left atrial free wall (Fig. 4.9b). Again, although it offers good access to the mitral and tricuspid valves (Fig. 4.9c), it can be difficult to close.

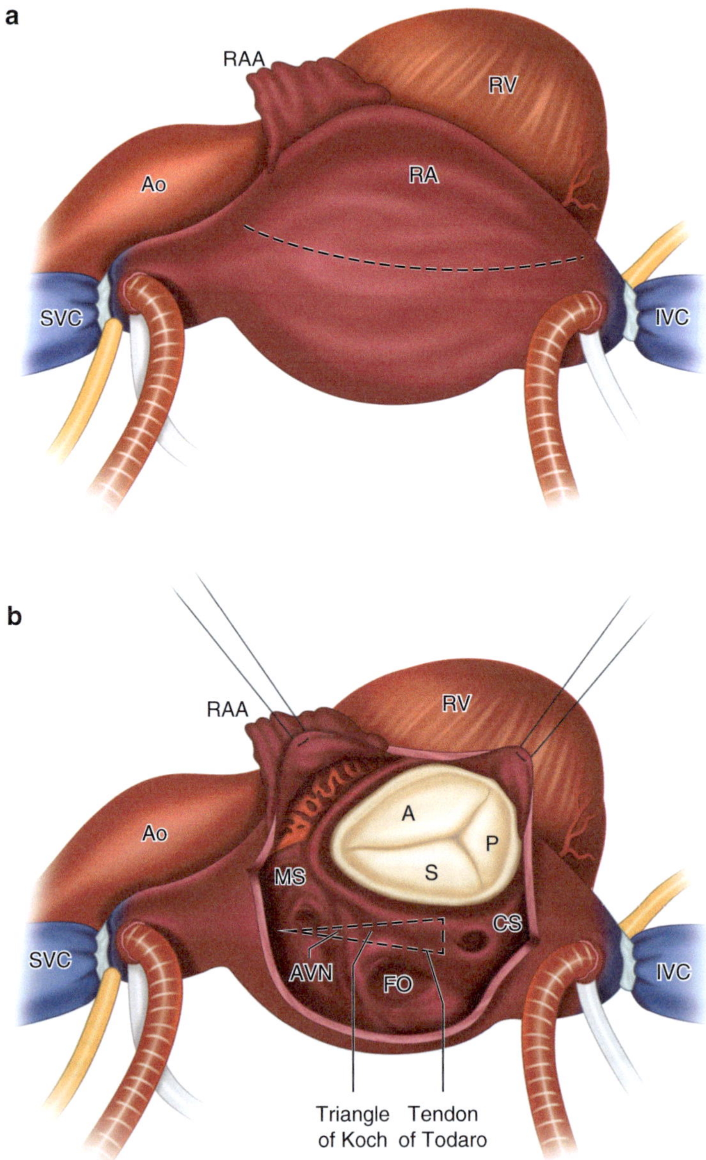

Fig. 4.10 Right atrial free wall incision for access to the tricuspid valve, with (**a**) an incision made from beneath the right atrial appendage towards the inferior vena caval cannula; and (**b**) giving excellent access to the tricuspid valve. SVC superior vena cava, Ao aorta, RAA right atrial appendage, RA right atrium, RV right ventricle, IVC inferior vena cava, MS membranous septum, AVN atrioventricular node, FO fossa ovalis, CS coronary sinus, A anterior tricuspid valve leaflet, P posterior tricuspid valve leaflet, S septal tricuspid valve leaflet

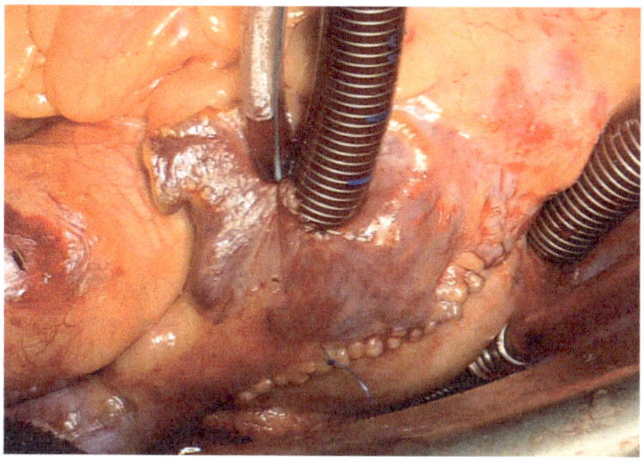

Fig. 4.11 Closure of the right atriotomy using 4/0 polypropylene suture

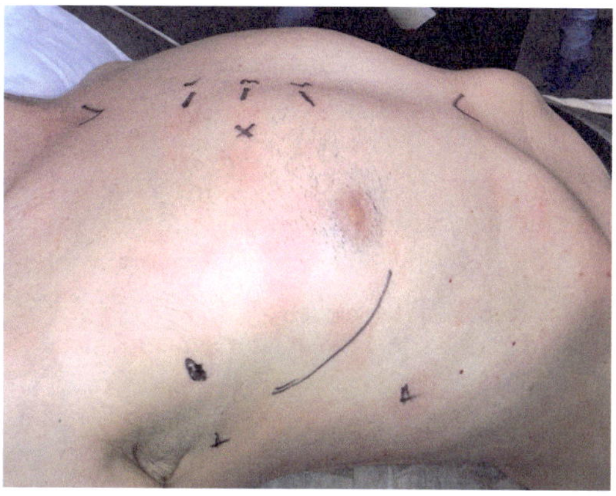

Fig. 4.12 Positioning of the patient prior to minimally invasive mitral valve surgery, with the skin incision and positioning of ports marked onto the anterior and lateral chest wall and the patient placed with the right chest elevated to 30°, using an inflated pressure bag

Right Atrial Free Wall Incision for Tricuspid Valve Access

An incision is made across the right atrial free wall from beneath the right atrial appendage towards the inferior vena caval cannula (Fig. 4.10a). Self-retaining retractor blades can then be inserted into the right atrium to give a very good view of the tricuspid valve (Fig. 4.10b).

Closure of the right atrial free wall is usually made with a one- or two-layered technique using a 4/0 polypropylene suture (Fig. 4.11).

Minimally Invasive Approach to the Mitral and Tricuspid Valves

Following general anaesthesia with a double-lumen endobronchial tube and placement of external defibrillation pads, the patient is positioned supine with slight elevation (30°) of the right chest, using an inflated pressure bag (Fig. 4.12).

The right femoral artery and vein are exposed through a 3 cm groin crease incision and cannulated using a Seldinger technique, supported by 5/0 polypropylene purse strings (Fig. 4.13). The arterial cannula sits in the common iliac artery, whilst the venous 3-stage cannula positioned in the inferior vena cava, right atrium and superior vena cava, under TOE guidance.

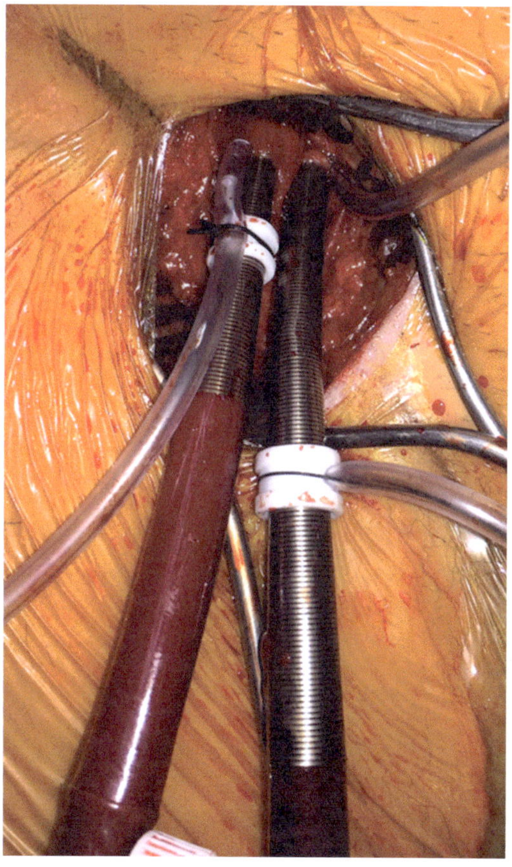

Fig. 4.13 Cannulation of the right femoral artery and vein

Additional venous drainage can be obtained with a second venous cannula inserted percutaneously through the right internal jugular vein, especially in patients requiring concomitant tricuspid valve surgery or with an increased body surface area. Vacuum-assisted cardiopulmonary bypass is used with mild hypothermia (32–34 °C).

There are a number of minimally invasive incisions described in the literature ranging from a right thoracotomy of vary sizes giving direct access to the mitral valve to a peri-areloar incision using a completely endoscopic technique. One example is performing a 5–7 cm right anterolateral thoracotomy in the fourth intercostal space in the submammary fold followed by insertion of a soft tissue retractor. A 10 mm thoracoport is then placed in the right fourth intercostal space in the mid-axillary line for insertion of the 30-degree camera and in the sixth intercostal space in the anterior axillary line for insertion of the pump sucker. Following initiation of cardiopulmonary bypass, an inverted C-shaped incision is made in the pericardium anterior to the right phrenic nerve and access to the heart is facilitated by pericardial and diaphragmatic retraction sutures, as required. An additional 3 mm stab incision is placed in the right second or third intercostal space in the anterior axillary line, through which a Chitwood aortic cross-clamp is inserted. Following aortic cross-clamping, antegrade cardioplegia is delivered through a long 35 cm cardioplegia cannula, inserted into the right lateral aspect of the ascending aorta (Fig. 4.14).

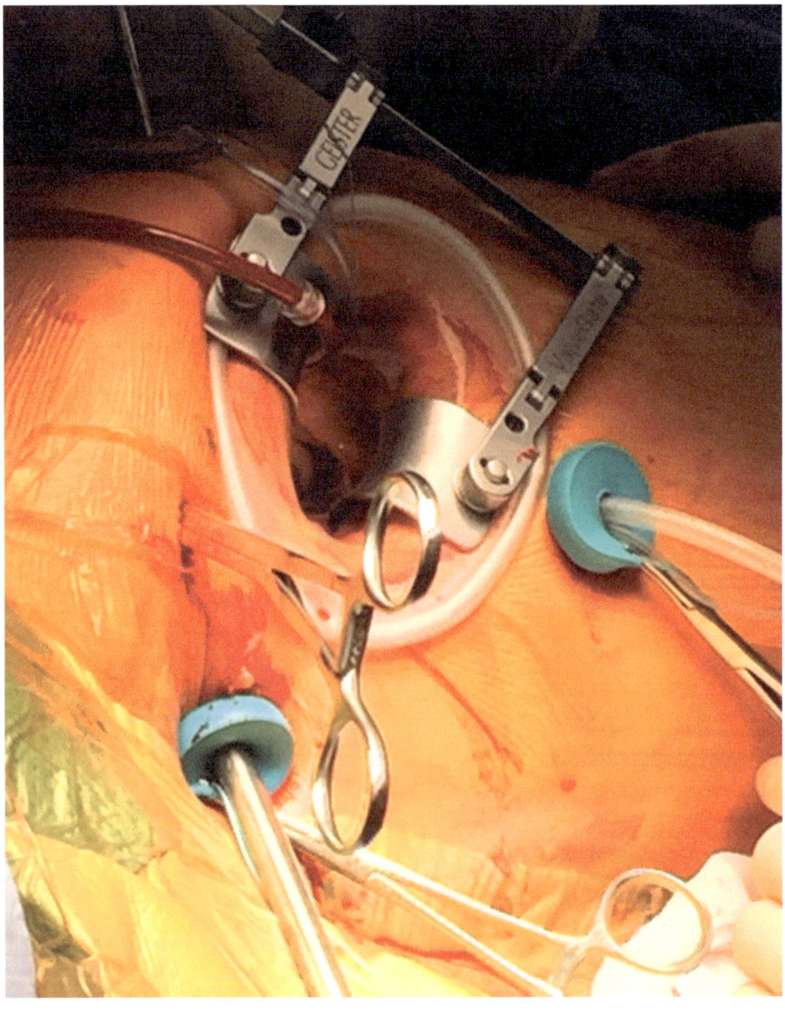

Fig. 4.14 Operative set-up for minimally invasive mitral valve surgery, following aortic cross-clamping and delivery of antegrade cold blood cardioplegia

Alternatively, an endoballoon can be used to occlude the ascending aorta, with an internal channel to deliver antegrade cardioplegia, which is passed via the femoral artery. In such instances, right radial artery monitoring is used to be certain that balloon migration and innominate artery obstruction have not occurred. Retrograde cardioplegia can also be delivered through a percutaneous trans-jugular catheter placed in the coronary sinus under TOE guidance. Carbon dioxide is administered at 2 L/min via the camera port throughout the procedure.

Access to the mitral valve can be obtained through a standard left atriotomy, or right atrial trans-septal approach if tricuspid valve disease is also present. Specialized surgical instruments, including a left atrial retractor, are then used to perform the majority of standard mitral valve surgical techniques. De-airing is performed using aortic root suction and by distending the left atrium with saline during closure, with TOE guidance.

Robotic Mitral Valve Surgery

Robotic mitral valve surgery can be performed either as port access surgery with robot assistance using a 3–4 cm right submammary incision, or as a robot-performed totally endoscopic procedure using a 15 mm 'working port', placed in the right fourth intercostal space in the anterior axillary line. The robotic camera is placed in the right fourth intercostal space just lateral to the mid-clavicular line. Otherwise, the initial setup for robotic surgery is similar to videoscopic mitral valve surgery with respect to femoral cannulation and antegrade intra-aortic cardioplegia. Following opening of the left atrium, the positions of the left and right robotic instrument arms are determined to provide optimal visualisation of the mitral valve. Commonly, the left trocar is placed in the third intercostal space in the anterior axillary line and the right trocar in the sixth intercostal space in the anterior axillary line, avoiding any internal and external arm conflicts. The 3-D high-resolution endoscope is placed through the medial portion of the mini-thoracotomy, with the other instruments passed through the remainder of the incision.

Robotic mitral valve surgery requires a number of components, including:

- An endoscope, which consists of two parallel cameras, channeled to each of the operator's eyes, providing up to 10× magnification in 3D
- Miniaturized standard surgical instruments, mounted on long thin shafts, which provide tremor-free movement through multiple degrees of freedom
- Bedside unit, with articulating arms that allow the endoscope and instruments to be electronically controlled at the surgeon's console
- Surgeon's console, which comprises of:
  - A viewing screen, which provides true 3-D vision with improved visualization
  - Two hand controllers, which directly translate the hand and finger motions of the surgeon to the instruments
  - A series of foot pedals, which allow camera focus, movement of instrument supports and electrocautery

Mitral and Tricuspid Valve Operative Techniques

5

Keywords
Annuloplasty · Annular decalcification and reconstruction · Leaflet plication · Leaflet resection · Leaflet augmentation · Edge-to-edge repair · Commissuroplasty · Valve replacement · Gore-Tex neo-chordae · Atrial fibrillation ablation · Left atrial appendage excision

Introduction

The complexity of the mitral valve and the fact that it can be afflicted by multiple pathologies means that the expert mitral surgeon must be practiced in a wide variety of surgical techniques. The most common lesion giving rise to mitral regurgitation is posterior leaflet prolapse, usually affecting the central P2 scallop. A potential mistake is to think that these are always simple and repair can follow a standard protocol. Whilst this may be true for many such valves, it is not uncommon to find secondary and tertiary lesions in these valves. Therefore, it is important to be flexible in approach and have a number of surgical options that can be utilised. For more complicated lesions, such as bi-leaflet prolapse, particularly the Barlow's valve, it is essential for the surgeon to be able to draw upon several surgical solutions to allow the best outcome. The rheumatic valve sets its own challenges and whilst prosthetic valve replacement is a very good option for most patients, a significant number of valves may be reconstructed. In the younger age group, especially women who may wish to become pregnant, reconstruction, if it can be performed well, is an excellent option. Another group in which reconstruction is commonly achievable are patients with endocarditis. Here, it is vital to debride all infected tissue prior to reconstruction. This will mean that the full range of surgical techniques may be required.

Mitral Valve Operative Techniques

Annular Techniques

Ring Annuloplasty (Fig. 5.1)
Ring annuloplasty is used to treat patients with annular dilatation and as an adjunct following most mitral repair procedures to support the annulus and prevent further annular dilatation. There are many varieties of annuloplasty rings, principally categorised by consistency (flexible, semi-rigid or rigid), shape (flat or saddle-shaped) and completeness (C-shaped partial band or complete ring). There is a great deal of myth and personal preference in the choice of ring. Evidence to support one choice over another is lacking.

Annuloplasty rings are used to reduce the orifice area of the mitral valve, stabilise the annulus and prevent further dilation in the future follow-

N. Moorjani et al., *Operative Mitral and Tricuspid Valve Surgery*,
https://doi.org/10.1007/978-1-4471-4204-1_5

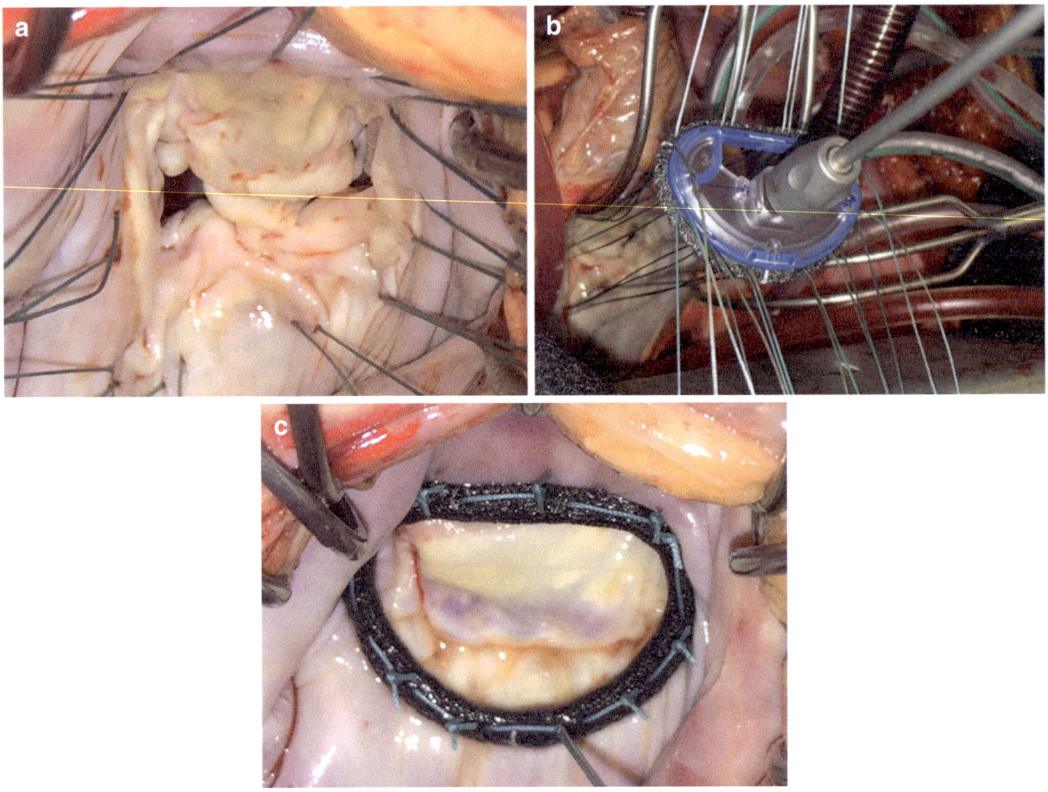

Fig. 5.1 Ring annuloplasty (**a**) insertion of interrupted horizontal mattress annuloplasty sutures, (**b**) placement of the sutures through the annuloplasty ring and (**c**) annuloplasty ring tied down in situ

ing surgical repair. There is little if any evidence to suggest that the mitral annulus stretches between the trigones at the aorto-mitral curtain; the left ventricular free wall is the region of stretch as a result of chronic ventricular volume overload. Hence, stabilising the annulus posteriorly between the trigones alone using a partial ring (band) is effective. In addition, allowing the inter-trigonal length of the annulus anteriorly to flex normally ensures that the natural saddle shape of the valve is retained. There is also an intuitive argument that a flexible band will allow some annular motion throughout the cardiac cycle acknowledging the significant change in orifice diameter between systole and diastole. It is also possible that the motion around a rigid ring may be more likely to result in ring dehiscence.

Horizontal mattress 2/0 Ethibond annuloplasty sutures are placed around the circumference of the mitral valve, with a 5 mm width and approximately 1 mm apart. An annuloplasty ring or band is then chosen according to the surface area of the whole mitral valve orifice, which represents the surface area of the anterior and posterior leaflets together. The sutures are tied and competency of the valve is assessed with static testing, by injecting cold saline into the left ventricle, using a bulb syringe to the point that the aortic root becomes tense. With the left ventricle distended, the depth of coaptation is measured by marking the atrial surface of the mitral valve leaflets with a sterile marking pen and the valve is assessed to make sure that there is no evidence of leaflet restriction or prolapse and that the coaptation height is >8 mm.

Reduction Annuloplasty (Fig. 5.2)

Reduction annuloplasty represents a technique used to treat patients with ischaemic mitral regurgitation, where a small mitral annuloplasty ring is implanted that is 1–2 sizes less than the normal ring size based on the anterior leaflet height and inter-trigonal distance. Traditionally, complete, rigid or semi-rigid annuloplasty rings are used, rather than a flexible ring or band, to reduce the anteroposterior (septal-lateral) diameter of the mitral valve orifice, thereby restoring mitral annular geometry and increasing the surface area of coaptation. In the setting of ischaemic mitral regurgitation, reduction annuloplasty relies on the tethered anterior leaflet to coapt with an essentially fixed posterior leaflet to maintain valve competency. Flat annuloplasty rings are thought to atrialise the commissures, which increases the distance between the posterior leaflet and the papillary muscles, thereby potentially increasing tethering of the posterior leaflet. In view of this, specifically designed ischaemic mitral rings have been introduced, which incorporate septo-lateral diameter reduction and have a saddle-shape to compensate for the tethered P2/P3 scallops of the posterior mitral valve leaflet. This restores the 3D shape of the annulus to normalise leaflet stress and allows the ring to be true-sized to the intercommissural distance and anterior leaflet height. Horizontal mattress 2/0 Ethibond ring annuloplasty sutures are placed around the circumference of the anterior and posterior annulus, with a 5 mm width and approximately 1 mm apart. The sutures placed in the region of the P2-P3 segment of the posterior annulus, however, are smaller (3 mm width) to reduce the tension on this part of the annulus, which is already tethered. The mitral valve annulus is then sized according to the intercommissural distance and height of the anterior leaflet, with no undersizing performed.

Annular Decalcification (Fig. 5.3)

In patients with extensive mitral annular calcification, it is often possible to strip out the calcium to allow either valve reconstruction or the insertion of a prosthesis which will then fit snuggly within a pliable annulus. First, the base of the posterior leaflet is incised, detached and retracted from the calcified annulus. The atrial endothelium is then incised at the border with the calcified bar. By keeping a sharp blade directly on the calcific bar next to the junction with the atrial tissue above and the ventricular tissue below, with tight control of the dissection plane, it is possible to excise the calcified bar without disruption of the atrioventricular junction. Excision of the calcified bar en bloc allows resection without fragmentation of the calcium. En bloc dissection is feasible because the calcific bar is usually encapsulated within a sheath of advancing fibrosis. Any residual calcification may be debrided using a rongeur. This process will leave the peri-vascular fat visible in the atrio-ventricular junction. It is important to appreciate that extensive debridement of the calcified mitral annulus is a technically complex procedure and can be associated with significant risks, including atrioventricular disruption, injury to the circumflex coronary artery and ventricular rupture.

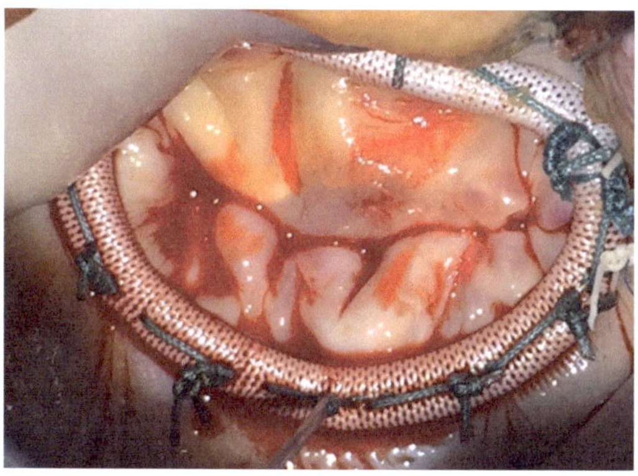

Fig. 5.2 Reduction annuloplasty in a patient with ischaemic mitral regurgitation using a Carpentier-McCarthy-Adams IMR ETlogix annuloplasty ring, which has reduced anteroposterior diameter and an asymmetric design with a reduced P2-P3 curvature

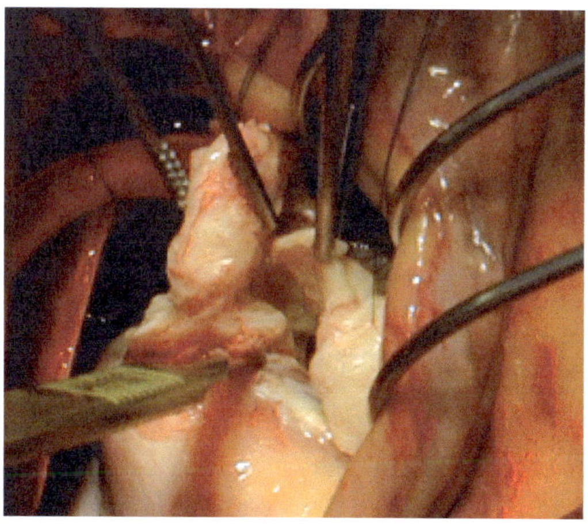

Fig. 5.3 En bloc resection of the mitral annular calcification, using a sharp blade to separate the calcific bar from the atrioventricular tissue

Annular Reconstruction (Fig. 5.4)
Following annular debridement in patients with extensive mitral annular calcification or annular destruction from infective endocarditis, the resultant anatomic separation between the left atrium, left ventricle and mitral annulus exposes the atrioventricular groove and necessitates annular reconstruction. At this stage, the fibrous edges of atrial and ventricular tissue can usually clearly be identified and used for annular reconstruction. This can be performed using a variety of different techniques, including direct annular suturing, atrial flap advancement or patch repair. These techniques help to preserve the integrity of the atrioventricular groove and reduce the risk of atrioventricular disruption.

If only a limited area of the atrioventricular groove has been exposed, direct annular suturing can be performed using either interrupted pledged sutures or figure-of-eight non-pledgeted sutures, placed into the atrial and ventricular fibrous edges.

Alternatively, the sliding atrium technique can be performed by undermining and mobilising the left atrial fibrous edge from the atrioventricular junction to form an atrial flap to use for annular reconstruction. In patients where the calcification process has extended from the annulus into the left atrial or ventricular wall, mobilisation of this tissue to effect a reconstruction can be difficult.

If a significant portion of the atrioventricular groove has been exposed, however, annular reconstruction using a patch repair technique is the safest way to reconstruct the atrioventricular junction. The patch allows the creation of a new annulus without tension on fragile tissues and helps to exclude the debrided atrioventricular junction from the high pressure left-sided circulation, thereby reducing the risk of tearing and subsequent atrioventricular disruption. Complete debridement and decalcification of the ventricular margin is an important prerequisite to reduce the risk of subsequent patch dehiscence. The choice of material used for the patch repair includes fresh or glutaraldehyde-fixed autologous pericardium, bovine pericardium or Dacron. It is imperative to use a generous over-sized patch, as a small patch will cause tension at the atrioventricular junction and risk tearing during cardiac contraction. The patch is attached to the atrial and ventricular free edges into the endothelium beyond the area of debridement, using a continuous 4/0 Prolene that is usually interupted at each end for security. Following annular reconstruction, mitral repair may be possible by reattaching the posterior leaflet to the pericardium. This depends entirely upon the amount of leaflet tissue that remains after the debridement. If repair is not possible, valve insertion can be performed. The sutures are placed from the ventricular side to the atrial side in the retained normal annulus in the usual way but through the patch at the level of the old annulus. By using a generously sized patch, these sutures will safely hold the valve in place.

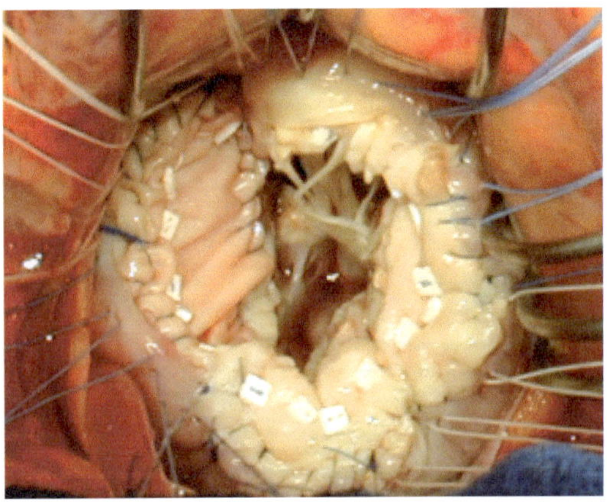

Fig. 5.4 Mitral annular reconstruction using pericardial patch repair

Leaflet Techniques

Leaflet Plication (Fig. 5.5)
Leaflet plication is used for patients with limited leaflet prolapse and involves using a series of interrupted 5/0 Prolene sutures to invert the redundant prolapsing segment. It produces a similar result to a limited triangular resection but without excising leaflet tissue. For patients with excess tissue associated with myxomatous degeneration, leaflet plication probably should not be used because of the bulk of tissue and a triangular leaflet resection

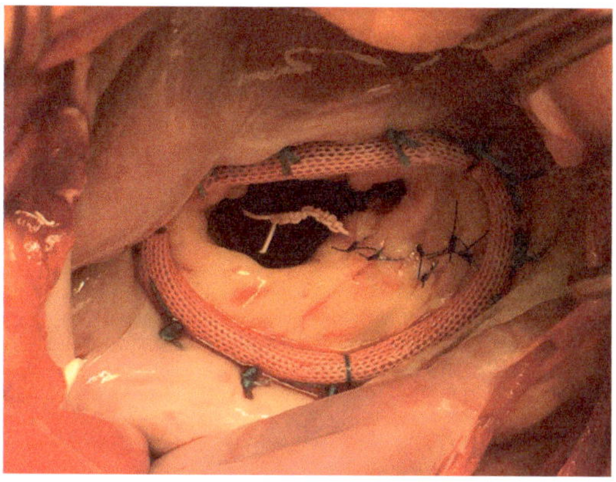

Fig. 5.5 Plication of the posterior mitral valve leaflet using interrupted 5/0 polypropylene sutures

is a better option in this situation. Leaflet plication is more commonly used on the posterior leaflet but can be used on the anterior leaflet if there is a small cleft, where the excess tissue can be tucked in under the opposing edge of the leaflet.

Leaflet Resection

Leaflet resection can be performed on the anterior and posterior leaflets but with different principles due the difference in shape of the two leaflets. Leaflet resection techniques for the posterior leaflet include triangular resection, quadrangular resection with or without sliding plasty, targeted wedge resection or detachment of the posterior leaflet from the annulus and resecting various amounts from the base of the posterior mitral valve leaflet from commissure to commissure. The choice between these resection techniques depends on the quantity of tissue in the posterior leaflet and specifically the height of the individual scallops, with the aim of repair to produce a symmetrical (all scallops equal in height) posterior leaflet <1.5 cm tall. For the anterior leaflet, resection is usually limited to a small triangular resection, not quadrangular resection, which is performed following the radial lines drawn from the centre of the anterior annulus. Resection of the anterior leaflet, however, is not very reliable with reports of early recurrence, and in practise, is usually only employed in patients with a large volume of the anterior leaflet billowing with chords of appropriate length.

Triangular Resection (Fig. 5.6)

Excision of a triangular segment of leaflet tissue represents the least extensive of the resection techniques used on the mitral leaflets. This was first described by Dwight McGoon as a modification of his imbrication technique for excessive tissue in the posterior leaflet, as described above. As compared to quadrangular resection, it is able to better preserve overall mitral valve geometry and physiology, as well as maintaining a larger mitral valve orifice area and surface area of coaptation. The first step when performing a triangular resection is to place 5/0 Prolene stay sutures around the normal chordae tendineae attached on either side of the prolapsed area. Gentle traction on these stay sutures allows the margins of resection of the prolapsing scallop to be clearly delineated. The extent of the triangular resection depends on the degree of prolapse, and amount and quality of the residual tissue, to ensure adequate tissue is left to reconstitute the leaflet without tension. Using a No 11 blade, the resection is performed with the base of the triangle at the free margin of the prolapsed segment and the apex of the triangle pointing towards but not reaching the annulus. In the posterior leaflet, additional wedge resections of the basal part of the prolapsing segment may also be required for patients with an asymmetrical or tall prolapsing scallop, so as to produce a symmetrical posterior leaflet, with a height of less than 1.5 cm. Approximately 5 mm of prolapsed tissue is left on either side of the resection margin to facilitate a tension-free reconstruction of the leaflet. Depending on the insertion points of the remaining native chords on either side of the resected portion and the degree of leaflet resection, implantation of Gore-Tex neo-chordae at the free edge of the reconstituted area may be necessary to give extra strength to the repair, especially in patients with insufficient chordal support. The residual segments of the posterior leaflet are then sewn together with a two-layered, tension-free anastomosis, using a continuous locking 5/0 Prolene suture, starting at the leaflet free edge and tying the knot at the annulus. It is also acceptable to use a single layer closure or interrupted sutures. In the presence of deep clefts on either side of the resected segment, excessive resection will open these and may lead to regurgitation

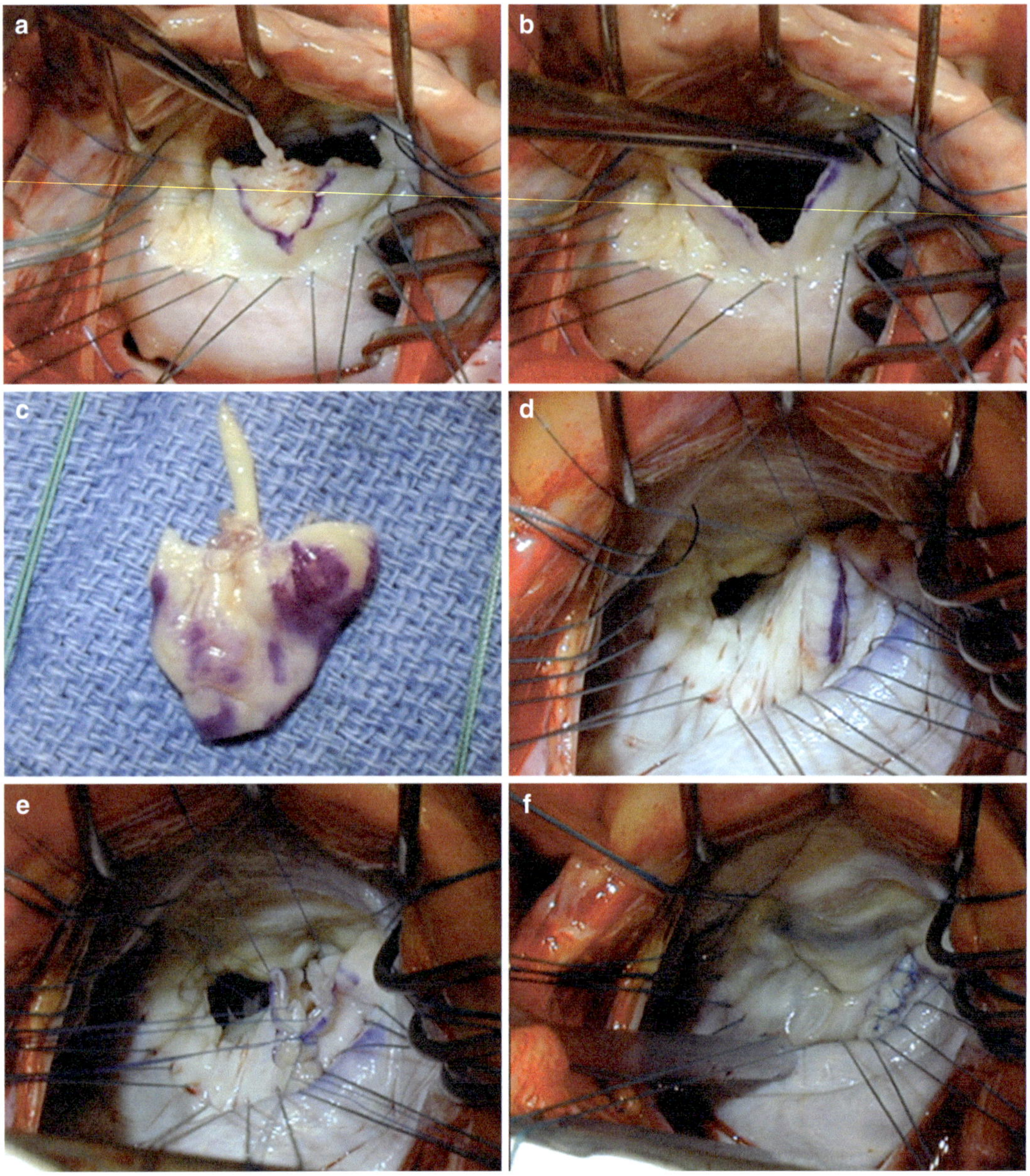

Fig. 5.6 Operative images illustrating triangular resection of the posterior leaflet. (**a**) Segmental analysis of the mitral valve demonstrating prolapse of the P2 scallop of the posterior leaflet caused by chordal rupture, (**b**) triangular resection of the prolapsed segment of P2, (**c**) excised segment of the P2 scallop, (**d**) apposition of the residual P2 leaflet tissue, (**e**) closure of the residual P2 leaflet tissue employing a two-layered tension-free anastomosis, using a continuous locking 5/0 Prolene suture and (**f**) static testing demonstrating a competent suture line

through them. It is therefore important not to over-resect tissue and to also bear this in mind as the edges are sewn together. These potential gaps may be overcome when the orifice is reduced with the annuloplasty ring. If, however, a residual leak is found on testing through the clefts between scallops of the posterior leaflet, then it may be desirable to partially close the clefts. This will also restore a more equal load distribution and energy sharing across the whole posterior leaflet. To allow the posterior leaflet to retain its normal functional mobility, these clefts are only closed to one half or two-thirds of their height, using an inverting suture on the ventricular side. In the majority of patients, most clefts, especially if shallow, are not closed as they contribute to the normal physiological movement of the mitral valve leaflets.

Small triangular resections on the leading edge of the anterior leaflet may be useful in Barlow type valves, where there is excessive leaflet tissue between chordal attachments. Larger anterior leaflet triangular resections are rarely used, as these repairs seem not to be stable and give rise to early recurrence of regurgitation.

Quadrangular Resection With or Without Sliding 'Plasty (Figs. 5.7 and 5.8)

Quadrangular resection is a technique used only on the posterior leaflet. Initially, the margins of the prolapsing segment are defined by passing a 5/0 Prolene suture around the adjacent normal chordae attached to non-prolapsing segments of the posterior leaflet. The prolapsing segment can then be excised as a quadrangle defined by imaginary lines drawn

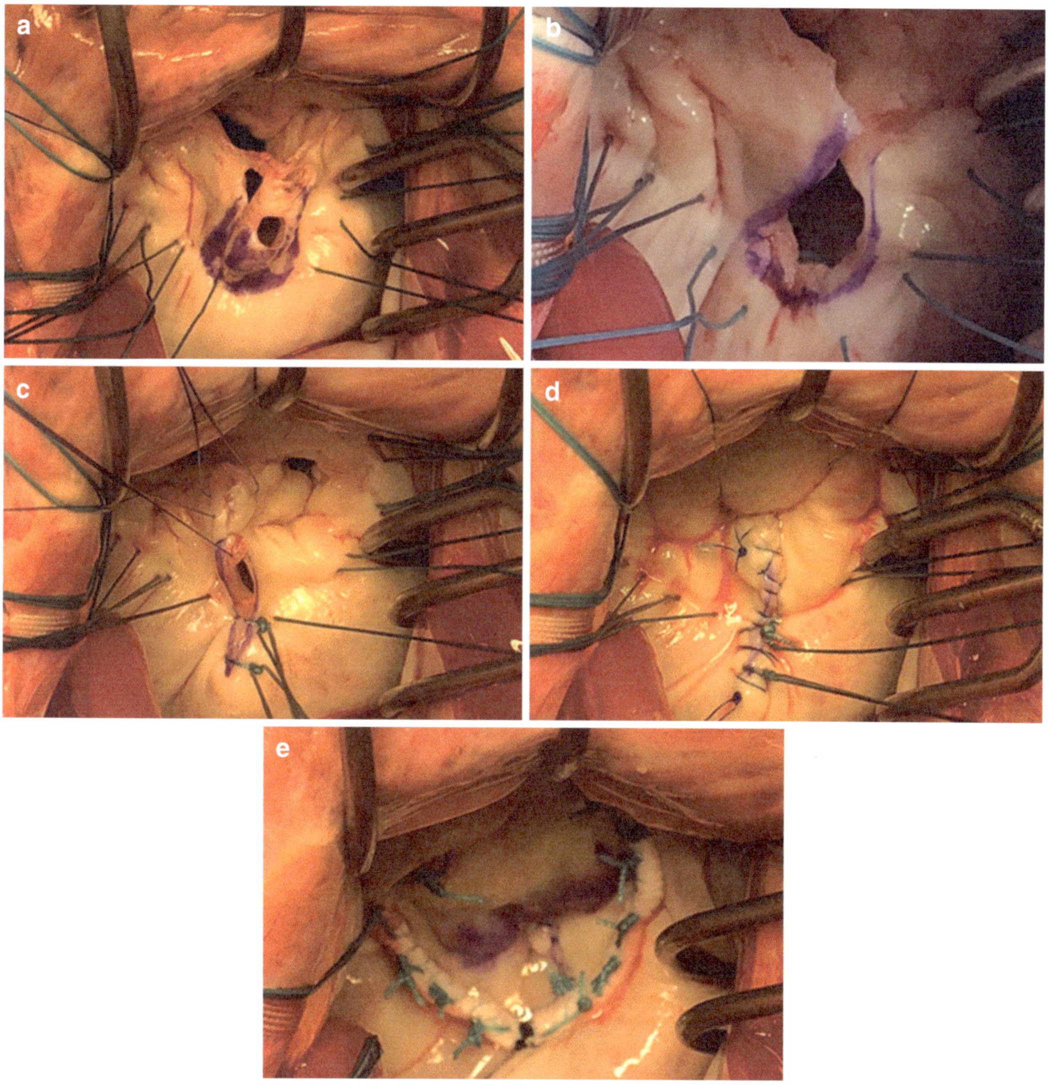

Fig. 5.7 Quadrangular resection without sliding plasty, with (**a**) demarcation of the quadrangular segment of P2 to be excised using a sterile marking pen, (**b**) residual gap in the posterior leaflet following quadrangular resection, (**c**) placement of 2/0 Ethibond horizontal mattress annular compression sutures to eliminate the defect in the posterior annulus, (**d**) suturing the edges of the residual posterior leaflet tissue together using 5/0 Prolene, and (**e**) implantation of an annuloplasty band

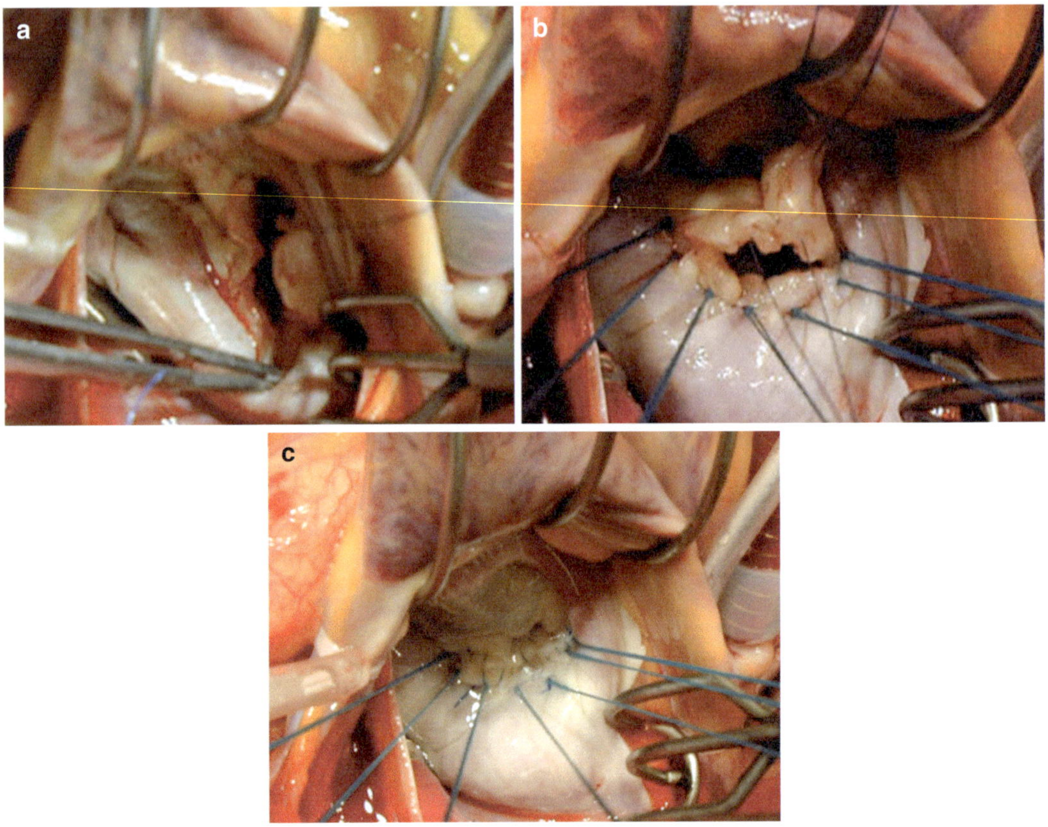

Fig. 5.8 Quadrangular resection of the posterior leaflet with sliding plasty, with (**a**) quadrangular resection of the P2 scallop of the posterior leaflet and detachment of the adjacent sections of the P1 & P3 scallops from the posterior annulus, (**b**) 2/0 Ethibond horizontal mattress compression sutures to plicate the posterior annulus, and (**c**) reattaching the posterior mitral valve leaflet to the annulus using 4/0 Prolene

from the top centre of the anterior annulus to the posterior annulus. This results in the segment to be resected having a shorter distance at the coaptation edge than at the annular margin. This is deliberate so as to eliminate tension on the leading edge of the leaflet when the edges of the resection are sewn together. The width of the residual gap between the resection margins will determine the need for either horizontal compression annuloplasty sutures or a 'sliding plasty'. Horizontal mattress 2/0 Ethibond annular compression plication sutures can be used to eliminate the defect in the posterior annulus. These are performed to bring the edges of the residual scallops together to obtain a tension-free union of the posterior leaflet. It is important to note that excessive plication in this way carries the risk of kinking the circumflex coronary artery.

If the excised portion is more than 1.5 cm, a sliding plasty is a better solution to restore leaflet approximation. To achieve this, the residual scallops are detached from the posterior annulus for approximately 2 cm in each direction. Horizontal mattress 2/0 Ethibond sutures are then placed along the resection margin. Tying these will then reduce the circumference of the posterior annulus and hence reduce the tension on the residual posterior leaflets. The leaflet edges are then sutured together using 4/0 Prolene sutures, with the annular margin suture also being passed through the neo-annulus at the geometrically correct point. These sutures can then be run along the neo-posterior annular margin, reattaching the leaflets to the neo-annulus. A second suture is begun at the lateral margins and run to the initial suture and then tied together. The posterior leaflet edges can then be sutured to each other using inverting interrupted sutures.

Leaflet Height Reduction (Fig. 5.9)

Leaflet height reduction can be used in isolation or in combination with leaflet resection and neochordal implantation. Horizontal mattress annuloplasty sutures (2/0 Ethibond) are placed around the circumference of the mitral valve and stay sutures (5/0 Prolene) are placed on the anterior and posterior leaflets. Using gentle traction on the posterior leaflet stay sutures and annuloplasty sutures, the heights of P1, P2 and P3 are assessed individually to determine whether any excess of tissue on the posterior leaflet would leave the

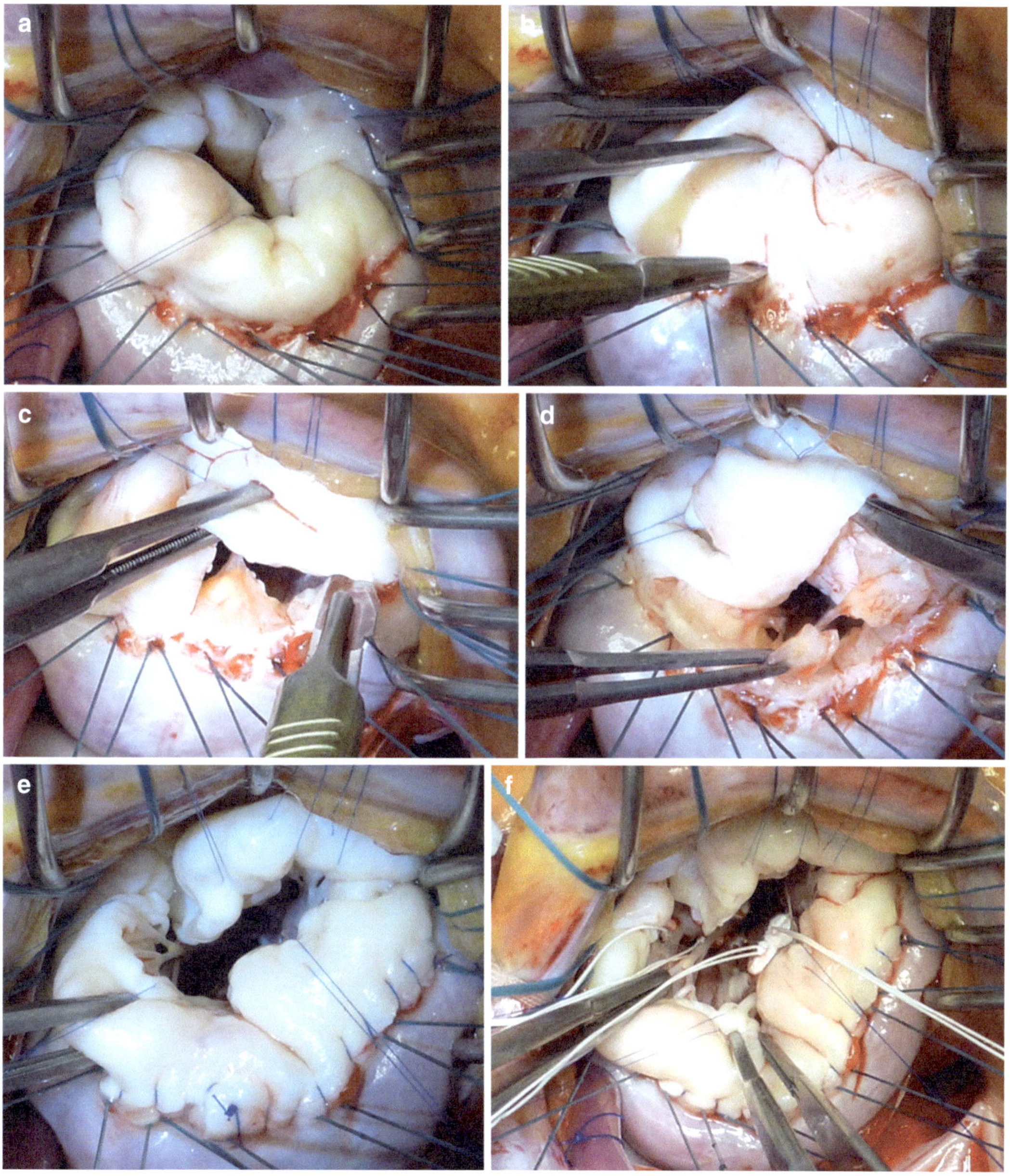

Fig. 5.9 Operative images illustrating leaflet height reduction used for repair of bileaflet prolapse. (**a**) Segmental analysis of the mitral valve, demonstrating marked bileaflet prolapse and excess of leaflet tissue, (**b**) incision at the centre of the annular attachment of the posterior leaflet, (**c**) extension of the incision just short of the anterolateral and posteromedial commissures, (**d**) excision of the basal portion of the posterior leaflet to reduce its height, (**e**) reattachment of the posterior leaflet using 4/0 polypropylene and (**f**) implantation of Gore-Tex neochordae to the anterolateral and posteromedial papillary muscles

valve at risk of systolic anterior motion (SAM) of the mitral valve. The posterior leaflet is incised horizontally, at the mid-point of its insertion to the annulus, using a No 11 blade. The incision is continued parallel to the posterior annulus, just short of both commissures, thereby detaching the posterior leaflet from the annulus. The base of the posterior leaflet is then resected, to reduce the height of the leaflet. The secondary and tertiary chords are preserved and if necessary, reattached to the annulus. The extent of resection depends on the degree of excess tissue of the posterior leaflet and its height in relationship to the anterior leaflet height. A ratio of approximately 2:1 (anterior to posterior leaflet height) is ideal. The frequent asymmetrical heights of the various segments of the posterior leaflet may require an asymmetrical excision of tissue to produce a symmetrical residual posterior leaflet following resection, although if this asymmetry is matched by that of the anterior leaflet, it is appropriate to keep them in proportion. Simply detaching and reattaching the posterior leaflet will reduce the height of the leaflet by 3–6 mm, depending on the depth of suture placement from the leaflet edge during reattachment. This brings the line of coaptation towards the posterior annulus, thereby reducing the risk of anterior displacement of the mitral valve during systole into the left ventricular outflow tract. The posterior leaflet is reattached to the annulus, using 4/0 Prolene. Any additional neo-chordae can then be implanted, as appropriate.

Leaflet height reduction can also be performed by making an incision from the leaflet free edge to the annular attachment, where the posterior leaflet is tallest. Both annular leaflet edges are then detached and an extended triangle of leaflet tissue is resected from the inferior portion (to the right of the valve from the surgeon's perspective) to reduce its height, so that it matches the height of the other side of the incision. The leaflets are then sutured back to the annulus and to each other. The degree of residual prolapse of the anterior and posterior mitral valve leaflets can then be reassessed with a reduced posterior leaflet height and neo-chordae implanted, as appropriate. Both of these techniques of leaflet displacement move the coaptation line posteriorly and thereby reduce the risk of SAM and subsequent left ventricular outflow tract obstruction.

Edge-to-Edge (Alfieri) Technique
(Fig. 5.10)

The edge-to-edge technique represents a functional rather than anatomical repair of the mitral valve and involves attaching the opposing coaptation edges of the leaflets at the central point of maximium prolapse. It is most frequently used for patients with bileaflet prolapse, a heavily calcified mitral annulus or as a rescue technique following failed repair. For optimal suture placement, the crucial step is to identify the origin of the regurgitant jet and to suture the anterior and posterior leaflets together at that point. It results

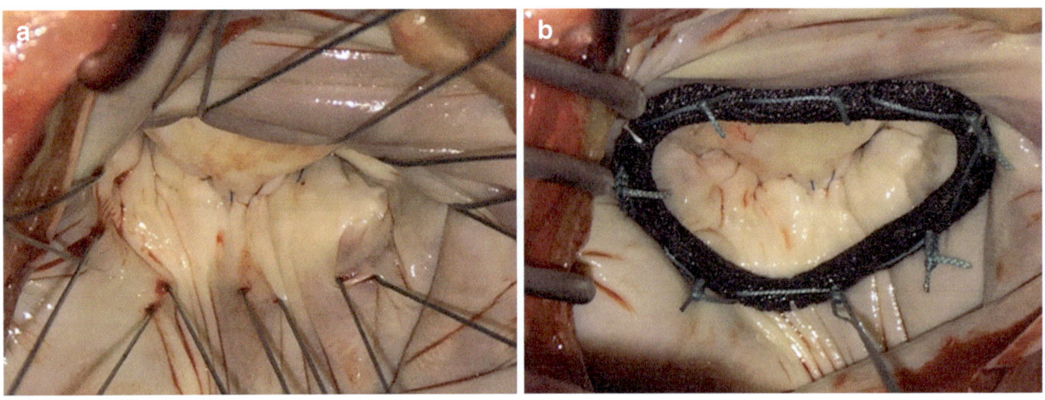

Fig. 5.10 Edge-to-edge repair of the mitral valve, with (**a**) two-layered 4/0 Prolene suture used to join the A2 and P2 scallops together, resulting in a 'double-orifice' mitral valve, followed by (**b**) implantation of an annuloplasty ring

in a ‘double-orifice’ mitral valve, with openings that are frequently asymmetrical. The sum of these two orifices must be greater than 2.5 cm^2 to avoid post-operative mitral stenosis. The valve can be tested for stenosis using Hegar dilators and for competency by static testing with saline distension of the left ventricle. This simple technique is reproducible and associated with short ischaemic and cardiopulmonary bypass times. The name of the technique is somewhat misleading, as the sutures are not placed at the edge of the leaflets but about 5–6 mm from the edge. It is more secure if it is done in two layers. This technique is supported with a ring annuloplasty to avoid future annular dilatation. A minimum ring diameter of 30 mm should be used to reduce the risk of post-repair mitral stenosis.

Commissural Closure (Fig. 5.11)

This technique, which is also known as a para-commissural edge-to-edge repair or modified ‘Magic’ suture, provides a simple functional (rather than anatomical) method for managing a patient with limited commissural prolapse, especially in patients with a large mitral valve orifice area. A suture is placed 5 mm from the free edge to imbricate the leaflet edges at the site of the commissural prolapse. More than one suture may be necessary. When using this technique, it is important to consider the resultant effective valve orifice area to avoid producing mitral stenosis.

Commissuroplasty (Fig. 5.12)

Prolapse of the A3 and P3 scallops is not an uncommon lesion and whilst it can be dealt with

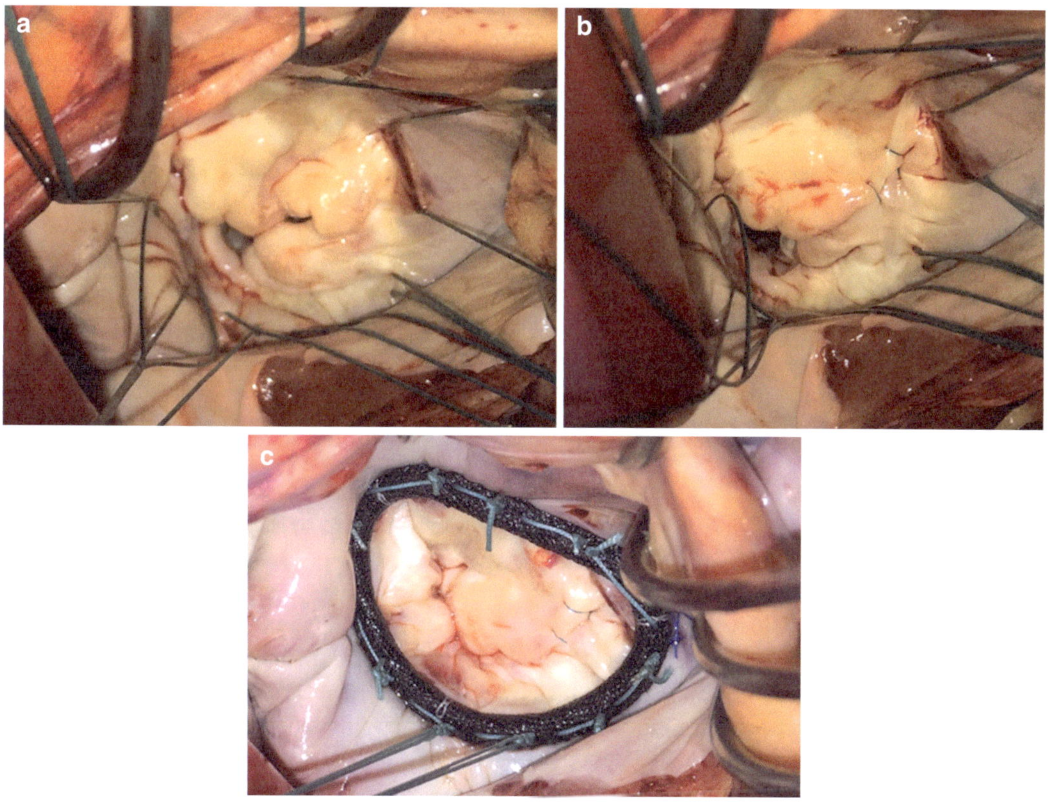

Fig. 5.11 Operative images illustrating (**a**) segmental analysis of the mitral valve, demonstrating isolated prolapse of the posteromedial commissure, (**b**) commissural closure using two 5/0 Prolene sutures to imbricate the leaflet edges at the site of the commissural prolapse, and (**c**) implantation of an annuloplasty ring

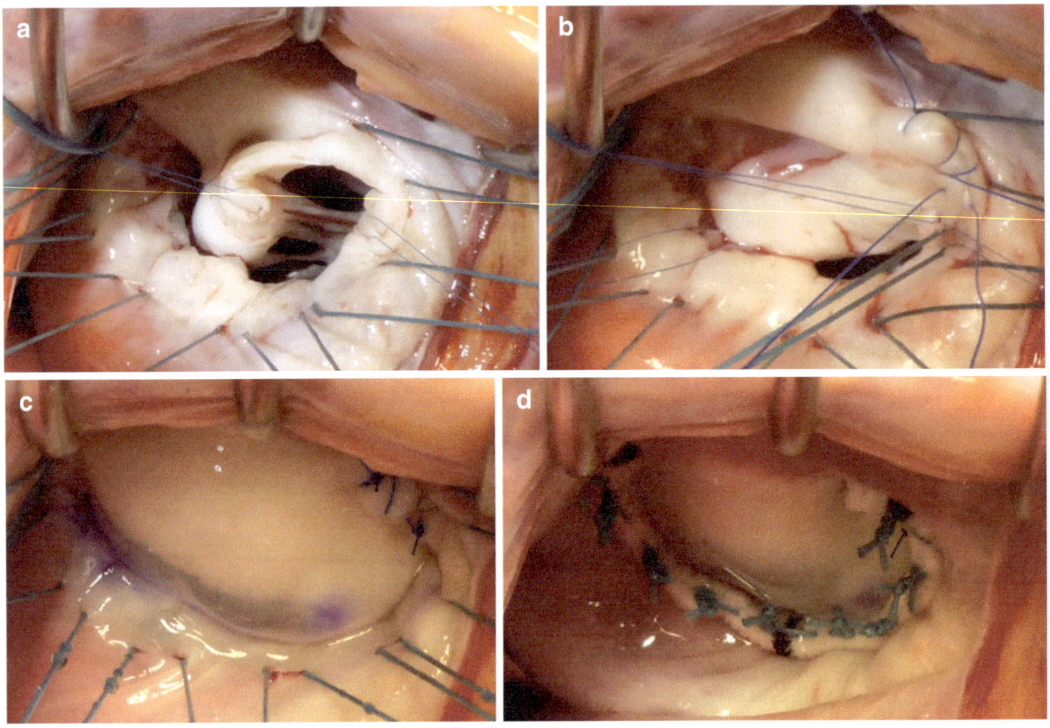

Fig. 5.12 Operative images illustrating (**a**) segmental analysis of the mitral valve, demonstrating isolated prolapse of the posteromedial commissure, (**b**) small quadrangular resection of the prolapsing leaflet tissue followed by reattachment of the leaflet tissue to the annulus, (**c**) saline distension of the left ventricle demonstrating a competent mitral valve, and (**d**) implantation of an annuloplasty band

as described above using an edge-to-edge technique, a more complete reconstruction is often possible. The underlying lesion is usually an abnormal papillary muscle arrangement, often with multiple short heads of the papillary muscles and short chordae, with an absence of the normal fan shaped chordae. At the time of presentation, ruptured chords may also be present but often they are stretched, with inadequately supported leaflets and apparent excess leaflet tissue. A quadrangular resection with undermining of the leaflets on either side of the excised tissue will leave more normal leaflet tissue, which can then be reconstructed. Horizontal mattress sutures are placed through the exposed annulus, which when drawn together and tied reduce the annular distance at that point. The leaflet edges can then be re-attached and sutured back to the annulus. A modification of this involves advancing the posterior leaflet behind the anterior leaflet and reattaching it. Neo-chords may be necessary to support the new commissural margins. An annuloplasty ring is then inserted in the usual way.

Commisurotomy

Commissurotomy represents a technique used for patients with commissural fusion caused by rheumatic mitral disease. It involves incision of the leaflet tissue at the commissures and is extended to within 2–3 mm of the annulus to ensure optimal mobilisation of the commissures. A commissurotomy, is usually done in combination with other techniques, which include peeling an inflammatory fibrotic layer from the surface of the thickened leaflets and splitting of the commissural fan chords and papillary muscles. In some cases, it will be necessary to perform chordal release of thickened and contracted secondary or primary chords. This will release the leaflet allowing greater mobility. Neo-chordae may be required to support the leaflet.

Leaflet Augmentation (Fig. 5.13)

In patients with hypoplastic leaflets or leaflet retraction secondary to extensive rheumatic or ischaemic mitral disease, leaflet augmentation can be used to improve mobility and pliability, thereby providing enough tissue to achieve a good depth of coaptation and increase the mitral orifice area. Posterior leaflet extension may be indicated in patients where severe retraction of the leaflet has caused the vertical height of the leaflet to be less than 10 mm, whereas anterior leaflet extension is performed if the vertical height or the surface area of the leaflet is less than that of a 26 mm annuloplasty sizer. Either glutaraldehyde-treated autologous pericardium or bovine pericardium can be used for leaflet augmentation. Although both may be subject to late calcification, the onset of this is delayed as compared to that when using untreated autologous pericardium. Other substitutes are available but lack long term follow up data.

The pericardial patch used for the posterior leaflet is usually suggested to be ovoid in shape but it is much better if it is trapezoid, otherwise the lateral limits fail to extend the leaflet far enough forwards towards the anterior leaflet. The patch should extend for most of the length of the posterior leaflet, from near commissure to commissure to allow complete mobilization of the entire restricted leaflet. An autologous pericardial patch can be trimmed, cleared of pericardial fat, soaked in 0.6% glutaraldehyde-buffered solution for 5–10 min at room temperature and then rinsed in 3 baths of normal saline for 5 min each. The glutaraldehyde treatment makes the pericardium stiffer and thereby easier to handle but prolonged treatment with glutaraldehyde leaves the pericardium at risk of increased fibrosis and excessive calcification.

The posterior leaflet is then detached from the annulus by making an incision 2 mm away and extending it from commissure to commis-

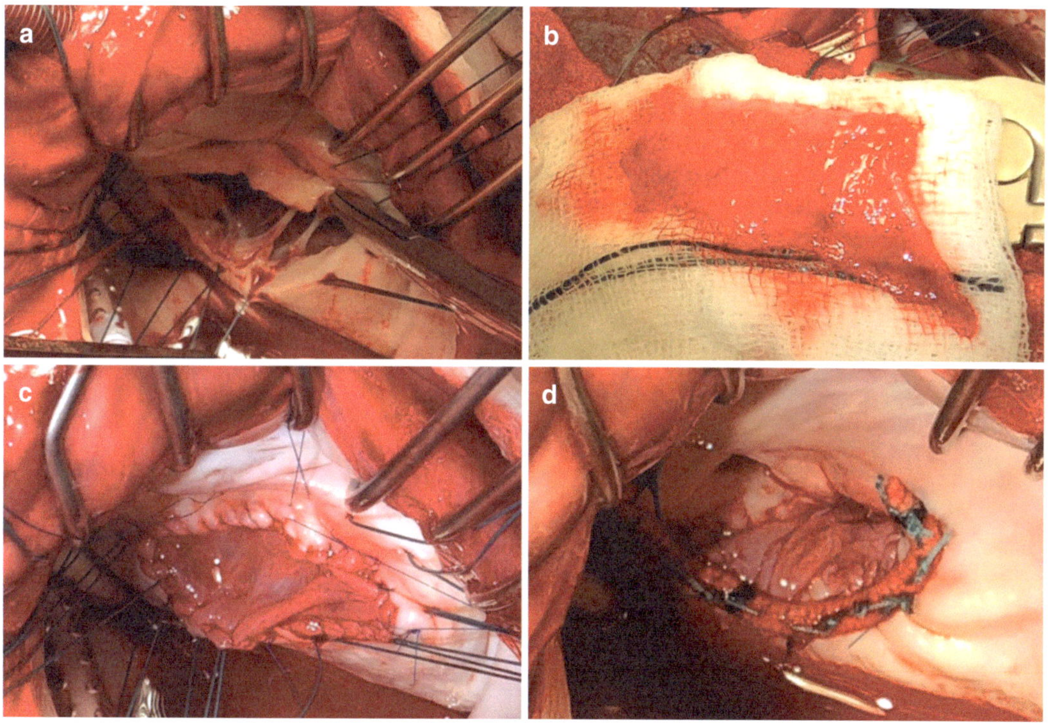

Fig. 5.13 Operative images demonstrating leaflet augmentation, with (**a**) detachment of the posterior leaflet from the annulus, (**b**) creation of a 'trapezoid' autologous pericardial patch, (**c**) attachment of the pericardial patch to the posterior annulus and leaflet, and (**d**) repaired mitral valve with the pericardial patch forming the atrial surface of the posterior leaflet

sure parallel to the annulus, preserving the free edge of the leaflet with the chordae attached (Fig. 5.13a). This allows great access to the left ventricular cavity and the sub-valvular apparatus, through which any additional chordal or papillary muscle releasing manoeuvres can be performed to further improve leaflet mobility and hence depth of coaptation. A patch is then fashioned in a trapezoid shape and sized so that the height of new posterior leaflet is 15–20 mm (5 mm is lost on either side due to the suturing effect) and that it would create a good depth of coaptation with the anterior leaflet (Fig. 5.13b).

The patch is attached to the annulus and the cut edge of the leaflet using a continuous locking 4/0 Prolene suture, to reduce the risk of 'purse-stringing' the patch, although this is not always necessary (Fig. 5.13c). The smooth side of the patch is placed on the atrial side to reduce the risk of thrombogenesis. As well as increasing the depth of coaptation, leaflet augmentation allows for the insertion of a larger annuloplasty ring, thereby reducing the risk of mitral stenosis. The pericardial patch essentially pushes the native retracted posterior leaflet tissue into the coaptation area with the pericardial patch being all that can be seen from the atrial aspect of the mitral valve (Fig. 5.13d). Following leaflet augmentation, any residual prolapse of the anterior or posterior leaflets can be supported with neo-chordal implantation.

Leaflet Reconstruction (Fig. 5.14)

In patients with leaflet perforation secondary to infective endocarditis, it is possible to reconstruct the native leaflet to provide a competent valve. Stay sutures (5/0 Prolene) are placed around the chordae tendineae attached on either side of the perforated area of the leaflet. Gentle traction on these stay sutures gives better access and visualisation of the leaflet. The vegetation and any residual infected leaflet surrounding the perforation are excised and sent for microbiological analysis. At this stage, it is important to assess the degree of destruction to the surrounding tissues to ensure that there is enough leaflet tissue and sub-valvar apparatus remaining intact and free from the infective process to produce a competent valve by repair. The defect in the leaflet body is usually repaired using fresh autologous pericardium, although glutaraldehyde-treated autologous pericardium or bovine pericardium can also be used. Although it is stiffer material, bovine pericardium is used if autologous pericardium is not available, such as in patients undergoing reoperation. Bovine pericardium, as well as glutaraldehyde-treated autologous pericardium, also have the advantage of being easier to handle and are used for more complex reconstructions. The pericardium is implanted using a continuous locking 5/0 Prolene suture, to avoid 'purse-stringing' the patch. It is important to oversize the patch to ensure that there is no tension on the leaflet causing restricted leaflet motion. In some

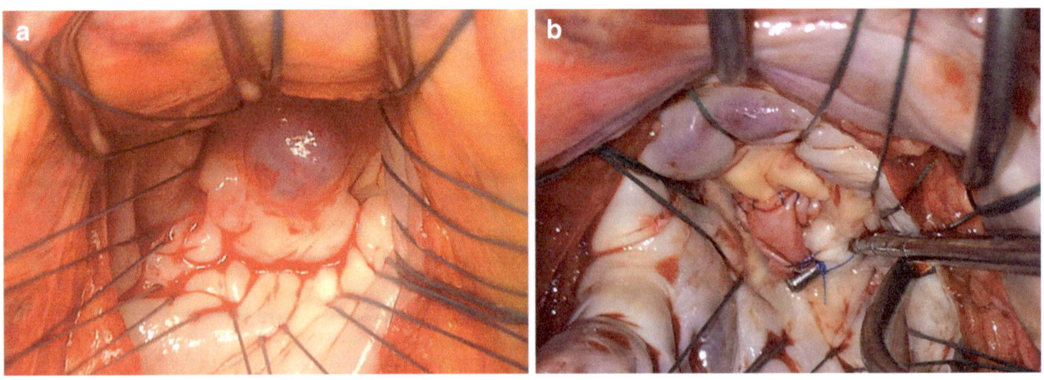

Fig. 5.14 Mitral valve leaflet reconstruction, with (**a**) infective endocarditic lesion on the A2 scallop of the anterior mitral valve leaflet, followed by (**b**) excision of the infected tissue and reconstruction with autologous pericardium

patients, additional Gore-Tex neo-chordae are required to support the free edge of the leaflet.

Chordal Techniques

Chordal Replacement (Figs. 5.15 and 5.16)

Chordal replacement involves the insertion of synthetic chordae, with Gore-Tex polytetrafluoroethylene (PTFE) sutures (W.L. Gore & Associates, Flagstaff, AZ, USA) most commonly used. This technique is primarily used for leaflet prolapse caused by chordal elongation or rupture. The major advantage of this technique is that it preserves the surface area of the leaflet and thus leaflet anatomy and mobility, thereby maximising the orifice area of the mitral valve. Stay sutures (5/0 Prolene) are placed around the normal chordae tendineae attached on either side of the prolapsed area of the leaflet and along the leading edge of the prolapsing segment. Gentle traction on these stay sutures allowed the margins of prolapsed segment of the leaflet to be clearly delineated, to assess the number of neo-chordae required and to identify the insertion point of the neo-chordae. The next step is gaining access to the papillary muscles, which can be improved by mechanical retraction of the leaflets using an additional retractor blade, leaflet retractor, large mechanical valve replacement sizer (Fig. 5.15a), Yankauer sucker tip or nerve hooks, as well as the 5/0 Prolene stay sutures on the leaflet edges (Fig. 5.15b).

When choosing which papillary muscle head to insert the neo-chordae, it is useful though not an imperative, to respect anatomy and to use the origin of elongated or ruptured chordae as a guide. In patients requiring multiple chordae to scallops on the leaflets, it is important to avoid crossing of these neo-chordae, by attaching those to the right of the midline of the leaflets onto the posteromedial papillary muscle and those to the left of the midline onto the anterolateral papillary muscle. The native chordae to A2 and P2 originate from both posteromedial and anterolateral papillary muscles and so if either papillary muscle head is small, the most robust looking one may be chosen.

Both limbs of a CV-4 Gore-Tex neo-chordae are passed through the fibrous part of the papillary muscle head, using a simple U stich. Although a suture can be supported with a pledget, there is no evidence to support its use and if the suture needs to be replaced, the pledget needs to be retrieved to avoid the risk of subsequent embolization. It is not necessary to tie a knot in the Gore-Tex suture at the papillary muscle level. Leaving the suture untied allows an equal distribution of tension in both limbs of the suture, otherwise if care is not taken to adjust their lengths appropriately one limb may become tense and the other loose. Each limb of the Gore-Tex suture is then passed through the prolapsing segment

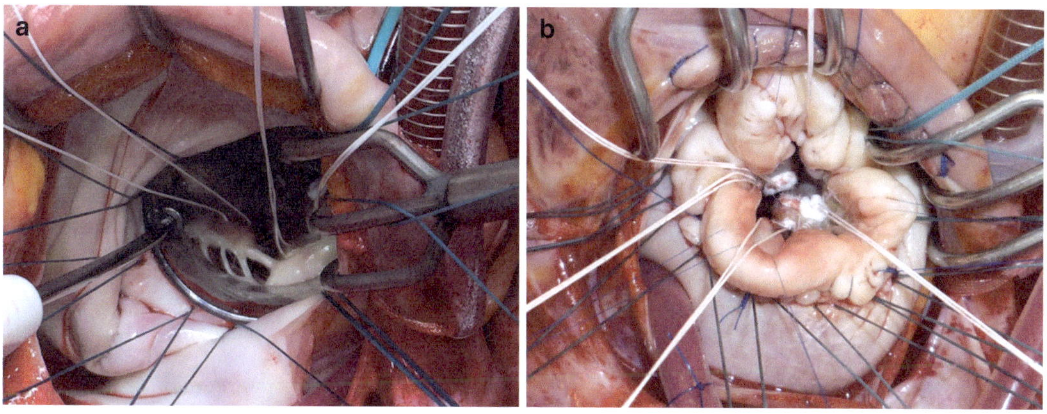

Fig. 5.15 Access to the papillary muscles by retraction of the mitral valve leaflets using (**a**) large mechanical valve replacement sizer and (**b**) 5/0 Prolene stay sutures on the leaflet edges

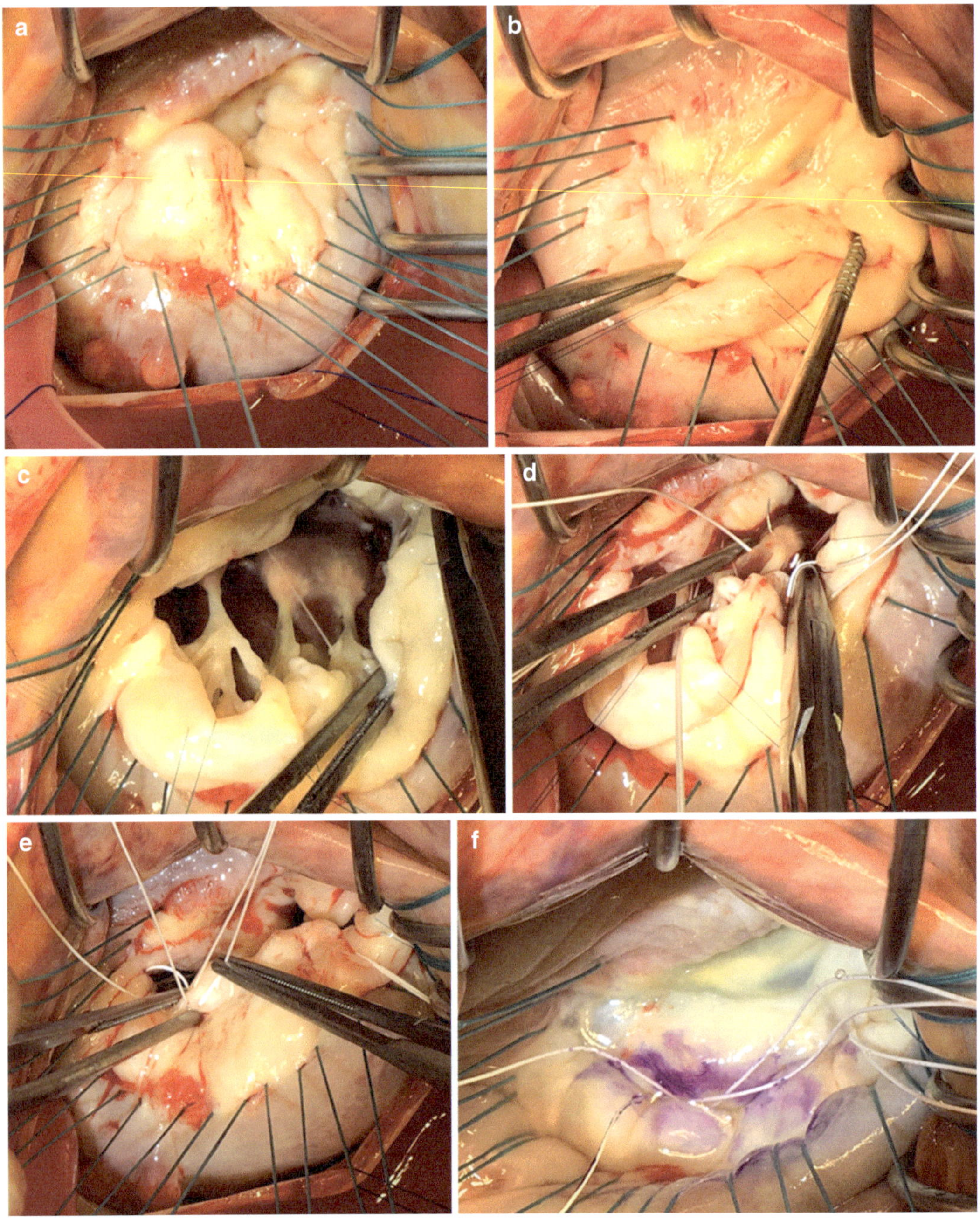

Fig. 5.16 Implantation of Gore-Tex neo-chordae using a single loop technique. The mitral valve is assessed using segmental analysis demonstrating (**a**) marked prolapse of the part of the P2 scallop of the posterior leaflet and (**b**) no significant prolapse of the anterior leaflet. (**c**) Access to the papillary muscles is gained by placing 5/0 polypropylene sutures on the leading edge of the posterior leaflet. (**d**) A pledgeted CV4 Gore-Tex neo-chordae is passed through the appropriate papillary muscles using a horizontal mattress suture. (**e**) Each limb of the Gore-Tex suture is then passed twice from the ventricular side to the atrial side through the free edge of the leaflet. (**f**) An ink test is then performed, which allows (**g**) the depth of coaptation to be assessed. (**h**) Once the optimal length of the neo-chord has been determined, the free ends of the Gore-Tex sutures are passed through the vertical limbs of the sutures and (**i**) tied on the ventricular side of the leaflet. (**j**) The repair procedure is completed by implanting an annuloplasty band from trigone to trigone

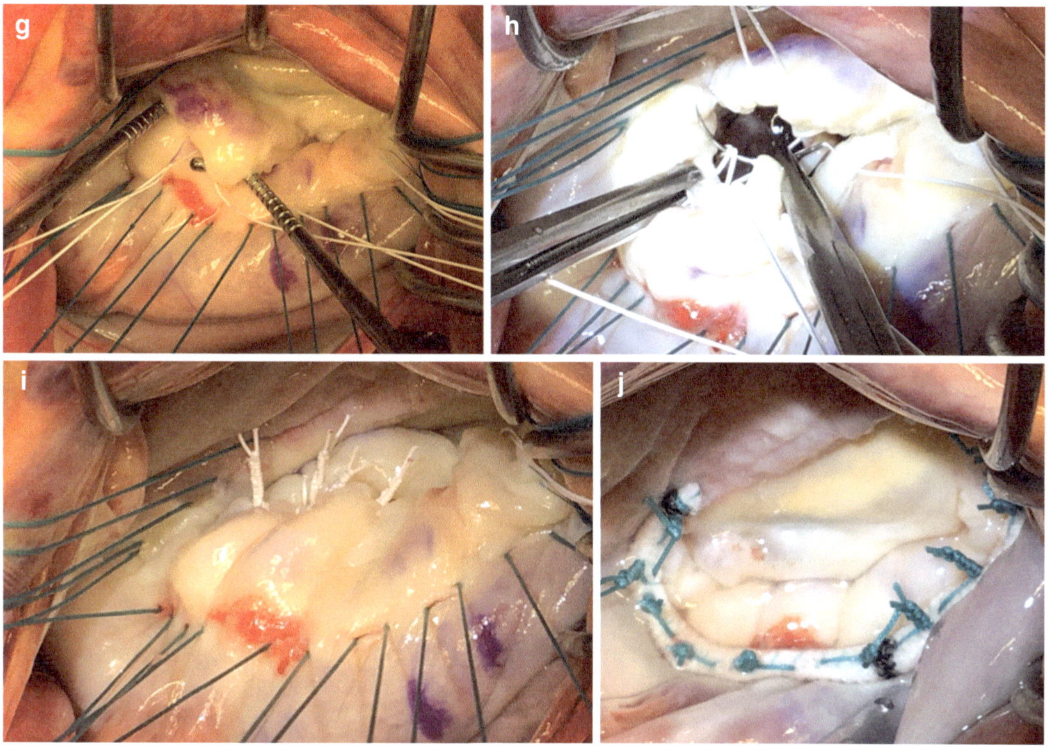

Fig. 5.16 (continued)

twice from the ventricular side to the atrial side about 5 mm away from the leaflet edge and 2–3 mm away from the boundary of normal leaflet.

Although implanting the Gore-Tex neo-chordae is relatively simple and reproducible, determining the length of the sutures can be challenging, as sutures that are too short result in restricted leaflet movement, whereas sutures that are too long result in residual leaflet prolapse, both of which are associated with persistent MR. Various techniques have been described to determine the height of the Gore-Tex neo-chordae, including using a functional assessment with saline inflation of the left ventricle to adjust the height of the neo-chord. An anatomical assessment can be made with pre-operative echocardiography by measuring the distance from the insertion point on the papillary muscles to the free edge of the prolapsing segment at the annular level or, intra-operatively, by using a graduated caliper. This distance can be used to select pre-made Gore-Tex loops. Alternatively, a fixed reference point can be used as a guide to the correct length and tension of the implanted neo-chord, including the anterior mitral valve annulus, non-prolapsing parts of the posterior leaflet (such as P1) or the hinge point of the posterior leaflet at the coaptation line (assessed with a methylene blue marker). Once the optimal length of the neo-chordae has been determined, the free ends of the Gore-Tex sutures are passed through the vertical limbs of the sutures to be tied on the ventricular side of the leaflet.

Chordal Transposition

This technique involves the transfer of normal posterior leaflet chordae to replace elongated or ruptured anterior leaflet chordae. It can also be performed by transferring a segment of normal posterior leaflet tissue in combination with the chordae tendineae. The advantage of this technique is that the prolapsing segment of the anterior leaflet is supported by naturally determined appropriate length native chordae, obtained from the opposite non-prolapsing segment of the posterior leaflet. This leaves a corresponding segment of posterior leaflet that will need to be repaired and can only be performed in patients with isolated anterior leaflet prolapse, associated with normal posterior leaflet and sub-valvular apparatus. In patients with elongated or ruptured primary free-edge chords, chordal transfer can be performed using a secondary chord sectioned at its implantation site on the base of the leaflet and sutured to the leaflet edge.

Flip-Over Technique

In this technique, a quadrangular segment of the posterior leaflet that lies directly opposite the prolapsing anterior leaflet segment is carefully cut away from the rest of the posterior leaflet and detached from the posterior annulus. It is then 'flipped-over' with its attached chords and sutured to the atrial surface of the prolapsing segment of the anterior leaflet segment. Any basal chords that are attached to the ventricular surface of the posterior leaflet segment can be preserved. As with chordal transposition, the main advantage of this technique is that the transferred chords are of appropriate length. The resulting gap in the posterior leaflet is repaired using annular plication sutures and reconstruction of the residual P1 and P3 segments of the posterior leaflet.

Chordal Shortening

Direct chordal shortening has been described and carried out in the past but the results are very poor, often with early recurrence of regurgitation. Chordal height reduction by reimplantation of the chords within the papillary muscle, however, allows a group of elongated chords to be shortened simultaneously. The technique involves performing a longitudinal incision, where the elongated chordae tendineae originates, from the tip towards the base of the papillary muscle. The elongated chordae can then be shortened by folding them into the deepest point of the incision and suturing them in position, to produce chordal length equal to the normal adjacent chordae. Although this technique directly addresses the underlying pathology, it also has unpredictable long-term results, with reports of chordal rupture and recurrent leaflet prolapse described.

Chordal Cutting

Normally, secondary chords remain tense during the cardiac cycle, thereby maintaining a constant papillary-annular distance. They carry three times the load compared to the primary chords and are responsible for maintaining the curvature of the leaflets. In patients with ischaemic mitral regurgitation, concomitant cutting of secondary chordae, arising from the affected papillary muscle, reduces tethering of the chordae tendineae on the leaflets, improves leaflet movement and increases the depth of coaptation. There are some concerns, however, about the effects of secondary chord cutting on left ventricular function, due to disruption of valvular-ventricular continuity and the potential for progressive left ventricular remodelling, especially in patients with severely impaired ventricles. In view of this, the secondary chords can be translocated to the free edge of the leaflet using 5/0 Prolene or replaced by Gore-Tex neo-chordae. The primary and tertiary chordae are also left in situ to preserve valvular-ventricular continuity.

Papillary Muscle Techniques

Papillary Muscle Shortening

Papillary muscle shortening is useful for patients with commissural prolapse caused by elongation of multiple chordae arising from the same papillary muscle head. Downward displacement of the papillary muscle head can be achieved by a small triangular wedge resection at the base of the head, using the prolapsing distance as a guide to the size of the wedge of tissue to be excised. The width of the resection will determine the degree of repositioning of the papillary muscle head and therefore the degree of retensioning. The papillary muscle head is then secured within the trench using a pledgeted 4/0 Prolene suture. An alternative technique is to make a longitudinal split in the papillary muscle and then resuturing the head to a lower point on the papillary muscle.

Papillary Muscle Splitting

Splitting of the papillary muscles and attached fan-chords that support restricted fused commissures involved in patients with rheumatic mitral disease can be used to increase mobility and pliability at the commissures.

Papillary Muscle Relocation

Papillary muscle relocation is based on the concept that the distance between the mitral annulus and the posterior papillary muscle is an important determinant of the leaflet tethering. The displaced posterior papillary muscle can be relocated using a transventricular suture to approximate it towards the mitral annulus and counteract the altered subvalvular geometry involved in ischaemic mitral regurgitation. Through an atriotomy, the papillary muscle can be approximated to the mitral annulus at the level of the posteromedial commissure using a Teflon-pledgeted 3/0 Prolene or CV4 Gore-Tex suture, which is placed from the fibrous head of the posterior papillary muscle through the mitral annulus at the level of the posteromedial commissure. The correct length of the papillary muscle relocation suture can then be determined and the suture tied down over a pledget on the atrial side of the annulus. This technique is supported with implantation of an annuloplasty ring.

An alternative technique is to access the head of the posterior papillary muscle via an aortotomy and pass the pledgeted 3/0 Prolene or CV4 Gore-Tex suture through the mid-point of the anterior annulus, which lies beneath the commissure between non-coronary and left coronary aortic cusps, and exteriorize it through the aortic wall. The suture can then be tied under echocardiographical guidance in the loaded beating heart to reposition the displaced posterior papillary muscle toward the mid-point of the anterior annulus.

Papillary Muscle Sling

This technique involves placing a 4 mm Gore-Tex tube around the base of both papillary muscles. The sling is then tightened to decrease the distance between both papillary muscles, thereby realigning the papillary muscles and reducing the tension on the chordae tendineae. An alternative to this technique involves simply suturing the heads of the papillary muscles together to reduce papillary muscle displacement and leaflet tethering.

Mitral Valve Replacement (Fig. 5.17)

Historically, mitral valve replacement was performed without preservation of the sub-valvular apparatus. This, however, is associated with very poor long-term outcomes, due to interference of the normal valvular-ventricular continuity and subsequent left ventricular enlargement and impaired contractility. Sub-valvular preservation involves maintaining the valvular-ventricular continuity and normal ventricular geometry by keeping the entire posterior leaflet and attached sub-valvular apparatus, whilst excising the anterior leaflet but reattaching the native chordae tendineae to the anterior annulus. If the native chordae tendinae cannot be preserved, such as with excessive thickening or calcification, Gore-Tex neo-chordae can be used to reattach the papillary muscles to the mitral annulus. It is thought that preservation of all the chordae results in reduced ventricular volumes and better systolic function compared with partial preservation.

Initially, a 2/0 Prolene suture is placed through the centre of the body of the anterior leaflet, which is used as traction to pull the leaflet away from the annulus to allow precise excision of the leaflet tissue. An incision is then begun approximately 2mm away from and parallel to the anterior annulus (Fig. 5.17a). The incision is extended in both directions towards the anterolateral and posteromedial commissures, thereby detaching the leaflet from the anterior annulus (Fig. 5.17b). The detached leaflet is then divided down its centre (Fig. 5.17c, d) and the triangles of excess tissue excised from each side (Fig. 5.17e). The remaining strips of leaflet, with inserted primary and secondary chordae tendineae, are reattached to the annulus using 2–0 Ethibond pledgeted sutures that will also secure the valve in the supra-annular position (Fig. 5.17f). This technique removes any chance of folded anterior leaflet remnant from being carried up into the left ventricular outflow tract causing obstruction. Simple plication of the anterior leaflet runs that risk and is unnecessary.

Attention is then turned to the posterior leaflet. Although, it is possible to retain the entire posterior leaflet along with its attached chordae tendineae, detachment of the leaflet from the annulus, excision of excess leaflet tissue and division through its centre with reattatchment to the annulus will again maximise the orifice area for optimal prosthetic valve size (Fig. 5.17g). Large masses of calcification and chordal fusion, however, will need to be excised to allow the valve prosthesis to be implanted and function efficiently. The posterior leaflet is therefore also resected approximately 2 mm from the annulus. The posterior mitral valve annulus is then debrided of calcific deposits if necessary. This allows the new prosthesis to sit more easily on the annulus. If decalcification is significant, it is very important to reinforce the atrioventricular continuity with a generous pericardial patch. This prevents the highly dangerous possibility of atrioventricular dissociation and also reduces the risk of a paravalvular leak following implantation of the mitral valve prosthesis. Once this is complete, the posterior leaflet chordae can be reattached to the annulus. Normal chordal insertion is fan-like to each side of the centre of the leaflet. By dividing the leaflet again in the centre and excising leaflet tissue, the remaining leaflet edge with attached chords can be again reattached to the annulus with the sutures that will be used to hold the valve in place.

Interrupted pledgeted non-everting 2/0 Ethibond sutures are then placed, with 5–8 mm between each limb of the suture and 1 mm spacing between adjacent sutures (Fig. 5.17 h). It is important to place the sutures through the thickened fibrous part of the annulus and not through the more friable myocardium. The depth of suture placement needs to be sufficient so that the suture

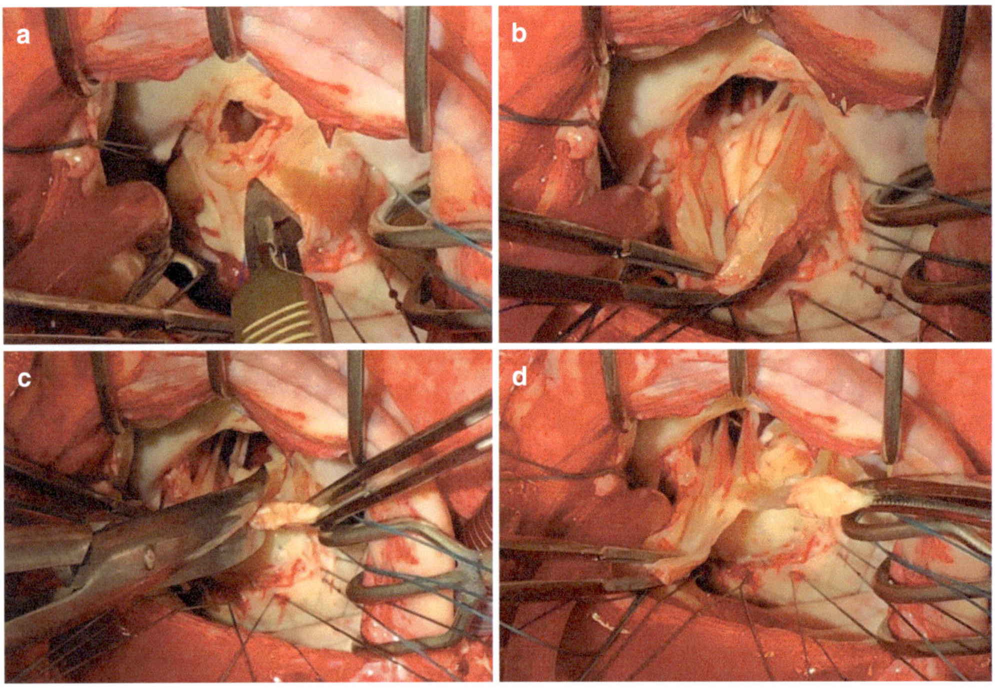

Fig. 5.17 Mitral valve replacement with preservation of the subvalvular apparatus. (**a**) Incision at the midpoint of the anterior leaflet; (**b**) extension of the incision in both directions towards the anterolateral and posteromedial commissures; (**c**) division of the anterior leaflet through its midpoint; (**d**) division of anterior leaflet is stopped just short of the attachment of the chordae tendineae; (**e**) excision of the majority of the anterior leaflet tissue leaving a rim of tissue attached to the chordae tendineae; (**f**) reattachment of the chordae tendineae to the anterior annulus using a valve replacement suture; (**g**) excision of the majority of the posterior leaflet tissue leaving a rim of tissue attached to the chordae tendineae; (**h**) implantation of the remaining valve replacement sutures, using non-inverting horizontal mattress 2/0 Ethibond sutures, plicating any residual leaflet tissue; (**i**) insertion of the sutures into the prosthetic valve sewing ring; (**j**) parachuting of the prosthetic valve down to the annulus, with the protective guard in situ to prevent the sutures getting caught around the struts; (**k**) implantation of the bovine pericardial prosthesis with preserved native chordae tendineae visible through the opening in the bioprosthesis; and (**l**) mitral valve bioprosthesis in situ

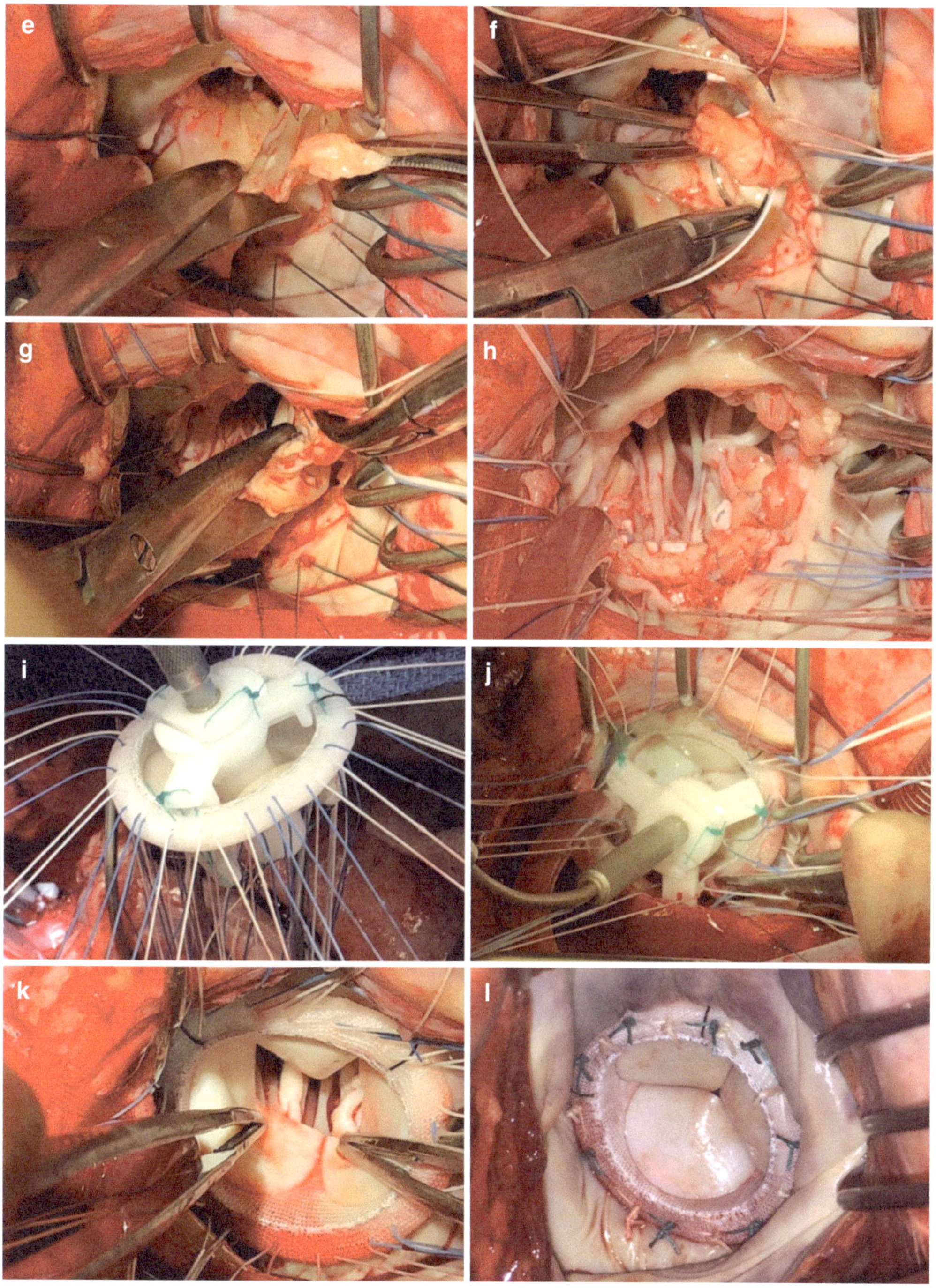

Fig. 5.17 (continued)

does not tear through but not so deep to injure nearby structures, such as the circumflex coronary artery, aortic valve, conduction tissue or coronary sinus. The valve orifice is then measured, using the sizers provided by the manufacturers. The sutures are placed through the sewing ring (Fig. 5.17i). It is helpful to divide the circumference of the valve ring into thirds and to place one suture at each of those three points and then evenly space the sutures in the thirds of the valve ring. When tying down the sutures for a stented biological valve, it is important to ensure that the sutures do not get trapped around the stents of the prosthesis. Certain bioprostheses come with a guard to reduce the risk of this occurring (Fig. 5.17j). The valve is then inspected from the left ventricular side to ensure that there are no suture loops (Fig. 5.17k) and then the prosthesis is the tied down in situ (Fig. 5.17l).

The choice of prosthetic valve depends on the patient's age, patient's wishes, and to some extent their need for warfarin therapy. Implantation of the mitral valve prosthesis is carried out using an interrupted, non-everting technique with horizontal mattress sutures from the ventricular side. This doesn't reduce the mitral orifice and this technique of sandwiching annular tissue between the pledgeted sutures, reattached leaflet and soft prosthetic sewing ring gives a very strong seal. Using this non-everting technique also allows the prosthesis to be implanted in a supra-annular position, thereby enabling a larger valve to be implanted as compared to an intra-annular valve technique. The use of interrupted sutures for mitral valve replacement has been shown to reduce the rate of paravalvular regurgitation, as compared to a semi-continuous valve implantation technique. Orientation of the implanted mitral valve prosthesis is particularly important for a bioprosthesis. The stents need to be aligned with the left and right trigones, so as to reduce their protrusion into the left ventricular outflow tract (LVOT) and reduce the risk of subsequent LVOT obstruction. For a mechanical prosthesis, the valve is orientated in an anti-anatomical position, so that the maximum flow is directed into the LVOT. It is also important to ensure that there is full motion of the mechanical leaflets, which are not impaired by the preserved native tissue.

In patients where there is excessive calcification, retraction or fibrosis of the mitral valve leaflets and sub-valvular apparatus, such that preservation of the entire sub-valvular apparatus is not feasible, Gore-Tex neo-chordae can be implanted. The Gore-Tex neo-chordae are implanted from the posteromedial papillary muscle to the 2 and 4 o'clock positions of the mitral valve annulus and from the anterolateral papillary muscle to the 8 and 10 o'clock positions, as required (Fig. 5.18).

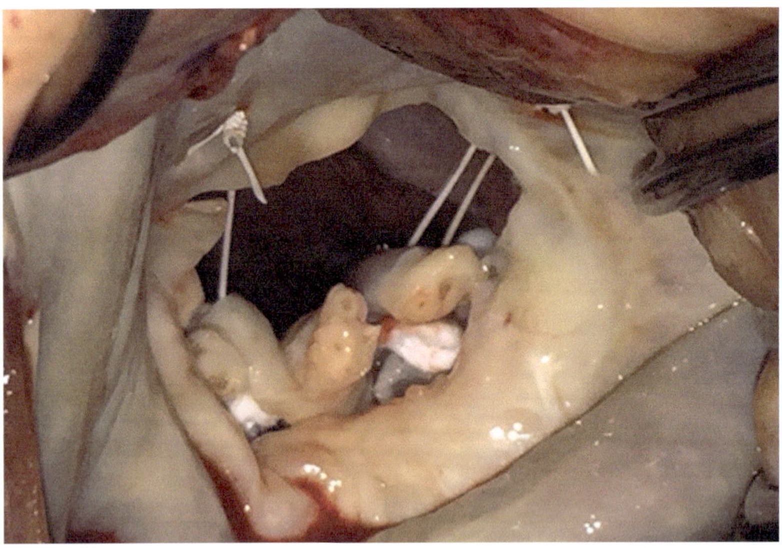

Fig. 5.18 Operative image demonstrating implantation of Gore-Tex neo-chordae from the posteromedial papillary muscle to the 2 o'clock position of the anterior annulus and from the anterolateral papillary muscle to the 10 o'clock position of the anterior annulus in a patient with a rheumatic mitral valve, where the sub-valvular apparatus to the anterior leaflet could not be preserved due to extensive fibrosis, shortening and calcification. The sub-valvular apparatus to the posterior leaflet, however, was preserved

Tricuspid Valve Operative Techniques

The tricuspid valve is positioned between two low pressure chambers, which have evolved to be very responsive to volume changes. Hence, there is a great deal of capacitance variation that can easily be catered for. The form of the tricuspid valve has evolved within this physiological environment. This gives rise to the difficulty in defining and understanding tricuspid valve regurgitation. Severe tricuspid regurgitation (TR) is the extreme form and is accompanied by significant atrial and ventricular dilatation. Just as with left-sided functional mitral regurgitation, once the right-sided chambers have dilated to the point where this obtends, it is irreversible and it is arguable that even with correction of the valvular regurgitation by reducing the orifice area, ventricular change is irreversable.

Mild TR is inconsequential in the absence of progressive pathology, such as untreated left-sided lesions or significant pulmonary hypertension. The very large grey area between mild and severe TR is difficult to assess both in terms of the likelihood of progression and functional implication. Deciding what to do and whom to treat is compounded by the fact that there is a significant recurrence of TR within 3–5 years after tricuspid surgery, even with a seemingly competent valve on leaving the operating room. Although parameters of valve dimension as predictors of outcome have been described, even these are open to challenge. This is particularly true in patients with Barlow's disease, where the orifice of both atrioventricular valves are significantly bigger than the average patient with other forms of non-functional mitral regurgitation.

The debate over which patients should have tricuspid valve repair continues to rage on, especially in the absence of level A evidence. If the TR is persistently moderate-severe or severe and, on exposing the heart, the right atrium is stretched and has a purplish hue instead of being of normal size with the soft pinkish hue of the normal chamber, then repair is a reasonable. The presence of correctable left-sided lesions will add to the likelihood of success in the mid-term.

The acquisition of meaningful data is always going to be difficult in these patients, as defining moderate TR in a consistent way in patients, where the degree of TR can vary significantly, is almost impossible. Volume and flow changes in response to exercise and levels of hydration, along with heart rhythm and rate can and does alter the situation constantly.

The current tendency to lower the threshold for repair of TR is as yet untested. Add to this, the multiplicity of ways of repairing the valve and the fact that few surgeons are very familiar with the techniques and perform tricuspid valve repair rarely, mean that we should proceed thoughtfully and with caution in these patients. An argument in the opposite direction is the fact that late TR surgery in redo cases with severe right ventricular dysfunction carries a significant mortality and morbidity.

Annular Techniques

Suture Annuloplasty (Fig. 5.19)
Suture annuloplasty can be performing using either the Kay technique (bicuspidisation) or the De Vega technique. The Kay annuloplasty technique involves using pledgeted horizontal mattress compression annuloplasty sutures to plicate the posterior tricuspid valve annulus, thereby effectively excluding the posterior leaflet from the functioning valve orifice and creating a 'bileaflet' tricuspid valve.

In the De Vega annuloplasty technique, two weaving 4/0 Prolene purse-string sutures are placed from the anteroseptal commissure to the posteroseptal commissure to cinch the anterior and posterior tricuspid valve annulus. This effectively downsizes the annulus to reduce the valvular orifice area, thereby increasing leaflet coaptation.

Although both techniques are relatively simple and quick to perform, they are less reproducible than ring annuloplasty. The Kay annuloplasty technique does not address progressive dilatation of the anterior annulus, whereas the De Vega

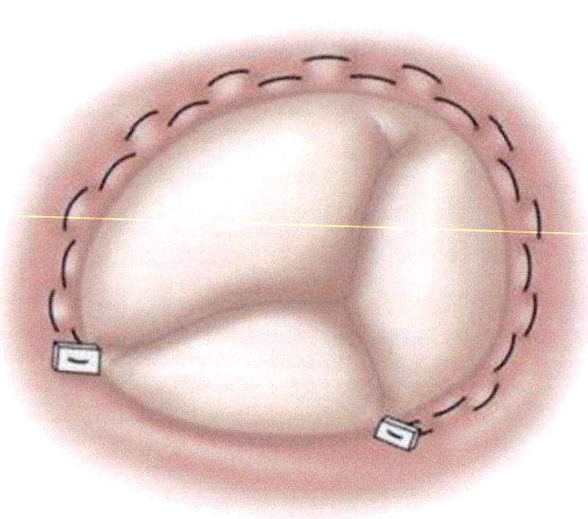

Fig. 5.19 The De Vega suture annuloplasty technique, where two weaving 4/0 Prolene purse-string sutures are placed from the anteroseptal commissure to the posteroseptal commissure to cinch the anterior and posterior tricuspid valve annulus

technique is associated with suture migration or dehiscence, thereby making both prone to progressive dilatation of the tricuspid annulus and recurrent regurgitation. Although suture annuloplasty techniques were previously the most frequent method of treating TR, they have recently been subject to significant criticism as a result of early failure.

Ring Annuloplasty (Fig. 5.20)

Ring annuloplasty is recommended as the treatment of choice for annular dilatation, in preference to suture annuloplasty, as it is a more reproducible and durable technique at reducing annular size and maintaining valvular competency. Tricuspid valve annuloplasty rings are usually incomplete to avoid the Bundle of His and the atrioventricular node that sit at the apex of the triangle of Koch, adjacent to the medial aspect of

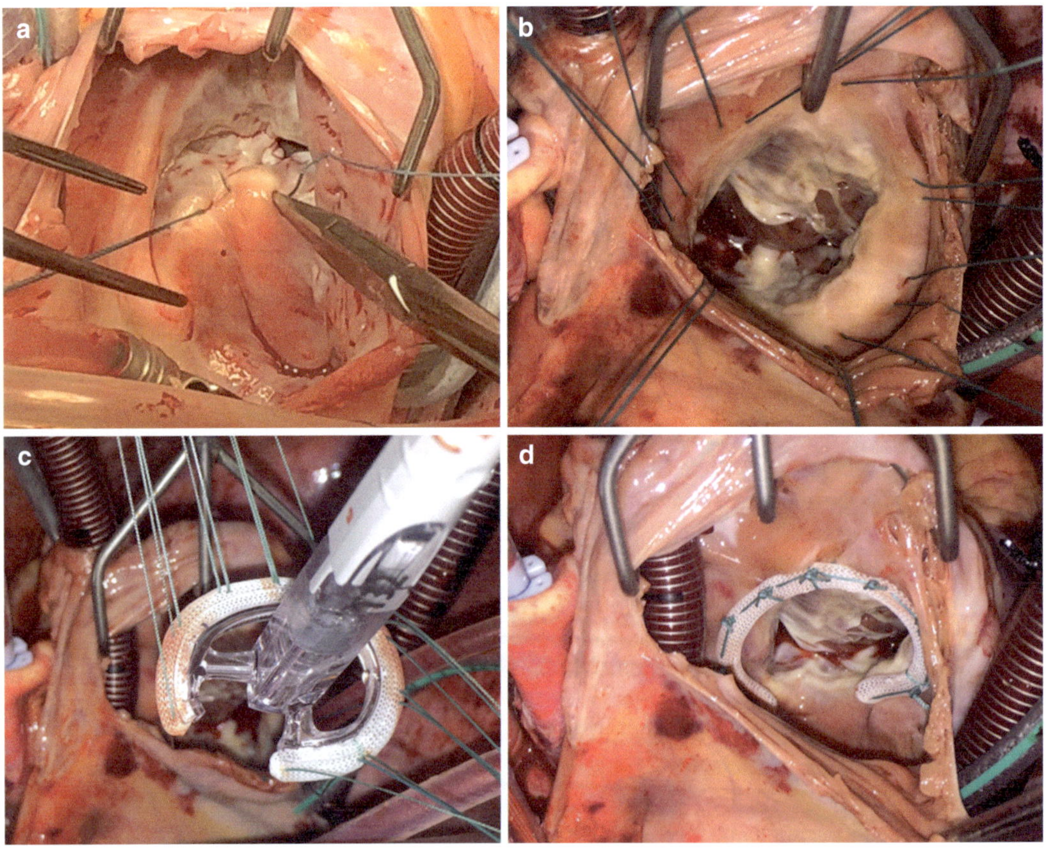

Fig. 5.20 Tricuspid valve ring annuloplasty, with (**a**) insertion of interrupted horizontal mattress annuloplasty sutures, starting from the mid-point of the septal annulus, (**b**) progressing anti-clockwise up to the anteroseptal commissure, (**c**) placement of the sutures through the annuloplasty ring and (**d**) annuloplasty ring tied down in situ

the septal annulus. The site of the conduction tissue can be seen in some patients, where it appears as yellow staining of the tissue in this area. As the majority of annular dilatation takes place in the anterior and posterior annulus, the use of these incomplete rings will achieve satisfactory reduction in annular size and valve competence for type I lesions. Horizontal mattress 2/0 Ethibond annuloplasty sutures are placed around the circumference of the tricuspid valve, with a 1 cm width and approximately 1 mm apart. These sutures are placed from the mid-point of the septal leaflet on the lateral half of the septal annulus, as well as the entire anterior and posterior tricuspid valve annulus.

There are various methods described to choose the correct size of annuloplasty ring. One is to measure the distance between the anteroseptal and posteroseptal commissures. Alternatively, the surface area of the anterior leaflet can be used, unless the other two leaflets are large, which is often the case in patients with Barlow's disease. In that situation, the surface area of the other two leaflets needs to be taken into account. Once chosen, the annuloplasty ring is sutured in place and competency of the valve is assessed with static testing, by injecting cold saline into the right ventricle, using a bulb syringe, whilst occluding the main pulmonary artery.

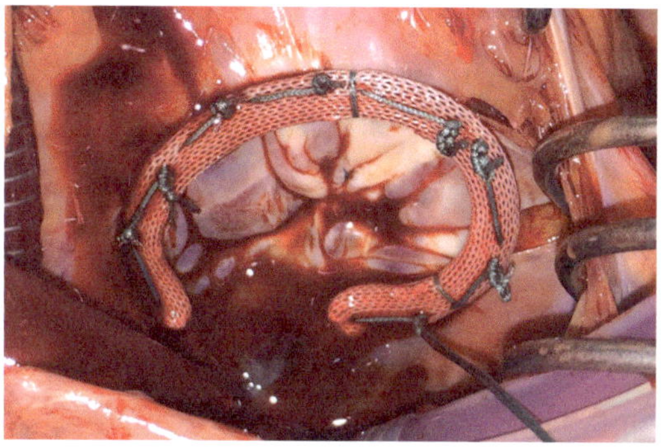

Fig. 5.21 Edge-to-edge repair ('clover' technique), where the free edges of the 3 leaflets are approximated using a 5/0 Prolene suture, producing a clover-shaped triple-orifice valve

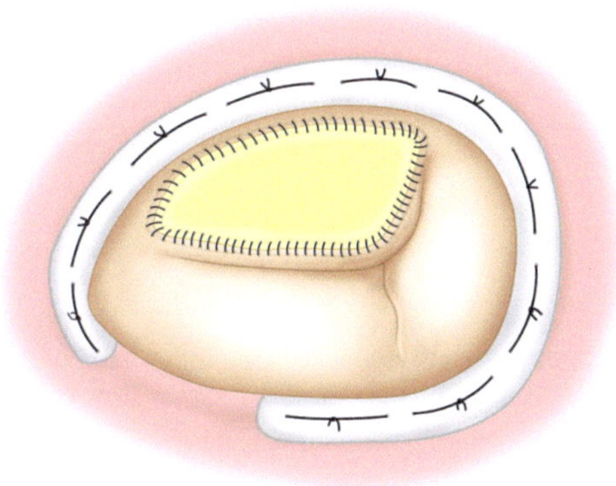

Fig. 5.22 Patch augmentation of the anterior tricuspid valve leaflet using bovine pericardium

Leaflet Techniques

Edge-to-Edge Repair (Fig. 5.21)

The edge-to-edge repair ('clover' technique) uses the same principles of the equivalent mitral repair technique by approximating the free edges of the valve leaflets, producing a clover-shaped triple-orifice valve.

Leaflet Augmentation (Fig. 5.22)

Leaflet augmentation is usually performed in patients with leaflet tethering, as an adjunct to increase the depth of coaptation. It is important all the leaflets are pliable, and that there is no leaflet or annular calcification. The affected leaflet is detached at its attachment to the annulus, from commissure to commissure. Annuloplasty sutures are then placed to enhance exposure, allowing a long oval-shaped autologous or bovine pericardial patch to be implanted, using a continuous locking 5/0 Prolene suture. It is important to slightly oversize the patch to ensure that there is no tension on the leaflet causing restricted leaflet motion.

Leaflet Reconstruction (Fig. 5.23)

In patients with leaflet destruction caused by infective endocarditis, leaflet reconstruction may be feasible if there is enough native tissue to form a competent valve following resection and debridement of the infected tissue with a clear margin. Repair of a defect in the leaflets is usually possible, even if up to 50% of the leaflet body is

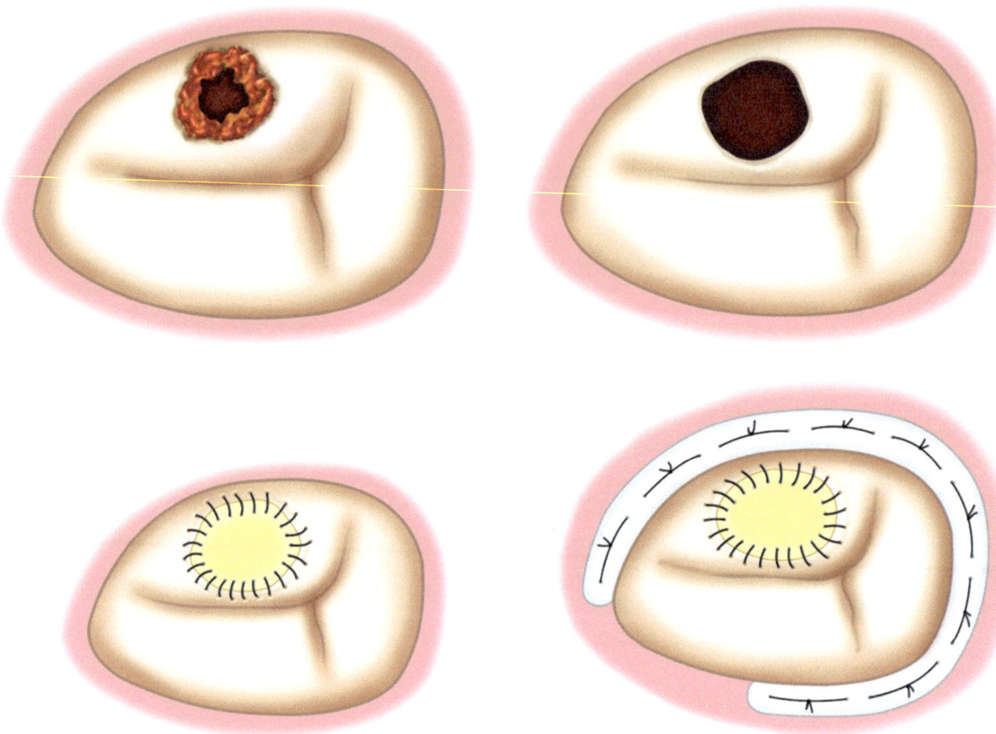

Fig. 5.23 Leaflet reconstruction following infective endocarditis destruction of the tricuspid valve. Once radical debridement of the anterior leaflet has been completed, reconstruction of the leaflet is performed using autologous pericardium, followed by implantation of an annuloplasty ring

involved, so long as the leading edge of the leaflet, along the coaptation line, is intact. Stay sutures (5/0 Prolene) are placed around the chordae tendineae attached on either side of the perforated area of the leaflet. Gentle traction on these stay sutures give better access and visualisation of the leaflet. If the valve is deemed repairable, any vegetations are resected, and all macroscopically infected and inflamed tissue is radically excised to ensure that the residual native tissue is free from infection and that the residual tissue will be strong enough to hold suture material. The defect in the leaflet body can then be repaired with glutaraldehyde-preserved autologous or bovine pericardium. The pericardium is implanted using a continuous locking 5/0 Prolene suture, to avoid purse-stringing the patch. It is important to slightly oversize the patch to ensure that there is no tension on the leaflet causing restricted leaflet motion. Once the repair procedure has been completed, the annulus is stabilised with an annuloplasty ring.

Chordal Techniques

Chordal Replacement

Chordal replacement is used in patients with a prolapsed tricuspid valve leaflet or flail leaflet due to chordal elongation or rupture, respectively. The diseased chordae are replaced with Gore-Tex polytetrafluoroethylene (PTFE) sutures (W.L. Gore & Associates, Flagstaff, AZ, USA). As it does not require the excision of valve tissue, it preserves leaflet anatomy, mobility and the maximal orifice area of the tricuspid valve. Chordal replacement is performed by passing both limbs of a CV-4 Gore-Tex neo-chord through the fibrous part of the papillary muscle head that was providing chordal support to the prolapsing leaflet. Both limbs of the neo-chord are then passed through the prolapsing segment approximately 5 mm from the free edge. The appropriate height of the Gore-Tex chordae is determined by functional assessment, using saline inflation of the right ventricle, whilst occluding the pulmonary artery. The height of the neo-chord can then be adjusted according to the desired height.

Tricuspid Valve Replacement (Fig. 5.24)

In patients with extensive disease of the valve where repair is not feasible, such as marked leaflet tethering, retraction or calcification with rheumatic valve disease (Fig. 5.24a) or carcinoid, replacement of the tricuspid valve is indicated. The choice between a mechanical or biological stented valve remains controversial. Although both have similar outcomes for survival, mechanical valves are prone to thromboembolic complications in the low-pressure right-sided circulation. Although mechanical valves are thought to have a greater durability, there is evidence of good long-term durability of a tricuspid valve bioprosthesis in the low-pressure right-sided circulation.

Interrupted pledgeted non-everting 2/0 Ethibond sutures are placed along the annulus, with approximately 1 cm between each limb of the suture and 1 mm spacing between adjacent sutures (Fig. 5.24b). It is important to place the sutures vertically upwards into the myocardium and not horizontally into the atrial or septal tissue. The depth of suture placement needs to be sufficient so that the suture does not tear through. Knowledge of the anatomical position of nearby structures, such as the right coronary artery, aortic valve, conduction tissue or coronary sinus is essential. At the supero-medial aspect of the septal annulus, sutures are placed through plicated septal leaflet tissue to avoid the conducting tissue, which lies at the apex of the triangle of Koch. The valve orifice is then measured, using the sizers provided by the manufacturers. The sutures are placed through the sewing ring and the prosthesis is the tied down. When tying down the sutures for a stented biological valve, it is important to ensure

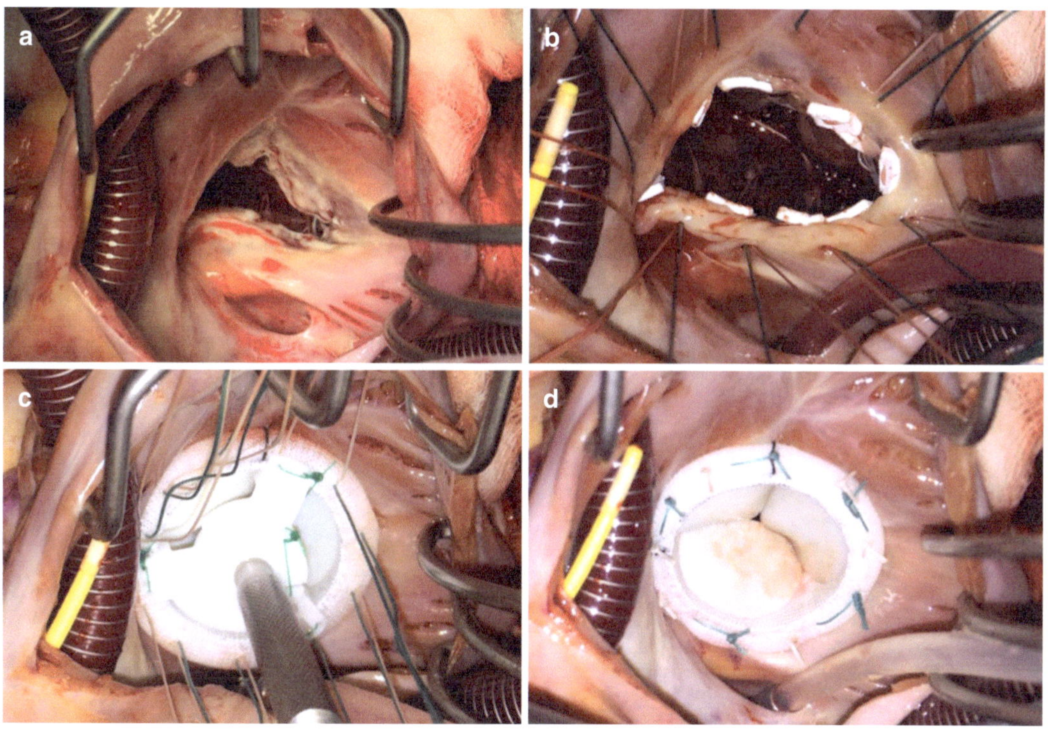

Fig. 5.24 Operative images demonstrating a tricuspid valve replacement, with (**a**) a rheumatic tricuspid valve characterised by fibrotic, retracted leaflets and rolled up free edges, (**b**) implantation of the valve replacement sutures, using non-inverting horizontal mattress 2/0 Ethibond sutures, plicating any residual leaflet tissue; (**c**) parachuting of the prosthetic valve down to annulus, with the protective guard in situ to prevent the sutures getting caught around the struts; and (**d**) tricuspid valve bioprosthesis in situ, following tying down of the sutures

that the sutures do not get trapped around the stents of the prosthesis. Certain bioprostheses come with a guard to reduce the risk of this occurring (Fig. 5.24c). A bioprosthtetic tricuspid valve is orientated with the stents aligned with the anteroseptal and posteroseptal commissures (Fig. 5.24d). A mechanical prosthesis is orientated in an anti-anatomical position, so that the maximum flow is directed into the right ventricular outflow tract.

Atrial Fibrillation Surgery

Before commencing atrial fibrillation ablation surgery, intra-operative trans-oesophageal echocardiography is used to ensure the absence of thrombus in the left atrium, especially in the left atrial appendage. Following initiation of cardiopulmonary bypass, the superior and inferior vena cava are mobilised. Pulmonary vein isolation is then performed on cardiopulmonary bypass with a decompressed beating heart to allow exit block to be determined by pulmonary vein pacing. The area between the right pulmonary artery and right superior pulmonary vein is then developed into the oblique sinus. Blunt dissection of the right superior and inferior pulmonary veins is performed to enable an umbilical tape to be passed around both veins together. Pacing thresholds are then measured from each pulmonary vein using a bipolar pacing probe. A bipolar radiofrequency clamp device (Atricure Inc., West Chester, OH) is then placed onto the left atrial tissue immediately adjacent to the junction with the right pulmonary veins (Fig. 5.25a). By placing the clamp on atrial tissue, it reduces the risk of developing pulmonary vein stenosis. The duration of the ablation is

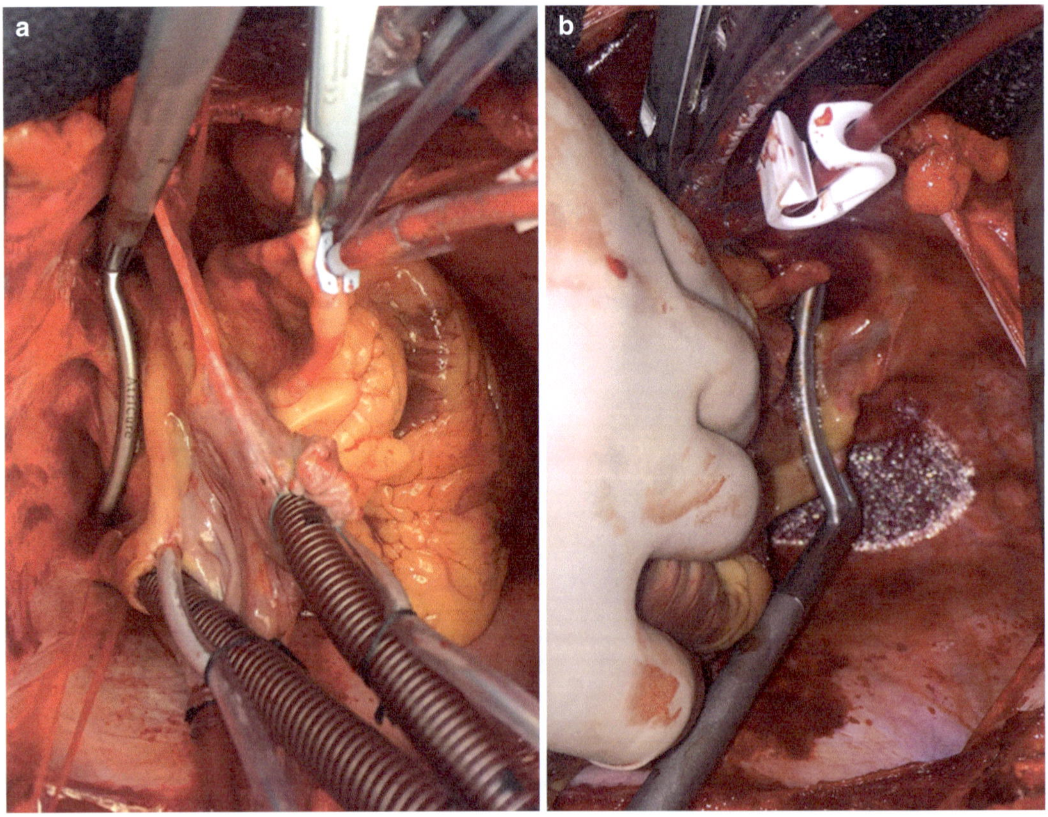

Fig. 5.25 Pulmonary vein isolation, which is achieved by placing a bipolar radiofrequency clamp device (Atricure Inc., West Chester, OH) on the left atrium adjacent to the (**a**) right and (**b**) left pulmonary veins

determined by the computed algorithms, calculated from the impedance monitoring. The lesion is repeated a second time by moving the clamp slightly to produce a parallel ablation line, thereby ensuring complete electrical isolation of the left atrium from the pulmonary veins is achieved. Isolation is confirmed by demonstrating exit block, which is evidenced by the inability to pace the atrium from either of the pulmonary veins. If exit block is not demonstrated, additional ablation lines are performed, as required.

Access to the left pulmonary veins is achieved by retracting the heart towards the right. Blunt dissection of the left superior and inferior pulmonary veins is performed, including dissection of the ligament of Marshall, again to enable a tape to be passed around both veins together. Once pacing thresholds are measured from each vein, the bipolar radiofrequency clamp device is passed around the left atrial tissue immediately adjacent to the junction with left pulmonary veins (Fig. 5.25b). The lesion is repeated with a second parallel ablation line and again isolation is confirmed by demonstrating exit block when pacing the pulmonary veins.

Following mobilisation of Sondergaard's inter-atrial groove anterior to the right pulmonary veins, a standard left atriotomy is performed. To achieve isolation of the entire posterior left atrium, the bipolar radiofrequency clamp device is first placed at the inferior aspect of the left atriotomy next to the right inferior pulmonary vein orifice across the floor of the left atrium towards the orifice of left inferior pulmonary vein (Fig. 5.26a), and then at the superior aspect of the left atriotomy next to the right superior pulmonary vein orifice across the roof of the left atrium towards the orifice of left superior pulmonary vein (Fig. 5.26b), to complete the box lesion set.

The next step of the left atrial lesion set is the mitral isthmus line, which requires a combination of bipolar radiofrequency and cryothermy, as the bipolar radiofrequency clamp device is unable to create a transmural lesion up to the mitral valve annulus due to the thickness of the tissue at that level. The bipolar radiofrequency clamp device is used to create an ablation line from the inferior aspect of the left atriotomy across the floor of the left atrium towards the mitral valve annulus (Fig. 5.27a). It is important to avoid the circumflex coronary artery, which runs parallel to the posterior mitral valve annulus, when creating this ablation line. The final 1-2cm up to the mitral annulus is then completed using a cryoprobe (Fig. 5.27b), followed by a separate application of the cryoprobe on the epicardial surface of the coronary sinus. The cryoprobe is applied for 2 min at -60 °C and thawed before removal, to avoid tearing of attached tissue. In patients with a right-dominant coronary artery system, the isthmus line is directed towards the junction of the P2 and P3 scallops of the posterior leaflet. In patients with a left-dominant coronary artery system, the isthmus line is directed towards the

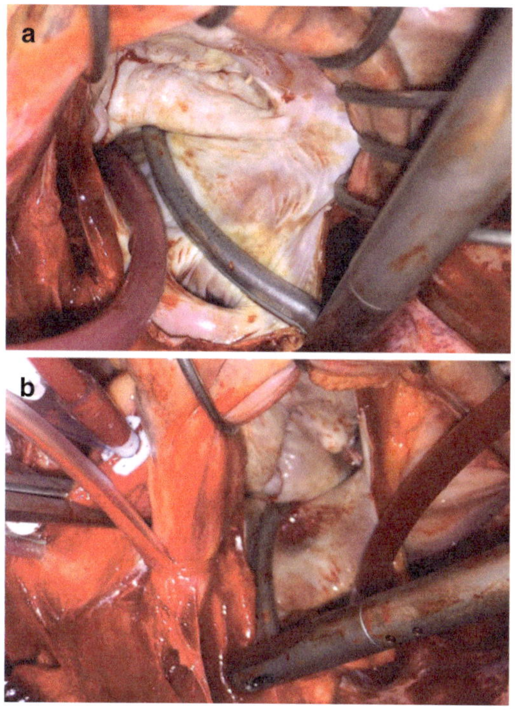

Fig. 5.26 Operative images illustrating completion of left atrial box lesion set, with (**a**) a connecting lesion from the right inferior pulmonary vein to left inferior pulmonary vein across the floor of the left atrium, and (**b**) a connecting lesion from the right superior pulmonary vein to left superior pulmonary vein across the roof of the left atrium

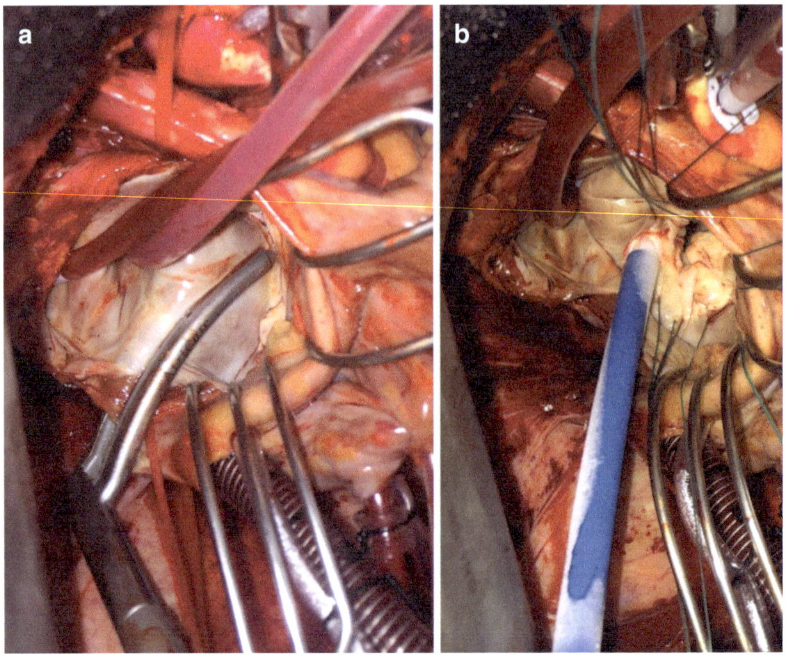

Fig. 5.27 Mitral isthmus line, created by (**a**) a lesion from the left atriotomy to the P2/P3 region of the posterior mitral valve annulus using a bipolar radiofrequency clamp device (Atricure Inc., West Chester, OH) and (**b**) completion of the final 1–2 cm up to the mitral annulus using a cryoprobe (Atricure Inc., West Chester, OH)

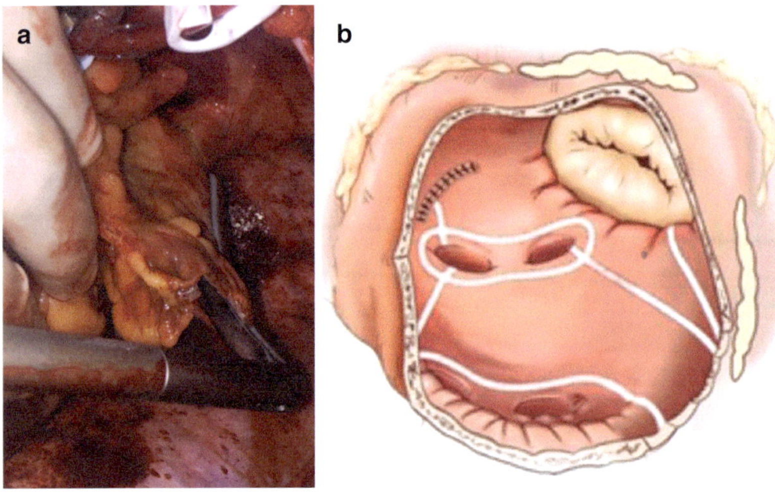

Fig. 5.28 (**a**) Operative image demonstrating the connecting lesion from the left atrial appendage to the lesion encircling the left pulmonary veins. (**b**) Illustration demonstrating the complete Cox-Maze IV left heart lesion set. (Reprinted with permission from Weimar et al. The Cox-maze IV procedure for lone atrial fibrillation: a single center experience in 100 consecutive patients. *J Interv Card Electrophysiol*. 2011;31(1):47–54.)

posteromedial commissure to avoid injury to the circumflex coronary artery.

The heart is then elevated again and the tip of the left atrial appendage excised. The bipolar radiofrequency clamp device is placed into the left atrial appendage stump to create an ablation line to connect with the one encircling the left pulmonary veins (Fig. 5.28a), to complete the left atrial lesion set (Fig. 5.28b)

The left atrial appendage stump is then excised using a stapling device (Fig. 5.29). If the left atrial appendage is excluded but not resected, any

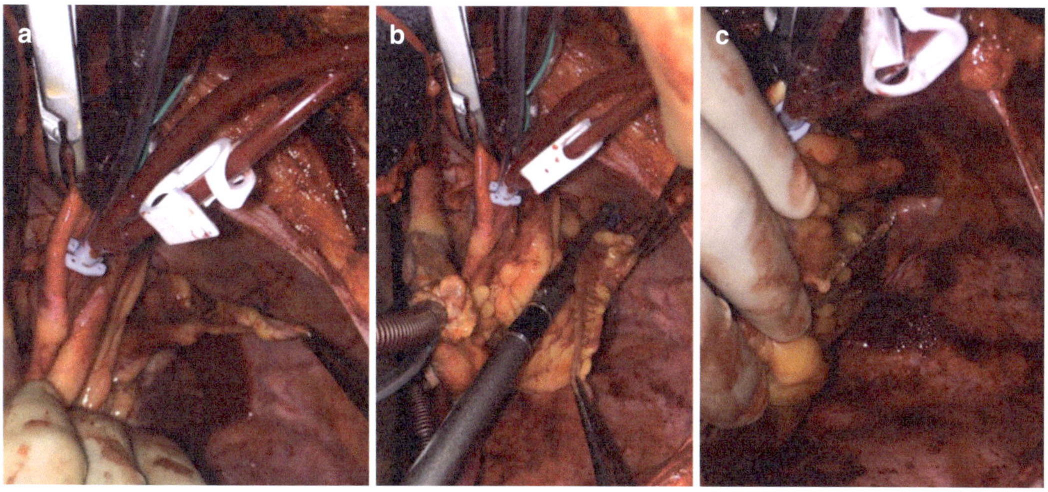

Fig. 5.29 Left atrial appendage excision. (**a**) Stretching of the left atrial appendage to identify the base, (**b**) excision of the left atrial appendage using an Echelon 60 triple-layer stapling device (Ethicon, Sommerville, NJ), and (**c**) assessment of the staple line for haemostasis

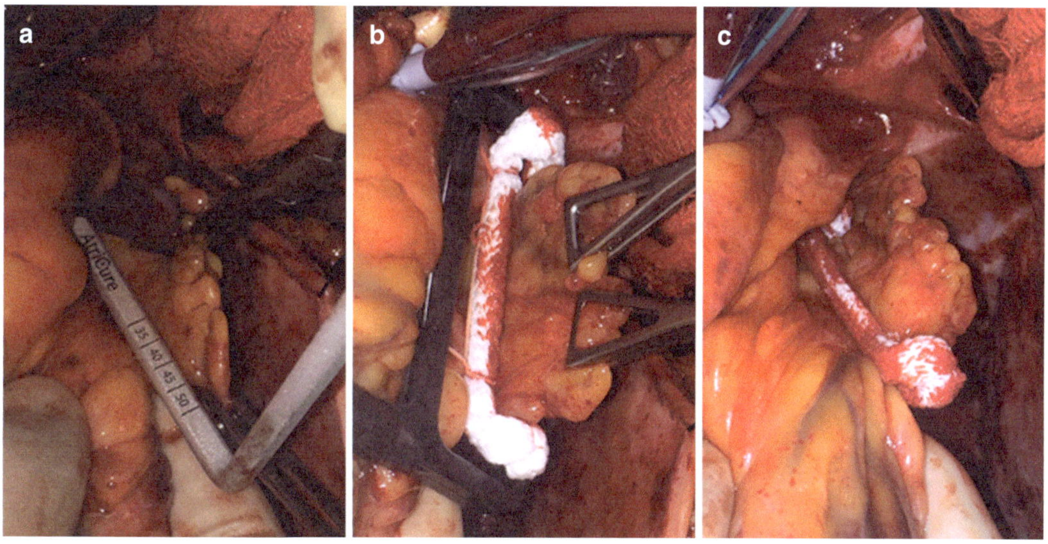

Fig. 5.30 Operative images demonstrating left atrial appendage exclusion, with (**a**) sizing of the left atrial appendage base, (**b**) positioning of the Atriclip device (Atricure Inc., West Chester, OH) at the base of the left atrial appendage, and (**c**) the deployed excluder device

residual flow should be checked using intra-operative trans-oesophageal echocardiography. For patients undergoing excision of the left atrial appendage, it is important to leave a residual stump less than 1 cm in size. The left atriotomy is then closed with a single-layer 3/0 non-absorbable monofilament polypropylene suture.

Alternatively, the left atrial appendage can be excluded using a specifically designed device. The base of the left atrial appendage is measured using a specific sizer (Fig. 5.30a). With the use of forceps or a Duval clamp, the excluder device is then carefully placed over the left atrial appendage (Fig. 5.30b). Once positioned at the base of

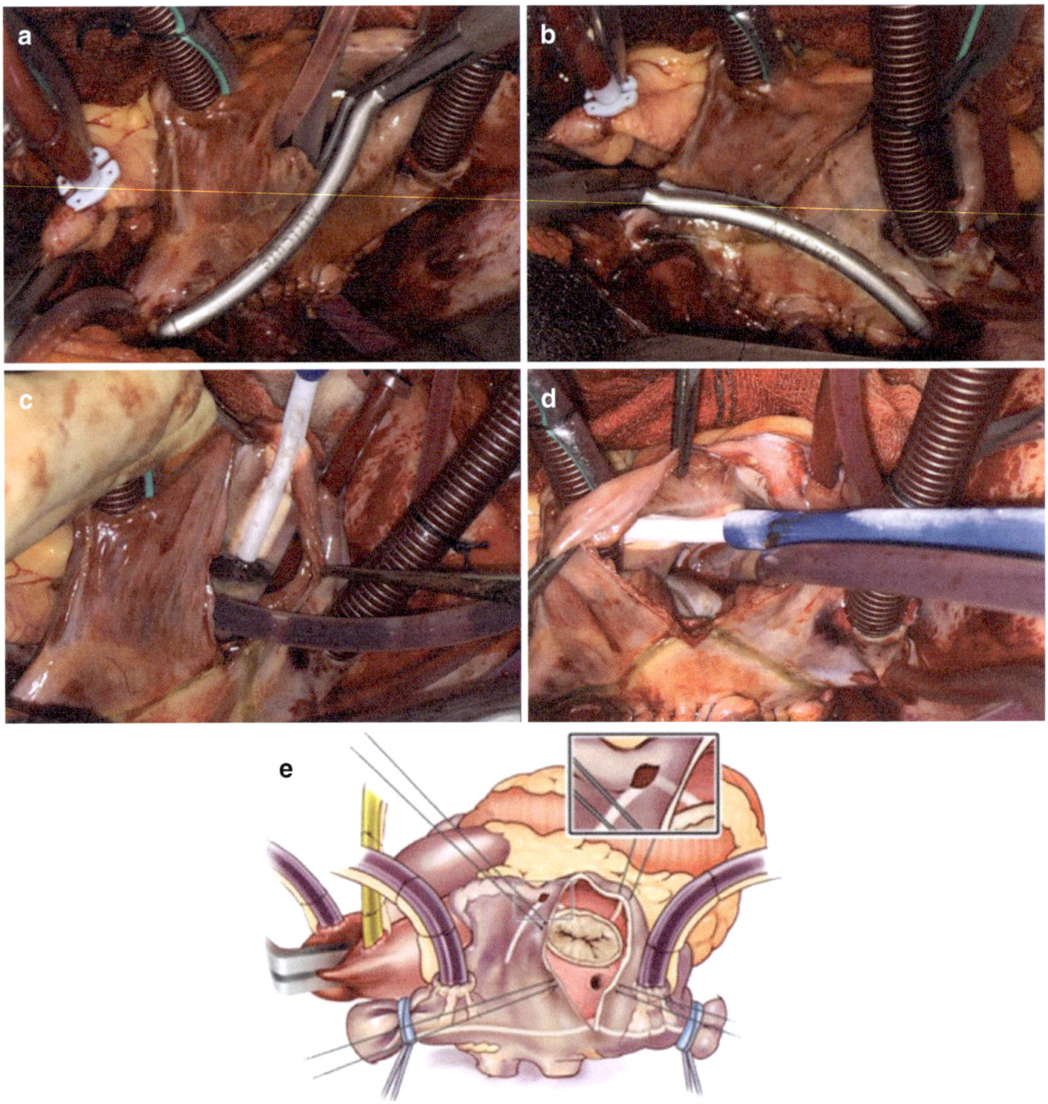

Fig. 5.31 Operative images illustrating the right atrial lesion set, with a (**a**) lesion from the right atriotomy to the superior vena cava using bipolar radiofrequency ablation, (**b**) lesion from the right atriotomy to the inferior vena cava using bipolar radiofrequency ablation, (**c**) lesion from the right atriotomy to the 2 o'clock position on the tricuspid valve annulus using a cryoprobe, and (**d**) lesion from the right atrial appendage to the 10 o'clock position on the tricuspid valve annulus using a cryoprobe. (**e**) Illustration demonstrating the Cox-Maze IV right heart lesion set. (Reprinted with permission from Weimar et al. The Cox-maze IV procedure for lone atrial fibrillation: a single center experience in 100 consecutive patients. *J Interv Card Electrophysiol*. 2011;31(1):47–54.)

the left atrial appendage, the device holder is released by cutting the holding sutures, allowing the device to deploy, thereby excluding the left atrial appendage from the circulation (Fig. 5.30c).

After snaring the cavae with tapes, a vertical right atriotomy is made from the intra-atrial septum up towards the right atrioventricular groove, at a level with the 2 o'clock position of the tricuspid valve. The bipolar radiofrequency clamp device is used to create ablation lines from the lateral aspect of the atriotomy towards the superior (Fig. 5.31a) and inferior venae cavae (Fig. 5.31b) onto caval tissue. The cryoprobe is then used to create a lesion from the medial aspect of the atriotomy towards the 2 o'clock position of the tricuspid valve annulus (Fig. 5.31c). A small incision is then made in the right atrial appendage and the cryoprobe is placed to create a lesion from the appendage towards the 10 o'clock position of the tricuspid valve annulus (Fig. 5.31d), to complete the right atrial lesion set (Fig. 5.31e). The right atriotomy and right atrial appendage incisions are closed with a double-layer 4/0 non-absorbable monofilament polypropylene suture.

6 Annular Dilatation

Keywords
Annular dilatation · Functional mitral regurgitation · Left atrial enlargement · Left ventricular enlargement · Atrial fibrillation · Idiopathic dilated cardiomyopathy · Ischaemic cardiomyopathy · Ring annuloplasty · Leaflet apposition · Failure of coaptation

Case History

A 52 year-old gentleman presented with a progressive history of increasing exertional dyspnoea, associated with intermittent palpitations. He had no prior history of rheumatic fever or infective endocarditis but was being followed up with atrial fibrillation. Medical management included amiodarone therapy and an electrical cardioversion, which had failed to provide sustained freedom from the atrial arrhythmia. Cardiac catheterisation had demonstrated no obstructive coronary artery disease.

Echocardiographical Findings

Trans-thoracic parasternal long-axis echocardiographic images revealed marked mitral annular dilatation, with normal movement of the mitral valve leaflets and no evidence of prolapse or restriction (Fig. 6.1a). This was also observed on the apical 4-chamber view (Fig. 6.1b), where both of the mitral valve leaflets can be seen to reach the annular plane during systole. Doppler flow across the mitral valve demonstrated a central jet of mitral regurgitation (MR), confirming annular dilatation as the dominant lesion and the absence of coaptation as the cause of the regurgitation (Fig. 6.1c).

Images derived from a trans-oesophageal probe allowed segmental analysis of the leaflets and showed no underlying structural disease of the leaflets and sub-valvular apparatus in the mid-oesophageal 4-chamber (Fig. 6.2a), 2-chamber (Fig. 6.2b) and long-axis (Fig. 6.2c) views. The mitral valve annulus was measured at 48 mm.

Quantification of the regurgitation, using the PISA method, revealed severe MR, with an regurgitant volume of 68 mL and regurgitant fraction of 59%, as well as a vena contracta of 0.77 cm. Associated with this, the left atrium was markedly dilated at 6.14 cm but the left ventricular size and function were preserved, with a left ventricular end-systolic diameter 3.7 cm, left ventricular end-diastolic diameter 5.2 cm and ejection fraction 67%. Three-dimensional (3D) echocardiographical images clearly demonstrate mitral annular dilatation with normal movement of the mitral valve leaflets (Fig. 6.3).

N. Moorjani et al., *Operative Mitral and Tricuspid Valve Surgery*,
https://doi.org/10.1007/978-1-4471-4204-1_6

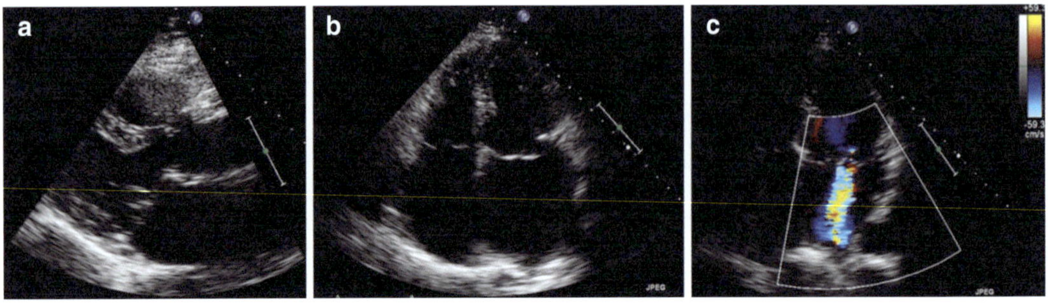

Fig. 6.1 Trans-thoracic echocardiographic images demonstrating left atrial enlargement and mitral annular dilatation with poor coaptation height on (**a**) parasternal long-axis and (**b**) apical 4-chamber views, resulting in (**c**) severe central mitral regurgitation on colour flow Doppler

Pathophysiology

Functional mitral regurgitation (FMR) is defined as valvular insufficiency in the absence of structural mitral valve disease. In this case, the cause was annular dilatation. Traditionally, mitral annular dilatation was only thought to develop following dilatation of the left ventricle as a result of ventricular pathology, which is most commonly secondary to ischaemic or dilated cardiomyopathy. More recently, however, enlargement of the left atrium, secondary to atrial fibrillation, has been described as a cause of annular dilatation and subsequent mitral regurgitation. The increasing mass of blood in the enlarging left atrium exerts considerable force on the atrioventricular junction pulling open the mitral orifice. The majority of dilatation occurs at the more flexible postero-inferior part of the annulus (Fig. 6.4). The fibrous skeleton of the heart limits dilatation of the anterior leaflet annulus.

As well as annular size, impaired contractility of the mitral annulus during the cardiac cycle may also play a role in the pathogenesis of functional mitral regurgitation. In functional mitral regurgitation, the regurgitant jet is observed throughout the line of coaptation, as opposed to a localised jet often seen with degenerative mitral valve disease.

Left Atrial Enlargement

Although mitral regurgitation is well documented as a trigger of atrial fibrillation, secondary to volume overload of the left atrium and subsequent chamber enlargement, atrial fibrillation has recently been implicated as a cause of functional mitral regurgitation. Atrial fibrillation causes a rise in left atrial wall tension and pressure, resulting in atrial remodelling and subsequent chamber enlargement, as a compensatory mechanism to restore normal intra-atrial pressures. There is fibrous infiltration of the atrial muscle, which in turn stretches more easily. For a time, the normal mitral valve can cope with a slowly dilating annulus as a result of the coaptation height of the apposing leaflets. With increasing left atrial volume, the mitral orifice enlarges causing loss of leaflet coaptation, thereby producing functional regurgitation in an otherwise structurally normal mitral valve. In addition, patients with longstanding AF may develop LV impairment, which is also associated with mitral annular dilatation.

Left Ventricular Enlargement

Functional mitral regurgitation more commonly occurs following dilatation of the left ventricle, associated most often with ischaemic heart disease or idiopathic dilated cardiomyopathy. Functional mitral regurgitation is thought to be present in over 50% of patients with a significantly impaired left ventricle and almost ubiquitous with end-stage cardiomyopathy. In these patients, progressive volume overload of the left ventricular results in chamber enlargement and subsequent stretching of the mitral annulus. As progressively more leaflet tissue is required to

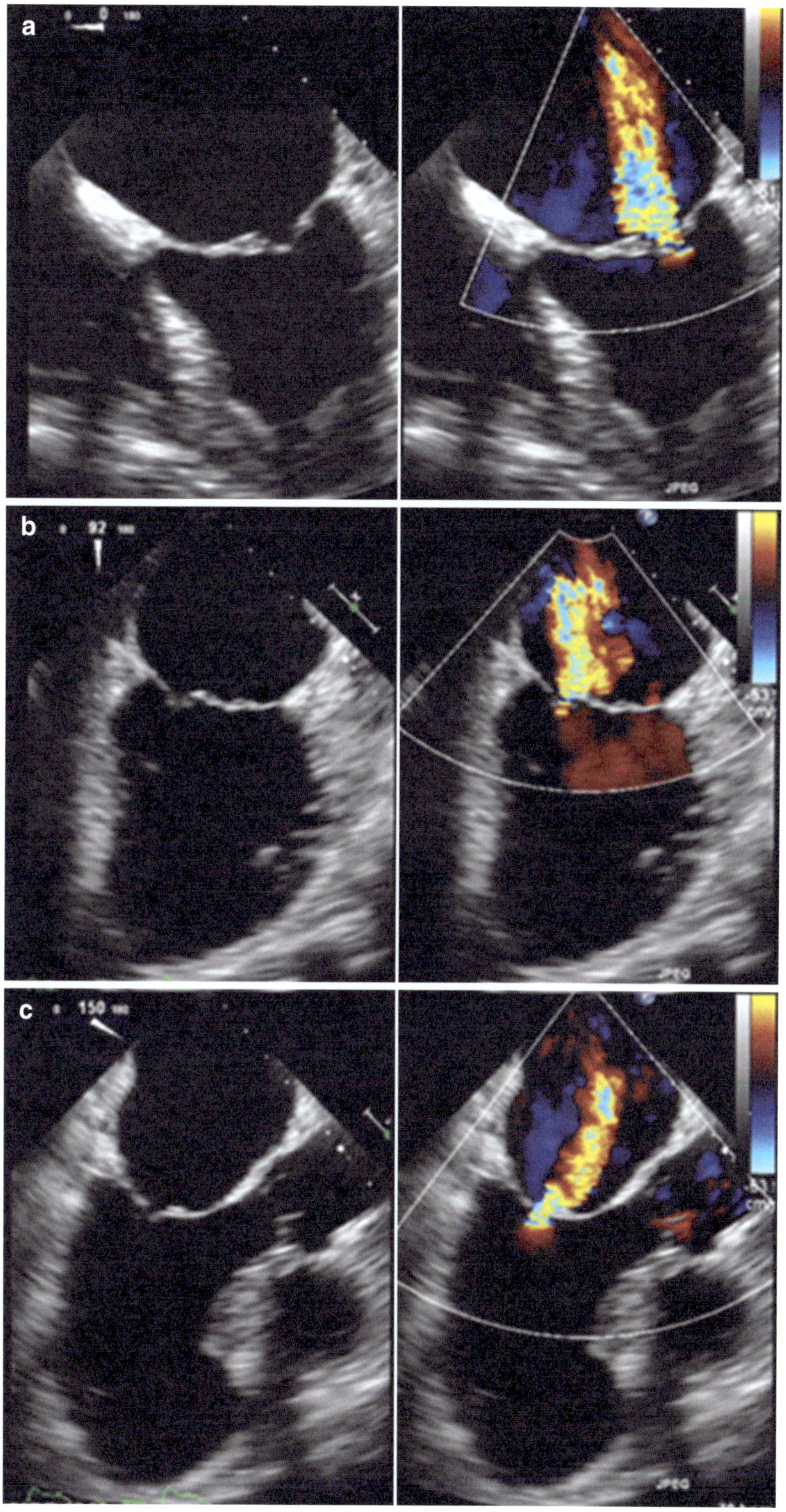

Fig. 6.2 Trans-oesophageal mid-oesophageal echocardiographic images (**a**) 4-chamber, (**b**) 2-chamber and (**c**) long-axis views demonstrating annular dilatation and flattening, resulting in reduced leaflet apposition and severe centrally directed mitral regurgitation on corresponding colour flow Doppler images

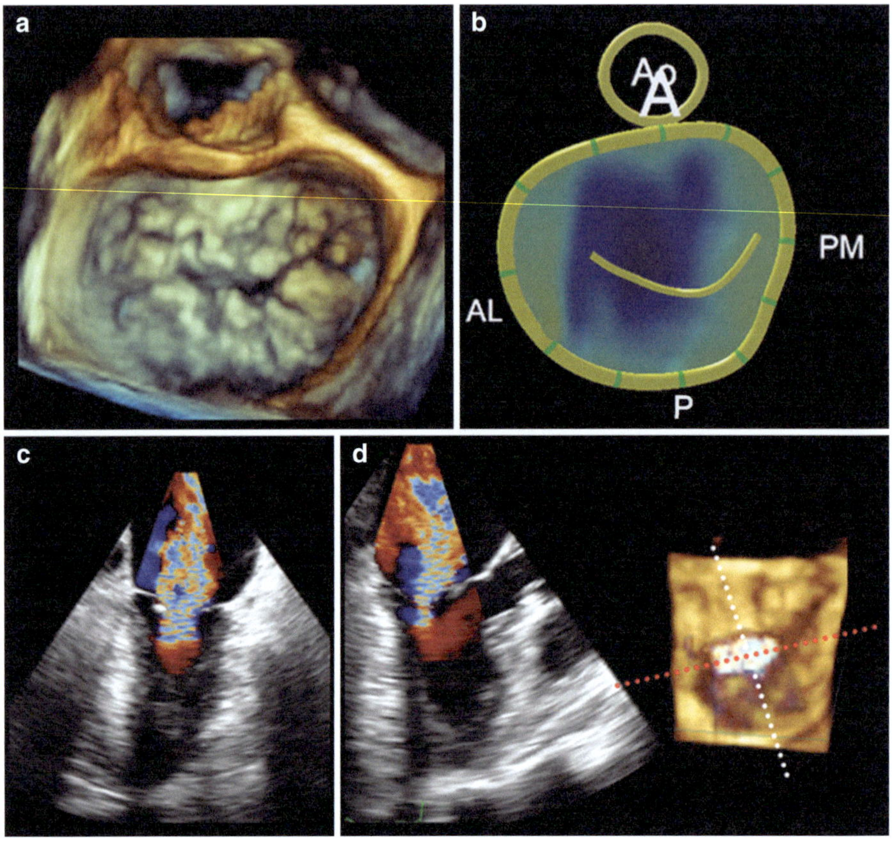

Fig. 6.3 Three-dimensional trans-oesophageal echocardiographical images demonstrating functional mitral regurgitation secondary to annular dilatation. (**a**) 3D surgical view showing minimal leaflet coaptation centrally; (**b**) 3D reconstruction of the mitral valve illustrating annular flattening and decreased leaflet movement (darker blue regions corresponding to leaflet position below the annular plane into the left ventricle); (**c–e**) 3D colour assessment of the elliptical regurgitant orifice seen from the left ventricular side obtained from 2 orthogonal planes, with the red dotted line corresponding to image c along the long-axis of the regurgitant orifice and the white dotted line corresponding to image d along the short-axis of the regurgitant orifice

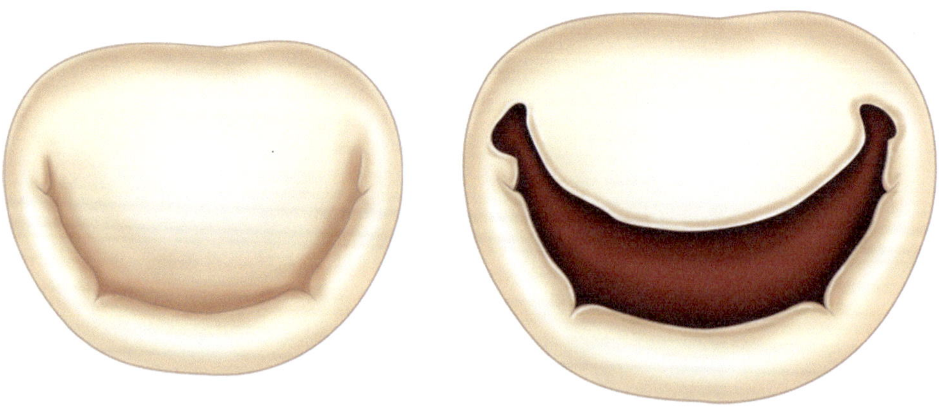

Fig. 6.4 Dilatation of the mitral valve annulus, especially of the posterior annulus

simply cover the orifice area, progressively less is available for the coaptation area. Eventually, there is loss of leaflet apposition and regurgitation ensues. In addition to mitral annular dilatation, the impaired left ventricle becomes more globular in shape moving away from the more complex cone shape of the normal ventricle. The ensuing loss of contractility results in reduced mitral annular fractional change and disturbs normal papillary muscle function that further contributes to functional mitral regurgitation. In patients with dilated cardiomyopathy, apical displacement of the papillary muscles results in tenting of both valve leaflets and subsequent impaired coaptation, which also contributes to the central functional mitral regurgitation. In patients with ischaemic cardiomyopathy, additional lateral displacement of the posteromedial papillary muscle causes asymmetrical tethering and restricted movement of the posterior mitral leaflet, with a resulting eccentric posterior directed jet of regurgitation (see Chap. 11). It has been suggested that functional mitral regurgitation associated with dilated cardiomyopathy is more related to mitral annular dilatation, whereas ischaemic cardiomyopathy related to ventricular enlargement, lateral displacement of the posteromedial papillary muscle and restricted posterior mitral valve leaflet movement.

The reduced forward stroke volume generated by the left ventricle associated with functional mitral regurgitation triggers neurohormonal activation and further LV remodelling in a progressive downward spiral characteristic of congestive heart failure, associated with a poor prognosis. It is important to note that the presence of functional mitral regurgitation leads to overestimation of LV ejection fraction, as it does not take into account the regurgitant volume of systolic flow into the atrium.

Surgical Strategy

In patients with functional mitral regurgitation, it is important to identify the underlying pathophysiological mechanism to plan the surgical intervention. If the aetiology of the regurgitation is related to pure annular dilatation secondary to atrial enlargement, reducing the annular size with implantation of an annuloplasty ring alone can result in excellent long-term results. If the aetiology is ventricular remodelling with apical or lateral displacement of the papillary muscles, such as with ischaemia, then repair techniques, including leaflet augmentation, chordal cutting or papillary muscle relocation (see Chap. 11), or ventricular remodelling, such as aneurysm plication or resection, may be needed. Increasingly, there has been an acceptance that chordal sparing valve insertion is a stable and satisfactory procedure. The now *passé* attitude that mitral valve replacement is bad in functional mitral regurgitation, based upon no meaningful evidence, has passed with the advent of randomised data. The caveat is that all sub-valvar connections should be preserved or reconstructed.

The primary goal of annuloplasty ring implantation is to restore leaflet apposition with a coaptation zone of 8–10 mm. In addition, implantation of an annuloplasty ring prevents further annular dilatation, restores annular geometry (3:4 ratio) and also reduces the tension on the valve leaflets, thereby preserving leaflet mobility (Fig. 6.5).

There are a number of valve prostheses available for implantation. Broadly, they are categorised by consistency (rigid, semi-rigid, flexible), shape (flat, saddle-shaped or with an exaggerated elevation of the posterior leaflet portion) and completeness (complete ring or a 'C' shaped band extending from trigone to trigone and not commissure to commissure). A frequently used example of a semi-rigid, complete ring is the Physio II annuloplasty ring (Edwards Lifesciences, Irvine, CA, USA), which has a rigid anterior part and a more flexible posterior part. Commonly used flexible partial rings are the Cosgrove band (Edwards Lifesciences, Irvine, CA, USA) or the Taylor ring (Abbott, St Paul, MN, USA), which is a complete flexible ring that can be divided to form a 'C-band'.

As the annuloplasty ring will determine the size, and in the case of a rigid or semi-rigid ring, the shape of the annulus following repair, it is important to choose the appropriate prosthesis size. Lengthy debates occur as to the most

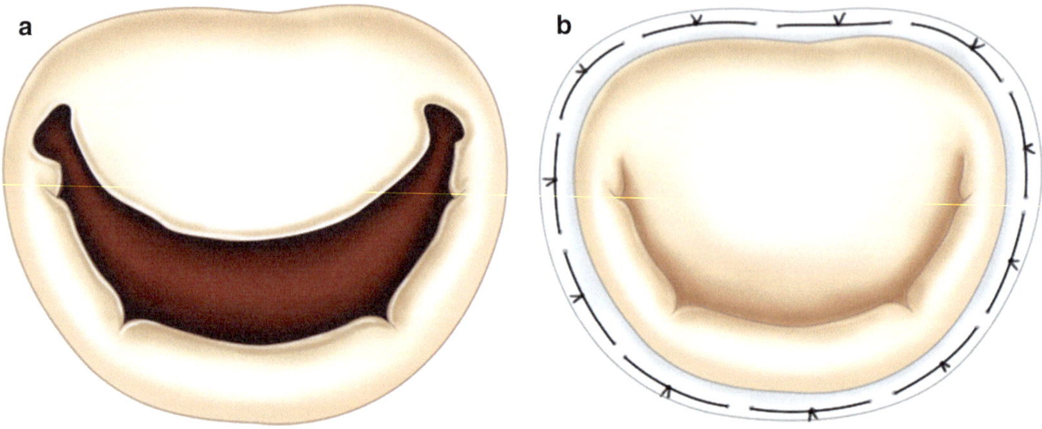

Fig. 6.5 (**a**) Distortion of mitral annular geometry with annular dilatation, especially of the posterior annulus. (**b**) Restoration of normal mitral annular geometry (3:4 ratio) following implantation of an annuloplasty ring

appropriate ring in relation to the aetiology of the mitral regurgitation but in truth this is virtually a 'data free zone'! Any data that does exist is at best level C evidence. Therefore, it is probably fair to state that at the present time there is no consensus on the most appropriate type of annuloplasty ring to use in each and every circumstance. A more detailed analysis of the rationale behind the reasons for the use of annuloplasty rings and the most appropriate choice can be found in Khamooshian et al., Innovations, 2014.

Although rigid rings are able to correct annular dilatation and restore coaptation, the fixed shape of a rigid or semi-rigid ring can affect the normal conformational changes of the mitral annulus that occur during the cardiac cycle. During exercise, these rigid rings are associated with an increase in peak velocity across the valve and hence may be more prone to producing some degree of mitral stenosis. Flexible annuloplasty rings cause less effect on normal MV motion by allowing the annulus to undergo changes in shape (non-planar) and size during the cardiac cycle, with decreased annular circumference and area in systole and increased orifice area in diastole. In addition, ring dehiscence is thought to be less likely due to the reduced tension on the sutures. It is suggested that semi-rigid rings may be able to provide a balance between the restoration of leaflet apposition of the rigid rings and dynamic changes of the annulus during the cardiac cycle allowed by flexible rings, although there is little hard evidence to support this.

If a rigid ring is to be used then, it is suggested that non-planar saddle-shaped rings may be better able to maintain normal annular geometry but whether this translates into improved clinical outcomes has yet to be established. Some non-planar annuloplasty rings, which have been specifically designed for functional mitral regurgitation caused by papillary muscle displacement, have a markedly reduced anteroposterior diameter and more saddle-shape to allow for an improved surface area of coaptation. There is, however, very little evidence to back up the claims.

Incomplete rings are thought to further minimise the interference on the conformational changes of the annulus during the cardiac cycle, as the band is attached to the trigones leaving the anterior annulus unbridled. Incomplete rings are particularly useful in patients where there is a risk of producing systolic anterior motion of the anterior mitral valve leaflet. Incomplete rings, however, may be less effective at reducing the annular dimensions, as even though attached to the fibrous skeleton, the anterior annulus is still capable of dilating. This is especially true for patients with ischaemic mitral regurgitation, where incomplete rings should not generally be used.

Choosing the Appropriate Size Ring

This step is of considerable importance and should not be taken lightly. The first thing to say is that the common usage of the term 'downsizing' ought to be ended and the concept of 'appropriate sizing' should be pre-eminent. There is a belief that the use of a small size ring will compensate for all manner of inadequacies in a repair and that by simply forcing greater coaptation all problems in incompetence may be solved. It is particularly heard in discussions on the correction of ischaemic mitral regurgitation but has been seen practiced in the repair of degenerative mitral regurgitation. Firstly, this will not work to solve inadequacies of leaflet repair if undertaken poorly or incompletely. Secondly, it will often produce mitral stenosis. Thirdly, it runs the real risk of forcing the posterior leaflet towards the septal annulus causing leaflet coaptation to occur too early, which in turn causes the anterior leaflet to retro-flex into the outflow tract, resulting in obstruction of flow through the aortic valve (systolic anterior motion of the anterior mitral valve leaflet, SAM).

The geometry of some hearts makes them very prone to this problem (see Chap. 15) and hence correct sizing of the annuloplasty ring is of vital importance. Again, there is considerable difference of opinion and stated presumed fact. Each of the manufacturers will describe the method that they feel is appropriate for their product. It is important to respect their descriptions but also to think about the validity of the information given, as different manufacturers employ a variety of sizing strategies, which are not always based on scientific evidence.

There are the following options for the sizing of the annuloplasty ring. It can be done using the notch-to-notch distance of the sizer to measure the inter-commissure distance; antero-posterior diameter of the sizer to measure the height of the anterior leaflet of the mitral valve or the anterior and posterior leaflets in end-systole with full coaptation, or by using the surface area of the sizer to measure the area of the anterior mitral leaflet or the area of the entire mitral valve orifice (i.e. the area of the anterior and posterior mitral valve leaflets combined). Sizing for some annuloplasty bands, however, necessitates using the inter-trigonal distance, hence the importance of reading the accompanying manufacturer's instructions with each ring.

Surgical Technique

In this case, the mitral valve was assessed using segmental analysis of the leaflets and the subvalvular apparatus and this information was correlated with the trans-oesophageal echocardiographical findings. Marked annular dilatation was observed with normal leaflets and no evidence of leaflet prolapse or restriction seen on echocardiography. Horizontal mattress annuloplasty sutures (2/0 Ethibond) were placed around the circumference of the mitral valve, with a 5 mm width and approximately 1 mm apart from trigone to trigone (Fig. 6.6a). A 29 mm Tailor flexible annuloplasty band (Abbott, St Paul, MN, USA) was then chosen, according to the surface area of the whole mitral valve orifice (i.e. the surface area of the anterior and posterior mitral valve leaflets together, Fig. 6.6b), having checked that the coaptation height with the line of coaptation delineated with a marker pen was 8–10 mm. The sutures were passed through the annuloplasty band (Fig. 6.6c), and tied in situ.

Competency of the mitral valve was assessed with static testing, by injecting cold saline into the left ventricle, using a bulb syringe. With a left ventricle distended (to the point that the aortic root became tense) with saline, the depth of coaptation was assessed by marking the atrial surface of the mitral valve leaflets with a sterile marking pen, which measured 9 mm. There was no evidence of leaflet restriction or prolapse (Fig. 6.6d).

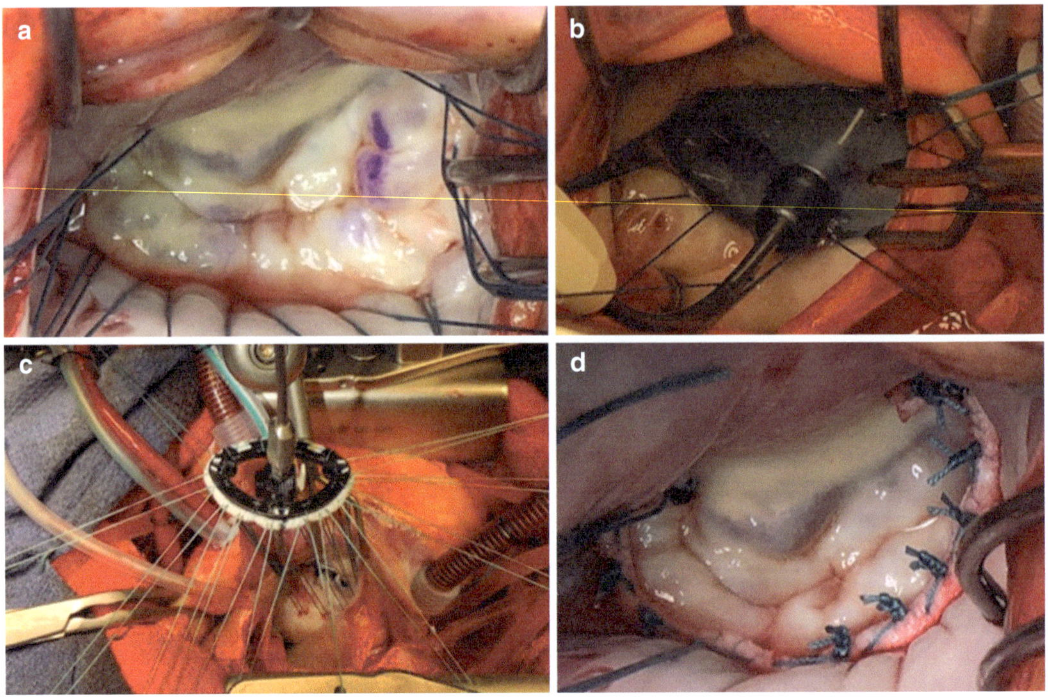

Fig. 6.6 Operative images demonstrating (**a**) isolated annular dilatation, with no evidence or leaflet prolapse or restriction, (**b**) sizing of the mitral valve annulus by measuring the surface area of the anterior and posterior mitral valve leaflets together, (**c**) passing the sutures through the 29 mm Tailor flexible annuloplasty band (Abbott, St Paul, MN, USA), and (**d**) competent mitral valve with static testing

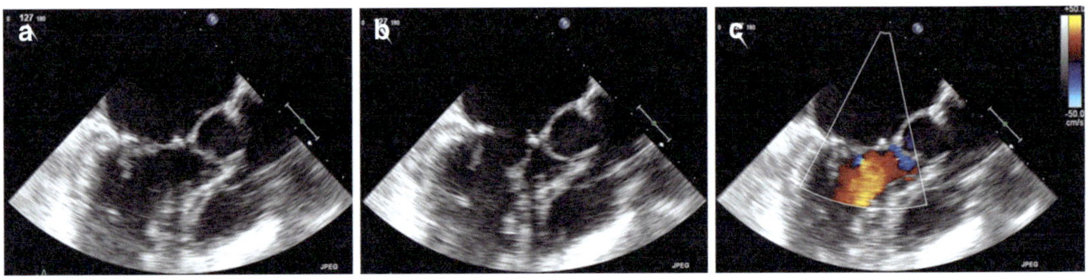

Fig. 6.7 Post-bypass intra-operative trans-oesophageal long-axis echocardiographical images demonstrating no SAM and a 9 mm depth of coaptation between the anterior and posterior leaflets in (**a**) systole and (**b**) diastole, and a competent mitral valve with no residual mitral regurgitation on (**c**) colour flow Doppler

Post-operative Echocardiogram

The post-repair trans-oesophageal echocardiogram (Fig. 6.7) confirmed:

1. Normal physiological functioning of the mitral valve complex with no residual mitral regurgitation.
2. The diameter of the mitral valve annulus reduced to 30 mm.
3. No evidence of mitral stenosis or systolic anterior movement of the mitral valve leaflets (SAM) into the left ventricular outflow tract, causing left ventricular outflow obstruction (LVOTO).
4. The depth of leaflet coaptation was 9 mm.

Surgical Tips

1. Identify the underlying pathophysiological mechanism to determine whether annuloplasty ring or band implantation alone will be sufficient
2. Appropriate choice of annuloplasty ring prosthesis according to underlying cause of the functional mitral regurgitation
3. Accurate sizing of the entire area of the mitral valve orifice
4. Obtaining an adequate depth of coaptation (>8 mm) is important for the long-term durability of the procedure.

Comment

Results of mitral valve surgery following annuloplasty ring implantation for functional mitral regurgitation are very dependent on the underlying aetiology. For patients with isolated mitral annular dilatation secondary to atrial fibrillation induced left atrial enlargement, annuloplasty ring implantation is associated with excellent outcomes, with an in-hospital mortality <1% and a low peri-operative complication rate. This is associated with excellent freedom from recurrent mitral regurgitation (100% with no or 1+ MR at 18 months), freedom from reoperation (100% at 18 months) and survival (100% at 18 months).

For patients with functional mitral regurgitation secondary to idiopathic dilated cardiomyopathy, short and long-term outcomes are significantly less favourable, as they are completely dependent on the underlying left ventricular function. For patients with an ejection fraction <30% at surgery, although symptoms status is improved in most patients, there is up to 30% mortality in the first year following surgery, with a recurrence rate of MR of up to 50% by 3 years and a mortality of upwards of 50% by 5 years (see Chap. 11).

Recommended Reading

Bothe W, Miller DC, Doenst T. Sizing for mitral annuloplasty: where does science stop and voodoo begin? Ann Thorac Surg. 2013;95(4):1475–83.

Khamooshian A, Buijsrogge MP, de Heer F, Gründeman PF. Mitral valve annuloplasty rings: review of literature and comparison of functional outcome and ventricular dimensions. Innovations (Phila). 2014;9(6):399–415.

Komeda M, Kitamura H, Fukaya S, Okawa Y. Surgical treatment for functional mitral regurgitation. Circ J. 2009;73(Suppl A):A23–8.

Manabe S, Kasegawa H, Fukui T, Tabata M, Shinozaki T, Shimokawa T, Takanashi S. Do semi-rigid prosthetic rings affect left ventricular function after mitral valve repair? Circ J. 2013;77(8):2038–42.

Ring L, Dutka DP, Wells FC, Fynn SP, Shapiro LM, Rana BS. Mechanisms of atrial mitral regurgitation: insights using 3D transoesophageal echo. Eur Heart J Cardiovasc Imaging. 2014;15:500–8.

Tanimoto M, Pai RG. Effect of isolated left atrial enlargement on mitral annular size and valve competence. Am J Cardiol. 1996;77:769–74.

Vohra HA, Whistance RN, Magan A, Sadeque SA, Livesey SA. Mitral valve repair for severe mitral regurgitation secondary to lone atrial fibrillation. Eur J Cardiothorac Surg. 2012;42:634–7.

Posterior Mitral Valve Leaflet Prolapse

7

Keywords
Posterior mitral valve leaflet prolapse · Myxomatous degeneration · Fibroelastic deficiency · Barlow's disease · Gore-Tex neo-chordae · Triangular resection · Quadrangular resection · Sliding plasty · Ring annuloplasty · Mitral regurgitation

Case History

A 78 year-old male patient presented with a short history of malaise and increasing dyspnoea on exertion. He had no history of rheumatic fever or infective endocarditis. He was being followed up with serial echocardiography after the recent discovery of a systolic murmur.

Echocardiographical Findings

A trans-thoracic apical 3-chamber echocardiographic image revealed prolapse of the posterior mitral valve leaflet (Fig. 7.1a). This was also observed on the apical 4-chamber view (Fig. 7.1b), where the posterior leaflet can be seen to override the annular plane during systole. Colour flow Doppler across the mitral valve demonstrated an anterior directed jet of mitral regurgitation (MR), confirming posterior leaflet prolapse as the dominant lesion (Fig. 7.1c).

Images derived from a trans-oesophageal probe allowed segmental analysis of posterior leaflet dysfunction and showed isolated prolapse of a tall P2 segment, in the mid-oesophageal 2-chamber (Fig. 7.2a), 4-chamber (Fig. 7.2b), long-axis (Fig. 7.2c, d) and trans-gastric short-axis (Fig. 7.2e) views, with associated anterior-directed mitral regurgitation on the corresponding colour flow Doppler images. Quantification of the regurgitation, using the PISA method revealed severe MR with an effective regurgitant orifice area of 51 mm^2, regurgitant volume of 65 mL and regurgitant fraction of 56%. The left atrium was dilated at 5.17 cm but the left ventricular size was preserved. The left ventricular end-systolic diameter (LVIDs) was 3.7 cm and left ventricular end-diastolic diameter (LVIDd) 5.2 cm, with an ejection fraction of 67%. Three-dimensional (3D) echocardiographical images clearly demonstrate the prolapsing P2 segment of the posterior leaflet with associated chordal rupture (Fig. 7.2f).

Pathophysiology

Mitral valve prolapse is characterised by excessive motion of the leaflet in systole beyond the plane of the annulus (atrioventricular junction), leading to mitral regurgitation. This is associated with excess leaflet tissue, often but not exclusively in both leaflets. Extensive posterior leaflet prolapse will lead to an unsupported anterior

N. Moorjani et al., *Operative Mitral and Tricuspid Valve Surgery*,
https://doi.org/10.1007/978-1-4471-4204-1_7

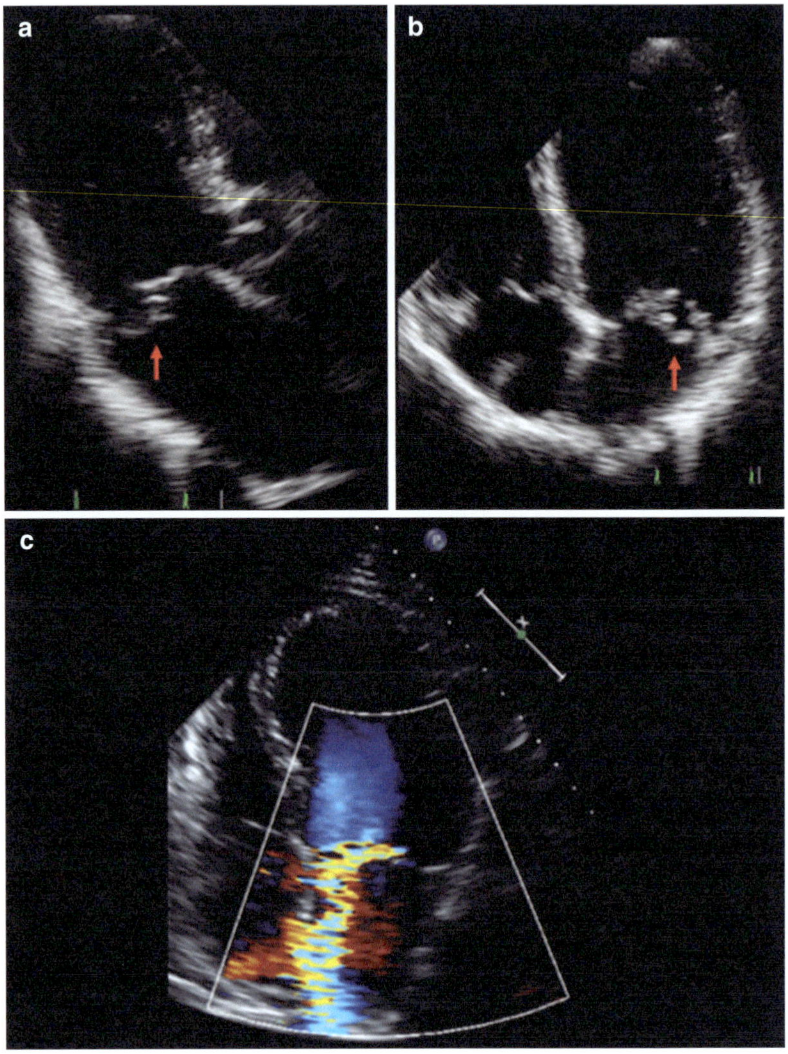

Fig. 7.1 Trans-thoracic echocardiographical images demonstrating prolapse of the P2 segment of the posterior mitral valve leaflet, secondary to ruptured chordae tendineae on (**a**) apical 3-chamber and 4-chamber views, resulting in (**c**) an anterior directed eccentric jet of severe mitral regurgitation, on colour flow Doppler

leaflet, which may function normally once the posterior leaflet pathology has been resolved. The leaflets are malformed in height and often with deep indentations that reach the annulus. They have never developed appropriately, as witnessed by chords arising from the edge of the leaflets in the depths of the indentations right up to the annulus. Histologically, the mitral leaflets are characterized by myxomatous degeneration, which consists of disrupted connective tissue and deposits of mucoid material between the collagen fragments. It is likely that these histological changes occur over time as the malformed valve is subject to abnormal stresses that cannot be properly distributed across the leaflet surfaces. Indeed, these histological changes are likely to be a result of prolonged trauma to the valve leaflets.

Chordal rupture is not always present in patients with degenerative mitral valve disease. If present, it may be secondary to mechanical weakening of the chordae because of the abnormal hemodynamic stresses arising from the redundancy of the valve leaflets and the deep indentations not allowing the normal sharing of the considerable systolic forces on the leaflets.

It has been suggested that histologically, degenerative mitral valve disease represents a spectrum of disease between two distinct phenotypes (Fig. 7.3), fibroelastic deficiency and that of Barlow's disease (diffuse myxomatous

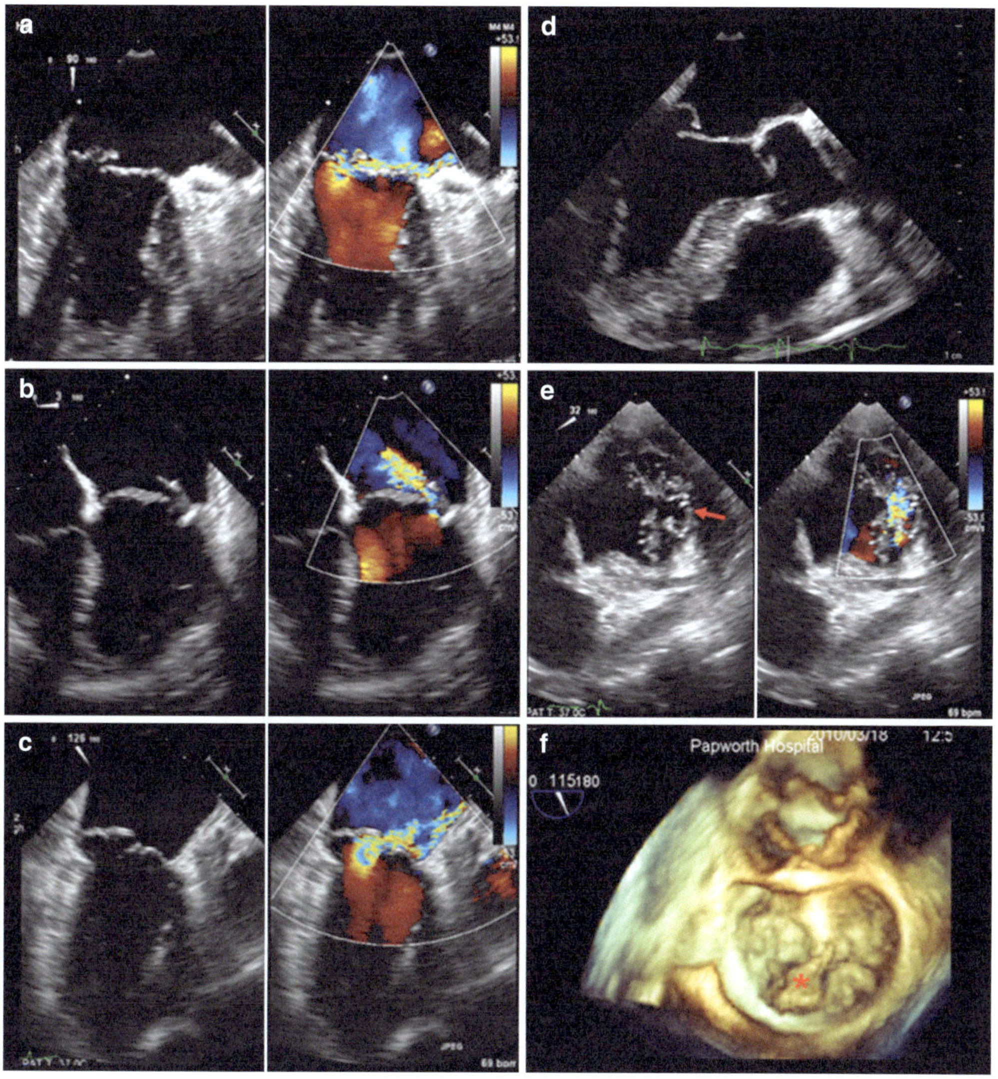

Fig. 7.2 Trans-oesophageal echocardiographical images demonstrating prolapse of the P2 segment of the posterior mitral valve leaflet, secondary to ruptured chordae tendineae on (**a**) 2-chamber, (**b**) 4-chamber, (**c**, **d**) long-axis and (**e**) trans-gastric views, resulting in an anterior directed eccentric jet of severe mitral regurgitation, on corresponding colour flow Doppler images, and (**f**) 3D surgical view with a P2 flail segment (red star) visible with two ruptured chords

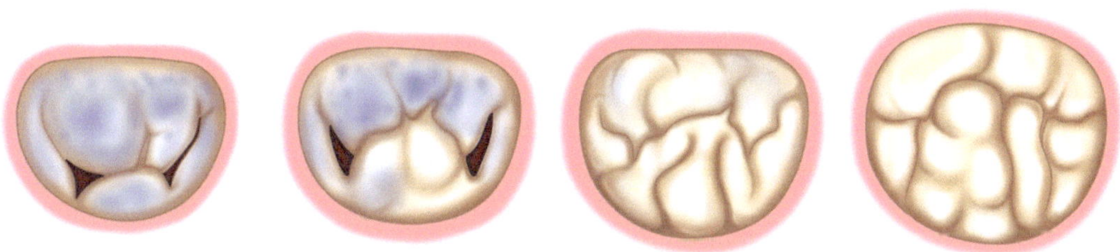

Fig. 7.3 Spectrum of degenerative mitral valve disease, with isolated fibroelastic disease (FED) through to Barlow's valve, with progressively increasing presence of secondary myxomatous changes affecting more than one leaflet and associated with an increased orifice size

degeneration). Fibroelastic deficiency is characterized by decreased connective tissue, deficient in collagen, elastin and proteoglycans, resulting in thin, smooth, translucent leaflets without excess tissue, thin, slightly elongated chordae and only moderate annular dilatation. It is interesting to note, however, that the portions of the valve leaflets that are affected contain the same myxomatous degenerative changes as in Barlow's disease. The characteristically slightly blueish tissue of this subset of valves are the parts that do not prolapse or suffer damage, namely the anterior leaflet. This suggests that there is a problem with this explanation. Indeed, characteristically in this group, there are deep indentations on either side of the prolapsed segment suggesting that this portion has been isolated from the rest of the valve and has had to bear the same force per square centimetre as the rest of the valve which has been able to distribute the forces acting upon it more satisfactorily. Abnormal load bearing on a deep clefted, poorly supported segment of the posterior leaflet over a period of time often results in the described secondary histological changes. It is characterised histologically by an increase in myxoid deposition, endothelial thickening and disruption of the collagen fibres, thereby producing a thickened and domed segment of the posterior leaflet. The non-prolapsing segments, however, do not exhibit these changes and are characterised by thin and translucent leaflet tissue.

If there is only one cleft, it is usually on the superior side of the prolapse (to the left as the surgeon sees it). If this is the case, then almost always there is abnormality of the posteromedial papillary muscle head, giving rise to the chords in this region. This all points to a congenital cause for these lesions.

Patients with chordal rupture and flail leaflet usually present at an older age after a shorter (if any) clinical history, suggesting prolonged trauma at the site giving rise to the lesion. Patients with Barlow's disease are usually significantly younger often with a long history of a murmur or known mitral regurgitation. Again this points towards a more diffuse congenital malformation of the valve. Although there are patients with extremes of bileaflet disease (Barlow's disease) and isolated posterior leaflet prolapse, patients may present with morbid anatomy anywhere along the spectrum between these two extremes, again supporting the notion that these are all variants of congenital malformation of a most complex structure.

In patients with mitral regurgitation, the most common lesion encountered is isolated prolapsed of the P2 segment of the posterior mitral valve leaflet, which accounts for about 60% of cases. In these patients, it is important to identify the underlying features that have resulted in a prolapsed segment of the leaflet, in order to achieve a physiological repair. If the mitral regurgitation is left uncorrected, subsequent ventricular and annular dilatation will ensue, secondary to volume overload of the left ventricle.

Surgical Strategy

The surgical manoeuvres available for the management of posterior leaflet prolapse can be divided into those at the level of the leaflet, including plication (McGoon technique) and resection (triangular resection, quadrangular resection, sliding plasty or wedge resection), or those at the level of the chordae tendineae, including chordal insertion/replacement (Gore-Tex© neo-chordae), chordal transfer and papillary muscle repositioning. The surgeon dealing with these lesions needs to be familiar with the whole armamentarium of techniques, as not all valves are amenable to just one technique and the surgical strategy will need to be tailored to suit each individual patient.

Chordal Insertion/Replacement (Fig. 7.4)

This manoeuvre involves the insertion of synthetic chords, with Gore-Tex© polytetrafluoroethylene (PTFE) sutures (W.L. Gore & Associates, Flagstaff, AZ, USA) most com-

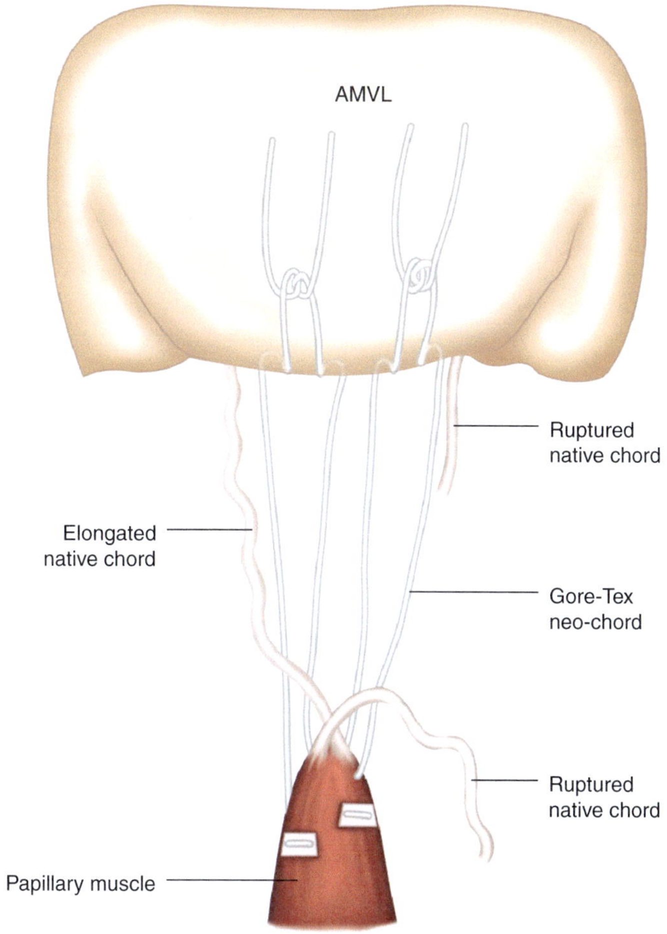

Fig. 7.4 Gore-Tex neo-chordae insertion to reduce prolapse caused by native chordal elongation or rupture. AMVL anterior mitral valve leaflet

monly used. The major advantage of this technique is that it does not require the excision of valve tissue. This preserves leaflet tissue and restores leaflet anatomy. Thus, the mobility and normal surface area of the posterior leaflet is restored, along with the maximal orifice area of the mitral valve compatible with valve competence. With time, these 'neo-chordae' may become covered with normal fibrosa and intima, and blood borne fibroblasts can insinuate themselves into the natural pores in this complex material. Chordal replacement is performed by passing both limbs of a CV-4 or 5 Gore-Tex neo-chordae through the fibrous part of the papillary muscle head that was providing chordal support to prolapsing segment of the posterior leaflet. Pledgets can be used on these sutures but should the neo-chordae need to be re-sited, these pledgets must be retrieved so as not to risk cerebral embolization if they escape into the ventricle. For this reason, many surgeons forgo their use. Both limbs of the neo-chordae are then passed through the prolapsing segment 5 mm from the free edge (Fig. 7.4). Although implanting Gore-Tex neo-chordae is relative simple and reproducible, determining the length of the sutures can be challenging, as sutures that are too short result in restricted leaflet movement, whereas sutures that are too long result in residual leaflet prolapse, both of which are associated with persistent MR. Various techniques have been described to determine the height of the Gore-Tex neo-chordae, including using:

(a) Functional assessment using saline inflation of the left ventricle to adjust the height of the neo-chord
(b) A caliper to measure the distance from the insertion point on the papillary muscles to the free edge of the prolapsing segment at annular level (the 'loop' technique).
(c) A fixed point as a reference to guide to the correct length and tension of the implanted neo-chord
   (i) Posterior annulus for patients with a normal length posterior leaflet
   (ii) Non-prolapsing parts of the posterior leaflet (P1 or P3) if the prolapsing segment is elongated. As P1 is closer to the fibrous skeleton than P3, it used as a reference point, as it less likely to prolapse
   (iii) Hinge point of the posterior mitral valve leaflet at the coaptation line

The authors' preference is to assess the height of the non-prolapsing portions of the leaflet and to match this for the prolapsed portion. This is then checked by distending the ventricle with saline and marking the coaptation line with a methylene blue marker.

Triangular Resection (Fig. 7.5)

Triangular resection represents a more limited approach to dealing with a prolapsing segment of the posterior leaflet. As opposed to quadrangular resection, triangular resection is better able to preserve mitral valve geometry and physiology, as well as maintain a larger valve orifice area and surface area of coaptation. The first step when performing a triangular resection is to place 5/0 Prolene stay sutures around the normal chordae tendineae attached on either side of the prolapsed area. Gentle traction on these stay sutures allows the margins of resection of the prolapsing scallop to be clearly delineated. This allows an assessment of the amount of residual tissue that will be left following resection. The extent of the triangular resection depends on the degree of prolapse, and amount and quality of the residual tissue, to ensure adequate tissue is left to reconstitute the posterior leaflet without tension. The resection is performed with the base of the triangle at the free margin of the prolapsed segment and the apex of the triangle pointing towards the annular aspect of the posterior leaflet. The apex of the triangle should not reach the annulus. Additional wedge resections of the basal part of the prolapsing segment may also be required for patients with an asymmetrical or tall prolapsing scallop, so as to produce a symmetrical posterior mitral valve leaflet, with a height of less than 1.5 cm. Approximately 5 mm of prolapsed tissue is left on either side of the resection margin to facilitate a tension-free reconstruction of the posterior leaflet.

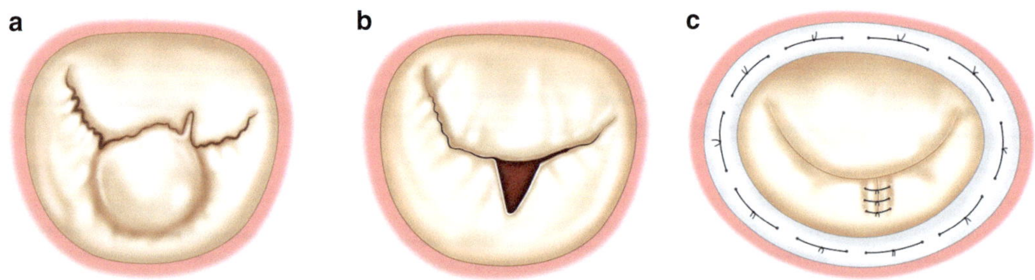

Fig. 7.5 (**a**) Posterior mitral valve leaflet prolapse, (**b**) treated with triangular resection of the prolapsing segment and (**c**) supported by implantation of an annuloplasty ring

Leaflet Plication (Fig. 7.6)

Leaflet plication (McGoon technique) was one of the first procedures described to treat a small area of prolapse on the posterior leaflet. It involves using a series of interrupted 5/0 Prolene sutures to invert the redundant prolapsing segment, producing a similar result to a limited triangular resection but without excising leaflet tissue. For patients with excess tissue associated with myxomatous degeneration, leaflet plication probably should not be used because of the bulk of tissue and triangular resection may be a better option in this situation.

Quadrangular Resection (Figs. 7.7 and 7.8)

Quadrangular resection of the prolapsing P2 scallop of the posterior leaflet combined with posterior annular plication is the classical approach described by Professor Alain Carpentier. It involves defining the margins of the prolapsing segment by passing a 5/0 Prolene suture around the adjacent normal chordae attached to non-prolapsing segments of the posterior leaflet. The prolapsing segment can then be excised as a quadrangle defined by imaginary lines drawn from the centre of the anterior annulus to the posterior annulus (Fig. 7.7). This results in the segment to be resected having a shorter distance on the coaptation edge than at the annular margin, which reduces tension on the leading edge of the leaflet when the edges of the resection are sewn together.

The width of the residual gap between the resection margins will determine the need for either horizontal compression annuloplasty sutures or a 'sliding plasty'. Horizontal mattress 2/0 Ethibond annular compression plication sutures can be used to eliminate the defect in the

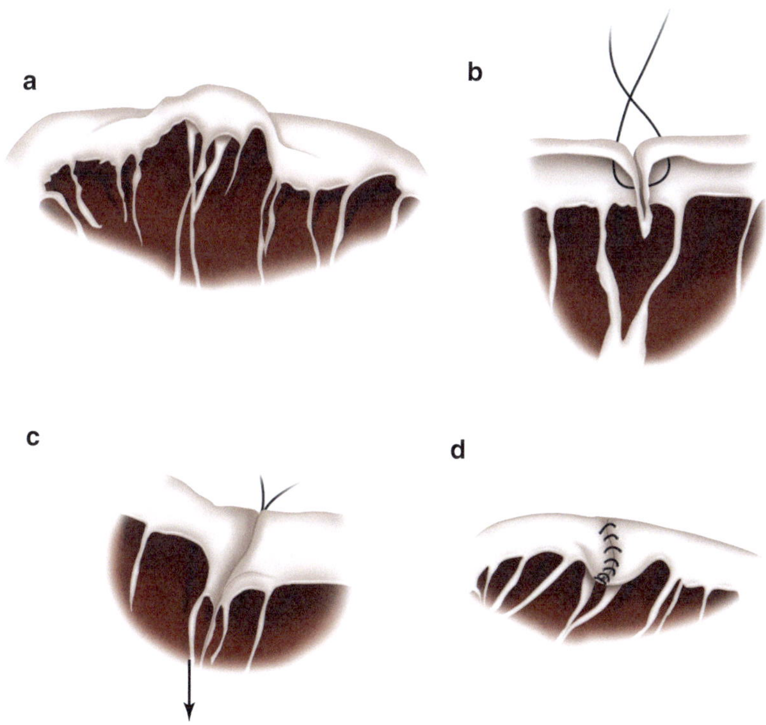

Fig. 7.6 (**a**) Prolapsed scallop of the posterior mitral valve leaflet treated with leaflet plication (McGoon technique), where (**b**) the excess tissue is inverted and (**c**) sutured in place. This results in (**d**) a non-prolapsing P2 scallop, equal in height to the adjacent posterior leaflet scallops

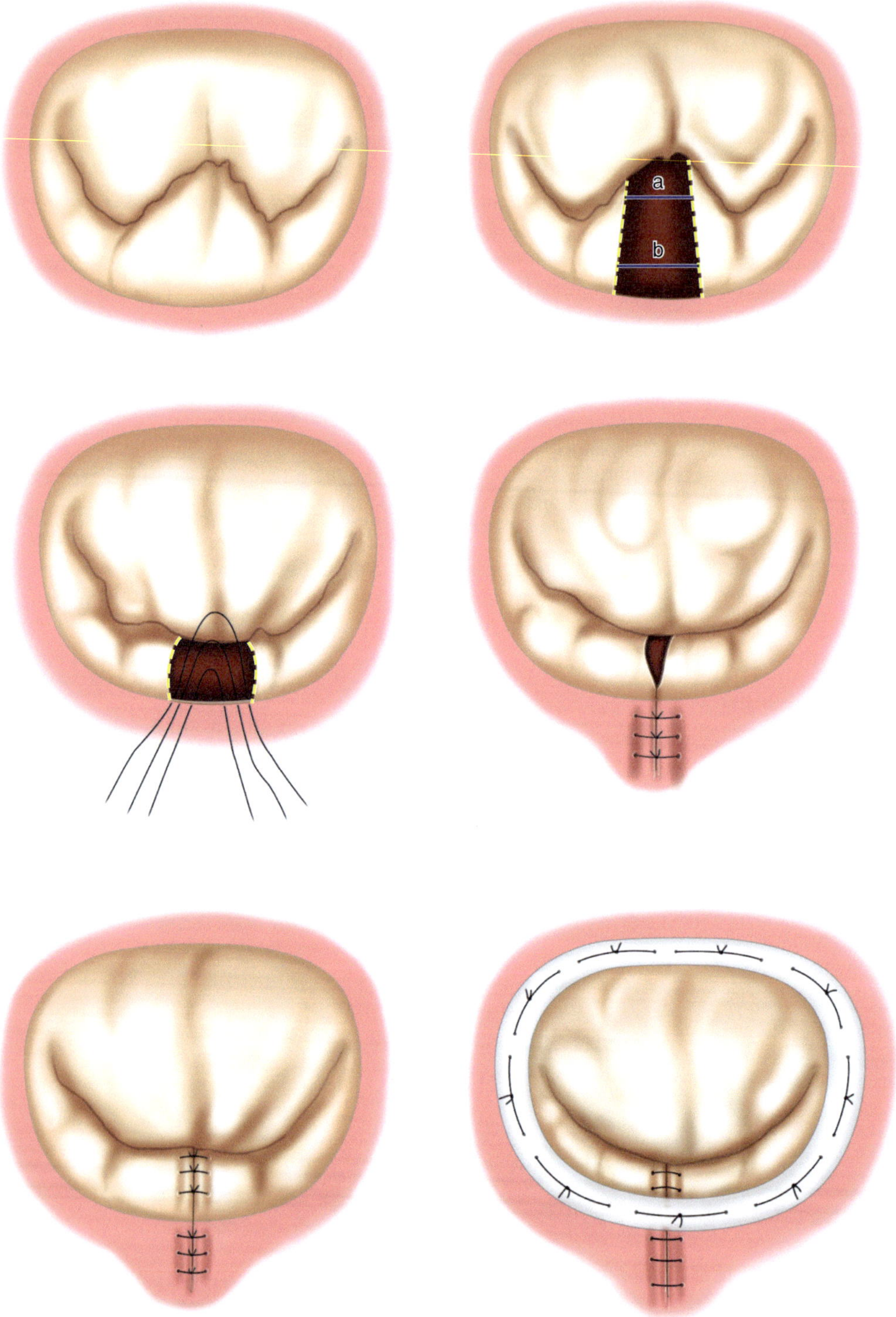

Fig. 7.7 Posterior mitral valve leaflet prolapse treated with quadrangular resection of the prolapsing segment, horizontal compression sutures and supported by implantation of an annuloplasty ring. Note the width of the quadrangular resection is wider at the base (b) of the leaflet than at the free margin (a)

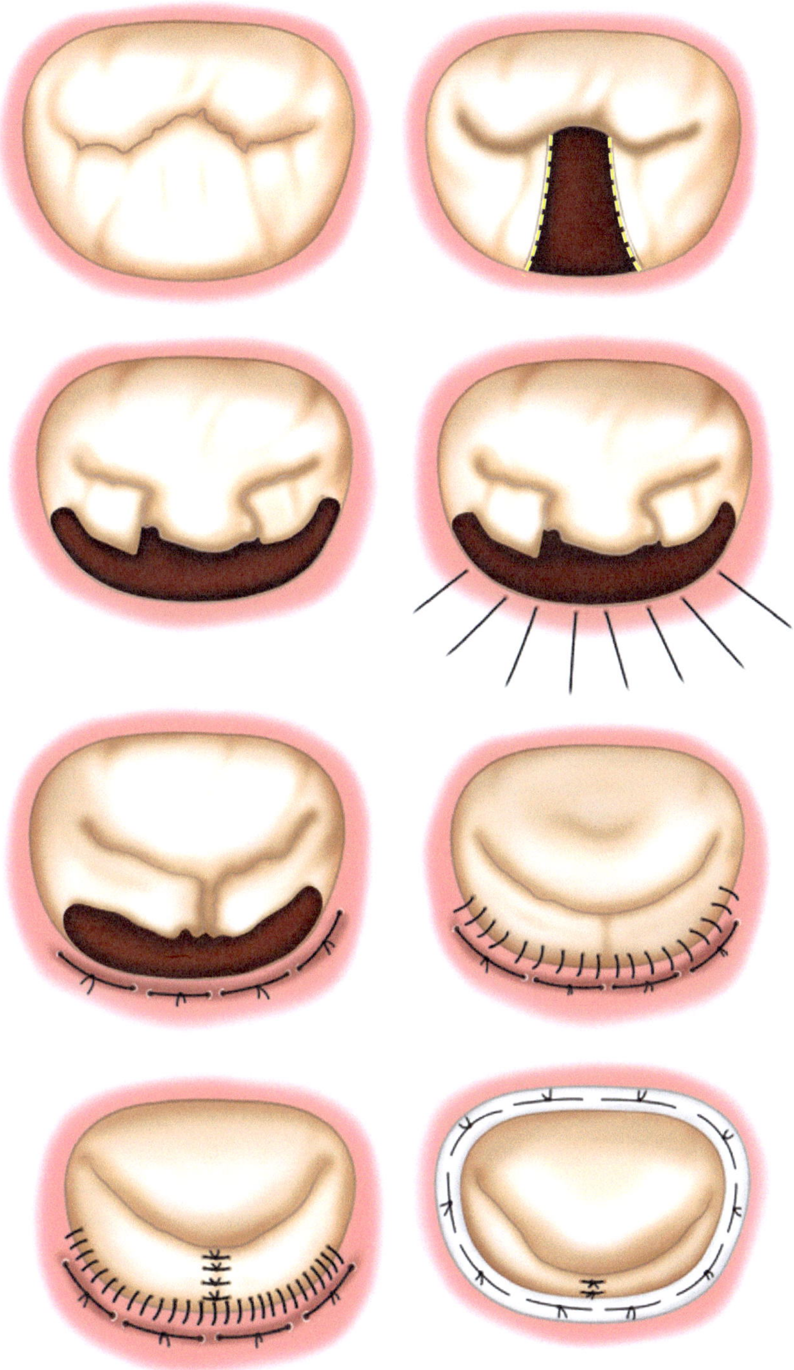

Fig. 7.8 Posterior mitral valve leaflet prolapse treated with quadrangular resection of the prolapsing segment, sliding plasty and supported by implantation of an annuloplasty ring

posterior annulus. These are performed to bring the edges of the residual scallops together to obtain a tension-free union of the posterior leaflet. It is important to note that excessive plication in this way carries the risk of kinking the circumflex coronary artery.

If the excised portion is more than 1.5 cm in width, a sliding plasty is a better solution to restore leaflet approximation (Fig. 7.8). To achieve this, the residual scallops are detached from the posterior annulus for approximately 2 cm in each direction. Horizontal 2/0 Ethibond sutures are then placed along the resection margin. Tying these sutures will then reduce the circumference of the posterior annulus and hence reduce the tension on the residual posterior leaflets.

The leaflet edges are then anastomosed together with 4/0 Prolene sutures with the annular margin suture also being passed through the neo-annulus at the geometrically correct point. These sutures can then be run along the neo-posterior annulus margin, reattaching the leaflets to the neo-annulus. A second suture is begun at the lateral margins and run to the initial suture and then tied together. The posterior leaflet edges can then be sutured to each other using a continuous locking 5/0 Prolene suture, starting from the free edge towards the annulus, or using inverting interrupted sutures. Interrupted sutures are better where there is a smaller leaflet height reducing the tendency to compression than a continuous suture can bring. This is minimised with a locking suture technique. The outcome of this procedure, however, is a frozen posterior leaflet and if excessive can impair normal anterior leaflet function. Indeed, mitral stenosis is not infrequent following this technique.

Although the advent of neo-chordal reconstruction has largely supplanted these types of resection, there will be circumstances where elements of them will be useful, including cases with destruction of leaflet tissue by endocarditis. The main advantages of neo-chordal insertion or a triangular resection are that they respect native mitral valve geometry maintaining normal valve physiology. They restore a normal surface area of coaptation and eliminate the risk of SAM if carried out correctly with the appropriate choice of annuloplasty ring size.

The principle goal of mitral valve reconstruction is to restore valve competence but the focus has shifted somewhat towards a desire to restore near-normal physiological movement of both leaflets. This re-assessment of the approach to repair has led to a rapid increase in the use of neo-chordae, first described by Robert Frater in 1982.

In making the decision between which technique to use, it is important to consider the quantity and quality of the native tissue, the size of the prolapsing segment and the likelihood of producing SAM. In practically all patients with posterior leaflet prolapse, competence can be restored using neo-chordae. The more leaflet tissue there is the easier it is to restore competence with good coaptation height. If the prolapsing segment is the same height as the opposing anterior leaflet or greater, it is wise to reduce the height of the leaflet, using the described techniques to reduce the risk of SAM. SAM can also be prevented by the use of neo-chordae alone simply by over-correcting the prolapse and drawing the leaflet almost to the tip of the papillary muscle with a very short neo-chord, although this will inevitably paralyse the movement of the leaflet. Occasionally, the papillary muscles are misplaced in the ventricle riding very high on the ventricular wall leaving inadequate distance between leaflet edge and the tip of the papillary muscle for adequate leaflet height reduction. In these cases, resection of the posterior leaflet to reduce its height becomes imperative. An additional attraction of neo-chord insertion is that the presence of deep indentations in the leaflet is not a problem. In resectional techniques, it is common to be left with a thin strip of leaflet with a deep indentation on the other side from the resection. This often makes reconstruction untidy and can lead to the need to resect more tissue than was initially desirable. Where there is a discrete excess of leaflet tissue, a triangular resection can give a very satisfactory result. It is wise to attach a neo-chord to the free edge of the repair to further stabilise it to enhance a good long-term result.

In larger valves, there is still a place for quadrangular resection, which will give a competent valve and a stable repair. Many surgeons are most comfortable with this technique and those whose use of neo-chordae is limited should embrace it. Likewise, with the use of sliding annuloplasty, this is an excellent technique giving the opportunity of reducing posterior leaflet height and restoring competence. Both of these procedures do produce a frozen posterior leaflet as discussed earlier and if the resection is too extensive they will produce mitral stenosis, especially if a smaller (<30 mm) ring size is used and this risk is greatest with a complete ring. It is important to emphasise that in all cases the selection of the annuloplasty ring size is crucial to prevent SAM and/or mitral stenosis.

Surgical Technique

The key principle in repairing any mitral valve is to identify and address all of the problems that exist. It is important to note that whilst current trans-oesophageal imaging is of the highest quality, it is still common for secondary lesions to be missed, either through echo drop-out or lack of recognition. Whilst interrogating the echocardiogram, it is easy to focus solely upon the area of leak and the associated prolapse, missing an area of relative prolapse that may not have an associated regurgitant jet but that will progress if not properly addressed. Also, it is wise to ensure preoperatively that the best quality echocardiogram has been obtained, as the information gleaned on the operating table is influenced by the fact that the patient is anaesthetised and relatively dehydrated; both factors in reducing filling volume and left ventricular afterload.

In this particular patient, the presence of deep clefts and insufficient chordal support had resulted in abnormal load sharing across the posterior mitral valve leaflet and subsequent prolapse of the isolated segment. Horizontal mattress annuloplasty sutures (2/0 Ethibond) were placed around the circumference of the mitral valve, with a 5 mm width and approximately 1 mm apart. They were placed at this stage as they provide much improved access and visualisation of the mitral valve leaflets and subvalvular apparatus for subsequent repair.

With the valve elevated into an even plane by the annuloplasty sutures, the mitral valve was assessed, using segmental analysis of the leaflets and the subvalvular apparatus, and correlated with the trans-oesophageal echocardiographical findings. In this patient, marked prolapse of the P2 segment of the posterior leaflet was observed associated with a ruptured chord that originated from the posteromedial papillary muscle. The P2 scallop of the posterior leaflet was excessively tall with a height of 3 cm, associated with a relative paucity of tissue in the remaining scallops of the mitral valve. In view of this, the patient underwent a limited triangular resection of the prolapsing P2 scallop of the mitral valve, in order to reduce the height of the posterior leaflet and to maintain a posteriorly positioned coaptation line. Alternatively, this could have been managed with neo-chordae alone or detachment from the posterior annulus, excision of approximately 25% of the height of the leaflet with reattachment to the posterior annulus. If necessary, any calcific deposits at the base of the resection area, in the posterior mitral valve annulus, can also be excised at this stage.

With an excess of tissue in the prolapsed segment, the first step is to resect a triangle of tissue. The extent of resection depends on the degree of prolapse, and amount and quality of the residual tissue, to ensure adequate tissue is left to reconstitute the posterior leaflet without tension. Stay sutures (5/0 Prolene) were placed around the normal chordae tendineae attached on either side of the prolapsed area of the P2 scallop. Gentle traction on these stay sutures allowed the margins of resection of the posterior leaflet to be clearly delineated and assessment of the amount of residual tissue that will be left following resection (Fig. 7.9a). The prolapsing P2 segment was resected in a triangular fashion using a No 11 blade and scissors (Fig. 7.9b). The base of the triangle was at the free margin of the prolapsed segment, with the apex of the triangle pointing towards the annular aspect of the posterior leaflet (Fig. 7.9c). The apex of the triangle should fall short of the annulus. Approximately 5 mm of prolapsed tissue was left on either side of the resection margin to facilitate a tension-free reconstruction of the posterior leaflet (Fig. 7.9d).

Depending on the insertion points of the remaining native chords on either side of the resected portion and the degree of leaflet resection, implantation of Gore-Tex neo-chordae at the free edge of the reconstituted area may be necessary to give extra strength to the repair, especially in patients with insufficient chordal support. In the presence of deep clefts on either side of the resected segment, it may be desirable to partially close these in order to restore a more equal load distribution and energy sharing across the whole posterior leaflet. To allow the posterior leaflet to retain its normal functional mobility, these clefts are only closed to one half or 2/3rd's of their height, using an inverting suture on the ventricular side. In the majority of patients, most clefts, especially if shallow, are not closed as they contribute to the normal physiological movement of the mitral valve leaflets. The residual segments of the posterior leaflet

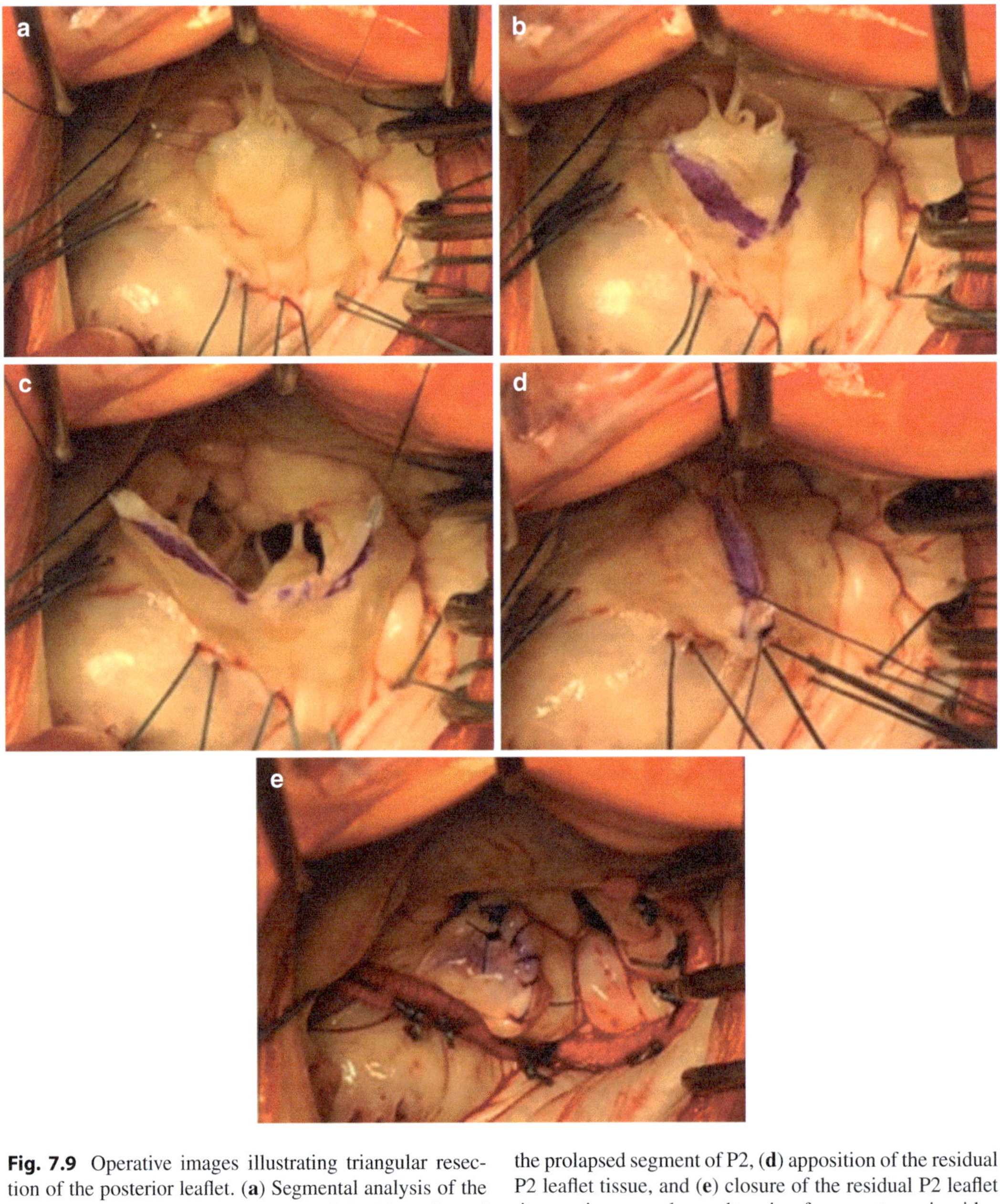

Fig. 7.9 Operative images illustrating triangular resection of the posterior leaflet. (**a**) Segmental analysis of the mitral valve demonstrating prolapse of the P2 scallop of the posterior leaflet caused by chordal rupture, (**b**) demarcation of the lines of resection, (**c**) triangular resection of the prolapsed segment of P2, (**d**) apposition of the residual P2 leaflet tissue, and (**e**) closure of the residual P2 leaflet tissue using a two-layered tension-free anastomosis with a continuous locking 5/0 Prolene suture and implantation of an annuloplasty band

were then sewn together restoring continuity of the posterior leaflet, with a two-layered tension-free anastomosis, using a continuous locking 5/0 Prolene suture, starting at the leaflet free edge and tying the knot at the annulus (Fig. 7.9e). It is also acceptable to use a single layer closure or interrupted sutures.

The next step is to assess competency of the mitral valve, which can be performed by injecting cold saline into the left ventricle using a bulb syringe to assess for any residual prolapse, restriction or regurgitation. The ventricle is filled until the aortic root feels quite tense indicating that the ventricle is well filled and is under some tension. Under-filling of the ventricle can mislead the surgeon into thinking that the repair is adequate when it may not be. With a left ventricle distended with saline, the depth of coaptation was assessed by marking the atrial surface of the mitral valve leaflets with a sterile marking pen and then evacuating the saline from the ventricle. The coaptation length can then be clearly visualized and, if necessary, increased to achieve at least 8 mm by the placement of additional Gore-Tex neo-chordae.

Once the posterior leaflet has been reconstructed, the annuloplasty ring or band is inserted. This is particularly important for patients with echocardiographical evidence of mitral valve annular dilatation. Sizing of the ring or band is based upon the surface area of both the anterior and posterior mitral valve leaflets, (with the ventricle tensioned and good coaptation height demonstrated), representing the surface area of the whole mitral valve orifice. This avoids reducing the short-axis of the mitral valve orifice, retaining the normal geometric relationships of the anterior and posterior leaflets in relationship with the natural valve orifice and reducing the subsequent risk of systolic anterior motion of the mitral valve. Furthermore, sizing in this way avoids producing a stenotic valve. Ring or band annuloplasty will prevent further annular dilatation and relieve the tension on the leaflets by optimizing the coaptation zone. The annuloplasty sutures are then passed through the ring or band which is then tied down in situ.

Following implantation of the annuloplasty band, injecting cold saline again allowed final assessment of the mitral valve for competency, and adequate depth (>8 mm) and evenness of coaptation. In the unlikely event of any residual regurgitation through indentations at the coaptation margin, these can be overcome by closing them using 5/0 Prolene.

Post-operative Echocardiogram

The post-repair trans-oesophageal echocardiogram (Fig. 7.10) confirmed:

1. Normal physiological functioning of the mitral valve complex with no residual mitral regurgitation.
2. The height of the posterior mitral valve leaflet was <15 mm.
3. No systolic anterior motion (SAM) of the anterior mitral valve leaflet into the left ventricular outflow tract, causing left ventricular outflow obstruction (LVOTO).
4. The depth of leaflet coaptation was >8 mm.

Surgical Tips

1. Prior to resection of mitral valve tissue in these patients, ensure that there is enough residual tissue to reconstruct the posterior leaflet with a tension free anastomosis and to maintain normal physiological movement of the posterior leaflet.
2. Closure of the deep clefts on either side of the resected segment to 2/3rd of their height will allow improved systolic load sharing across the whole leaflet.
3. Ensure that the height of the posterior leaflet is no more than 50% of the height of the anterior leaflet, to reduce the risk of post-repair systolic anterior motion (SAM) of the mitral valve.
4. If necessary, support the triangular resection leaflet repair with neo-chords, as well as an annuloplasty band or ring.
5. Obtaining an adequate depth of coaptation (>8 mm) is important for the long-term durability of the procedure.

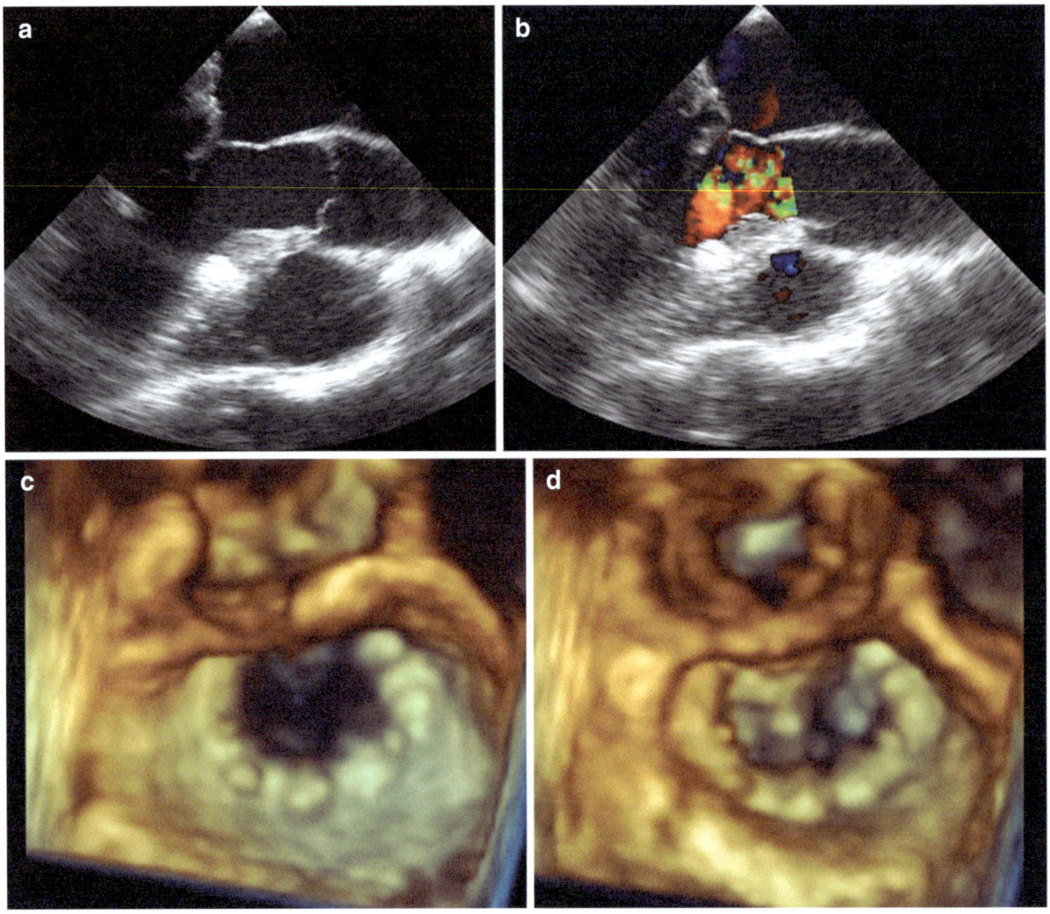

Fig. 7.10 Post-bypass intra-operative trans-oesophageal echocardiographical images demonstrating (**a**) 10 mm depth of coaptation between the anterior and posterior leaflets, and no SAM on the mid-oesophageal long-axis view, with (**b**) a competent mitral valve with no residual mitral regurgitation on the corresponding colour flow Doppler image. Three-dimensional views in (**c**) diastole and (**d**) systole demonstrating the annuloplasty band in situ, with the plane of leaflet coaptation drawn down below the level of the annulus into the LV and no residual P2 prolapse

Comment

Results of mitral valve surgery following triangular resection for posterior leaflet prolapse have shown excellent outcomes, with an in-hospital mortality <1% and a low peri-operative complication rate. Mid to long term outcome measures have also demonstrated excellent freedom from recurrent mitral regurgitation (95% with no or 1+ MR at 5 years), freedom from reoperation (99% at 5 years) and survival (98.5% at 5 years).

Recommended Reading

Gazoni LM, Fedoruk LM, Kern JA, Dent JM, Reece TB, Tribble CG, Smith PW, Lisle TC, Kron IL. A simplified approach to degenerative disease: triangular resections of the mitral valve. Ann Thorac Surg. 2007;83(5):1658–64.

George KM, Mihaljevic T, Gillinov AM. Triangular resection for posterior mitral prolapse: rationale for a simpler repair. J Heart Valve Dis. 2009;18(1):119–21.

Milano A, Codecasa R, Le-Carlo M, Nardi C, Tartarini G, Verunelli F, Bortolotti U, Wells FC, Northrup W. Mitral valve annuloplasty for degenerative disease: assessment of four different techniques. J Heart Valve Dis. 2000;9(3):321–6.

Moorjani N, Viola N, Janusauskas V, Livesey S. Adjusting the length of artificial polytetrafluoroethylene chordae in mitral valve repair by a single loop technique. J Thorac Cardiovasc Surg. 2009;138(6):1441–2.

Padala M, Powell SN, Croft LR, Thourani VH, Yoganathan AP, Adams DH. Mitral valve hemodynamics after repair of acute posterior leaflet prolapse: quadrangular resection versus triangular resection versus neochordoplasty. J Thorac Cardiovasc Surg. 2009;138(2):309–15.

Ring L, Rana BS, Ho SY, Wells FC. The prevalence and impact of deep clefts in the mitral leaflets in mitral valve prolapse. Eur Heart J Cardiovasc Imaging. 2013;4:595–602.

Anterior Mitral Valve Leaflet Prolapse

8

Keywords
Anterior mitral valve leaflet prolapse · Chordal replacement · Chordal transposition · Posterior leaflet 'flip-over' · Leaflet resection · Leaflet plication · 'Edge-to-edge' technique · Papillary muscle repositioning · Gore-Tex neo-chordae

Case History

A 63 year-old man presented with a prolonged history of increasing exertional dyspnoea associated with lethargy. He had no history of rheumatic fever or infective endocarditis. He was being followed up with serial echocardiography over several years with known mitral regurgitation.

Echocardiographical Findings

Trans-thoracic apical 3-chamber echocardiographic images revealed prolapse of the anterior mitral valve leaflet (Fig. 8.1a). This was also observed on the parasternal long-axis and apical 4-chamber views (Fig. 8.1b, c), where the anterior leaflet can be seen to override the annular plane during systole. Colour flow Doppler across the mitral valve demonstrated an eccentric posteriorly directed wall-hugging jet of mitral regurgitation that reaches the pulmonary veins (Fig. 8.1d).

Using trans-oesophageal echocardiographical, segmental analysis of the anterior leaflet demonstrated isolated prolapse of the A2 segment, in the mid-oesophageal 5-chamber, bicommissural and long-axis views (Fig. 8.2a–c). Doppler flow across the mitral valve in these views demonstrated a posterior directed jet of mitral regurgitation (MR), confirming anterior leaflet prolapse as the dominant lesion (Fig. 8.2a–c). Quantification of the regurgitation, using the PISA method, revealed severe MR, with an effective regurgitant orifice area of 48 mm^2, regurgitant volume of 68 mL and regurgitant fraction of 59%, associated with a vena contracta of 0.78 cm. The left atrium was dilated at 5.24 cm but the left ventricular size and function were preserved, with a left ventricular end-systolic diameter 3.9 cm, left ventricular end-diastolic diameter 5.4 cm and ejection fraction 63%. Three-dimensional (3D) echocardiographical images clearly demonstrate the prolapsing A2 segment of the anterior leaflet (Fig. 8.2d).

N. Moorjani et al., *Operative Mitral and Tricuspid Valve Surgery*,
https://doi.org/10.1007/978-1-4471-4204-1_8

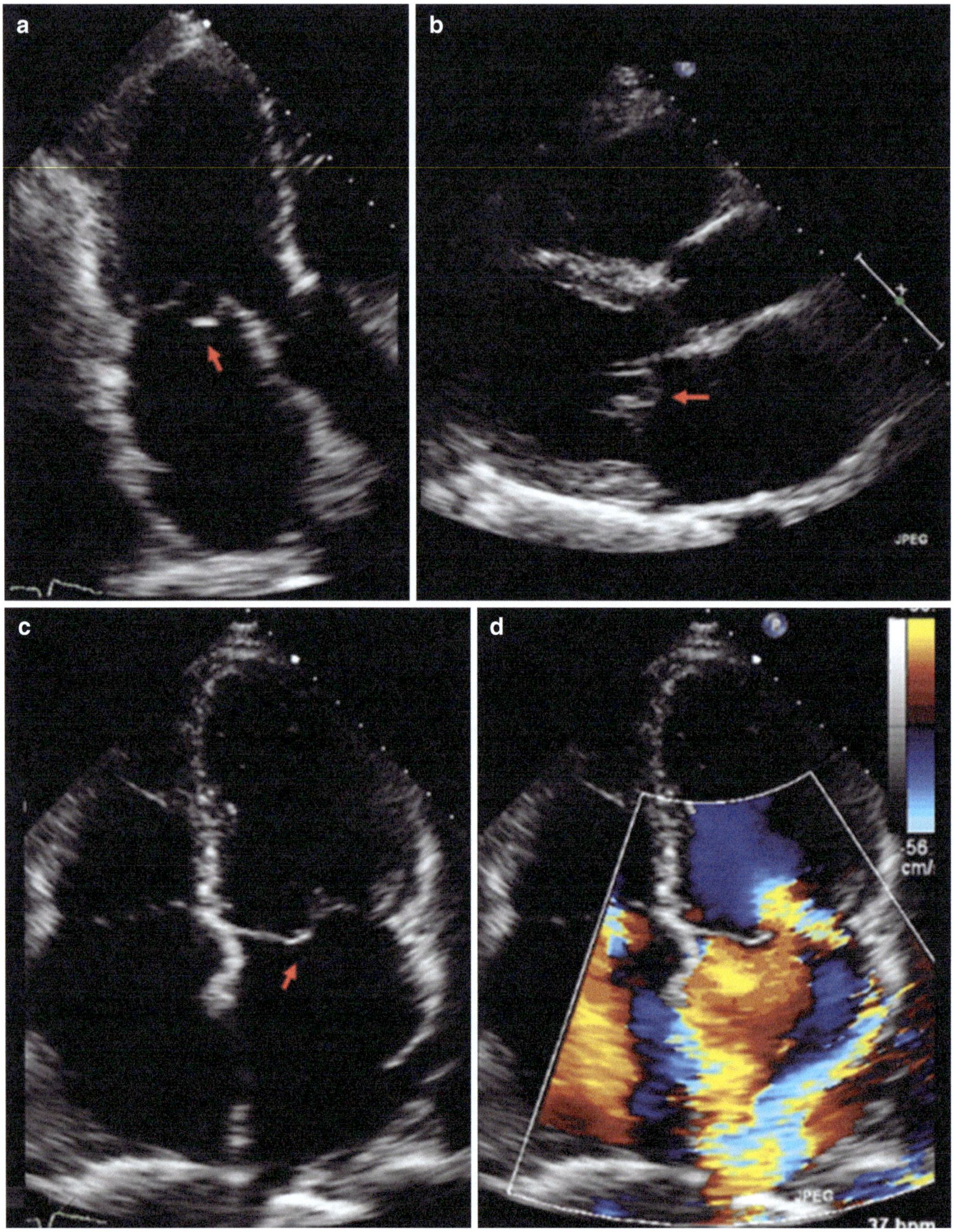

Fig. 8.1 Trans-thoracic echocardiographical images demonstrating prolapse of the A2 segment of the anterior leaflet, secondary to ruptured chordae tendineae, on (**a**) apical 3-chamber, (**b**) parasternal long-axis and (**c**) apical 4-chamber views, resulting in (**d**) an eccentric posteriorly directed 'wall-hugging' jet of mitral regurgitation, which is seen to extend into the right pulmonary veins using colour flow Doppler on the apical 4-chamber view

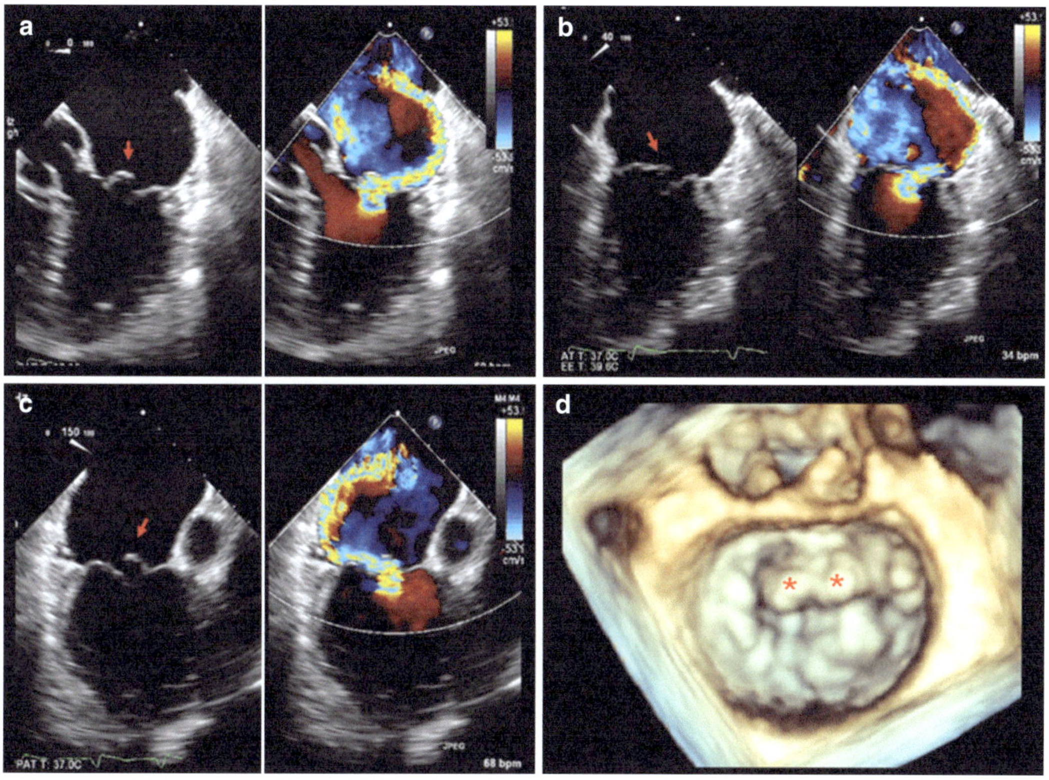

Fig. 8.2 Trans-oesophageal echocardiographical images demonstrating prolapse of the A2 segment of the anterior leaflet, secondary to ruptured chordae tendineae (red arrow) on (**a**) mid-oesophageal 5-chamber, (**b**) bicommissural and (**c**) long-axis views, resulting in a posterior directed jet of severe mitral regurgitation on corresponding images using colour flow Doppler. (**d**) Three-dimensional surgical view confirms the presence of extensive A2 prolapse (red stars)

Surgical Strategy

Anterior leaflet prolapse is more difficult to treat than that of the posterior leaflet. By the nature of the large surface area of the leaflet with a much greater leaflet height, it is of utmost importance to create a deep and even coaptation margin. As this is more difficult to obtain, it is not surprising that the long-term results are not as good as for posterior leaflet pathology. There are a number of techniques that can be used to correct the prolapse. They can be categorised as follows:

(a) Chordal replacement, chordal transposition and posterior leaflet 'flip-over'.
(b) Leaflet resection, leaflet plication and the 'edge-to-edge' technique
(c) Papillary muscle repositioning

Techniques involving the papillary muscle or chordae tendineae avoid resection and address the pathology at the level of the subvalvular apparatus. The techniques most frequently used to correct anterior leaflet prolapse in contemporary practice is chordal replacement (most common), chordal transposition and the 'flip-over' technique.

Chordal Replacement

Chordal replacement focuses on replacement of the diseased, elongated or ruptured chordae tendineae with Gore-Tex polytetrafluoroethylene (PTFE) sutures (W.L. Gore & Associates, Flagstaff, AZ, USA). The advantage of this technique is that it preserves the surface area of the leaflet and thus leaflet anatomy and mobility, thereby maximising the orifice area of the mitral valve. Over time, Gore-Tex neo-chordae have been shown to maintain their flexibility (even after 10 years from implantation), as they become covered in fibrous tissue and endothelium but in the absence of calcification. Implanting Gore-Tex neo-chordae is relatively simple and reproducible but the key to success is in determining the correct length of the sutures (Fig. 8.3). Various techniques have been described to determine the height of the Gore-Tex neo-chordae, including using:

(a) Saline inflation of the left ventricle with adjustment of the height of the neo-chord to give an even coaptation height across the whole of the leaflet.
(b) Pre-measured Gore-Tex loops (the 'loop' technique), using pre-operative echocardiography and an intra-operative graduated caliper to measure the distance from the fibrous head of the papillary muscles to the free edge of the prolapsing segment at annular level.
(c) The anterior annulus to act as a guide to the correct length and tension of the implanted neo-chord.

Chordal Transposition

This technique involves the transfer of normal posterior leaflet chordae to replace the elongated or ruptured anterior leaflet chordae. It can also be performed by transferring a segment

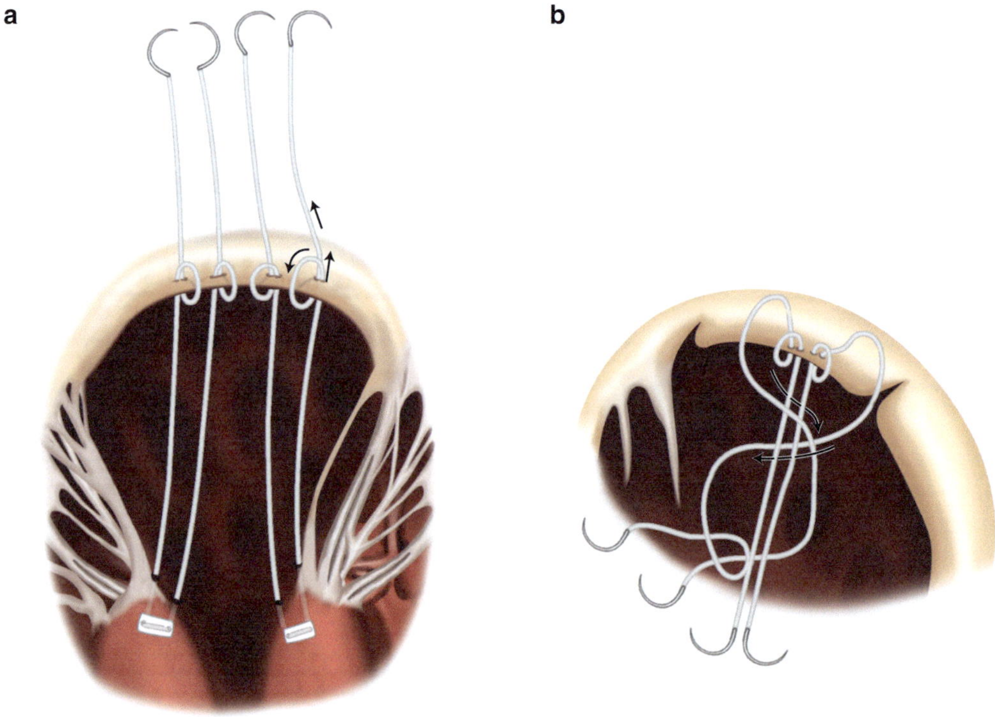

Fig. 8.3 Implantation of Gore-Tex neo-chordae using a single loop technique. (**a**) A pledgeted CV4 Gore-Tex suture is passed through the appropriate papillary muscles using a horizontal mattress suture. Each limb of the Gore-Tex suture is then passed twice through the free edge of the anterior leaflet, from the ventricular side to the atrial side. (**b**) Once the optimal length of the neo-chord has been determined, the free ends of the Gore-Tex suture are passed through the vertical limbs of the suture to be tied on the ventricular side of the leaflet

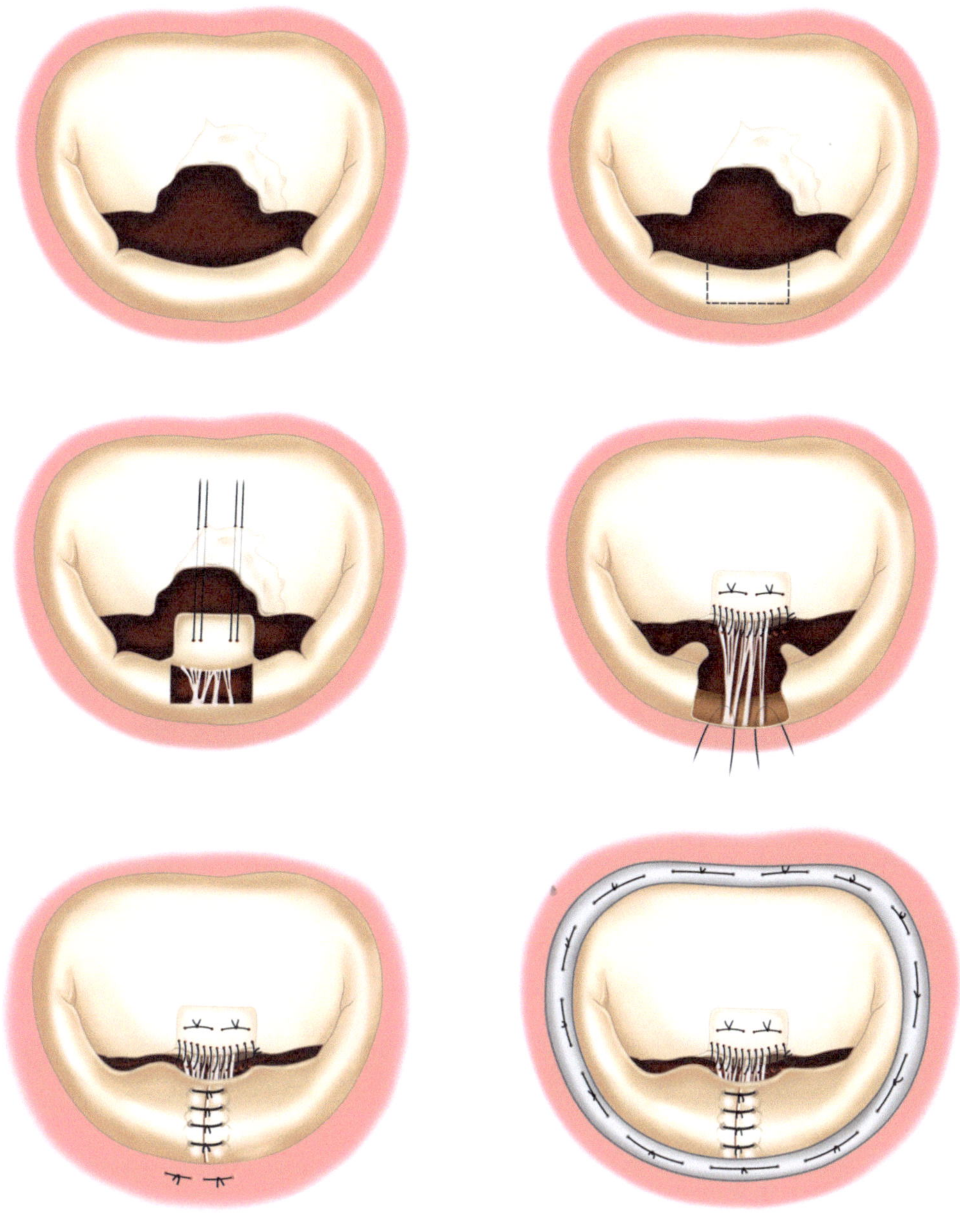

Fig. 8.4 Chordal transposition, which is performed by transferring a segment of normal posterior leaflet tissue in combination with the chordae tendineae and suturing it to the ventricular side of the prolapsing segment of the anterior leaflet using 5/0 polypropylene suture. The defect in the posterior leaflet is repaired using a quadrangular resection and horizontal compression annuloplasty sutures, followed by ring annuloplasty

of normal posterior leaflet tissue in combination with the chordae tendineae (Fig. 8.4). The advantage of this technique is that the prolapsing segment of the anterior leaflet is supported by naturally determined appropriate length native chordae, obtained from the opposite non-prolapsing segment of the posterior leaflet. This leaves a corresponding segment of posterior leaflet that will need to be repaired and can only be performed in patients with isolated anterior leaflet prolapse, associated with normal posterior leaflet and sub-valvular apparatus. In patients with elongated or ruptured primary free-edge chords, chordal transfer can be performed using a secondary chord sectioned at the implantation site on the base of the leaflet and sutured to the leaflet edge.

Flip-Over Technique

In this technique, a quadrangular segment of the posterior leaflet that lies directly opposite the prolapsing anterior leaflet segment is carefully cut away from the rest of the posterior leaflet and then detached from the posterior annulus (Fig. 8.5). It is then 'flipped-over' with its attached chords and sutured to the atrial sur-

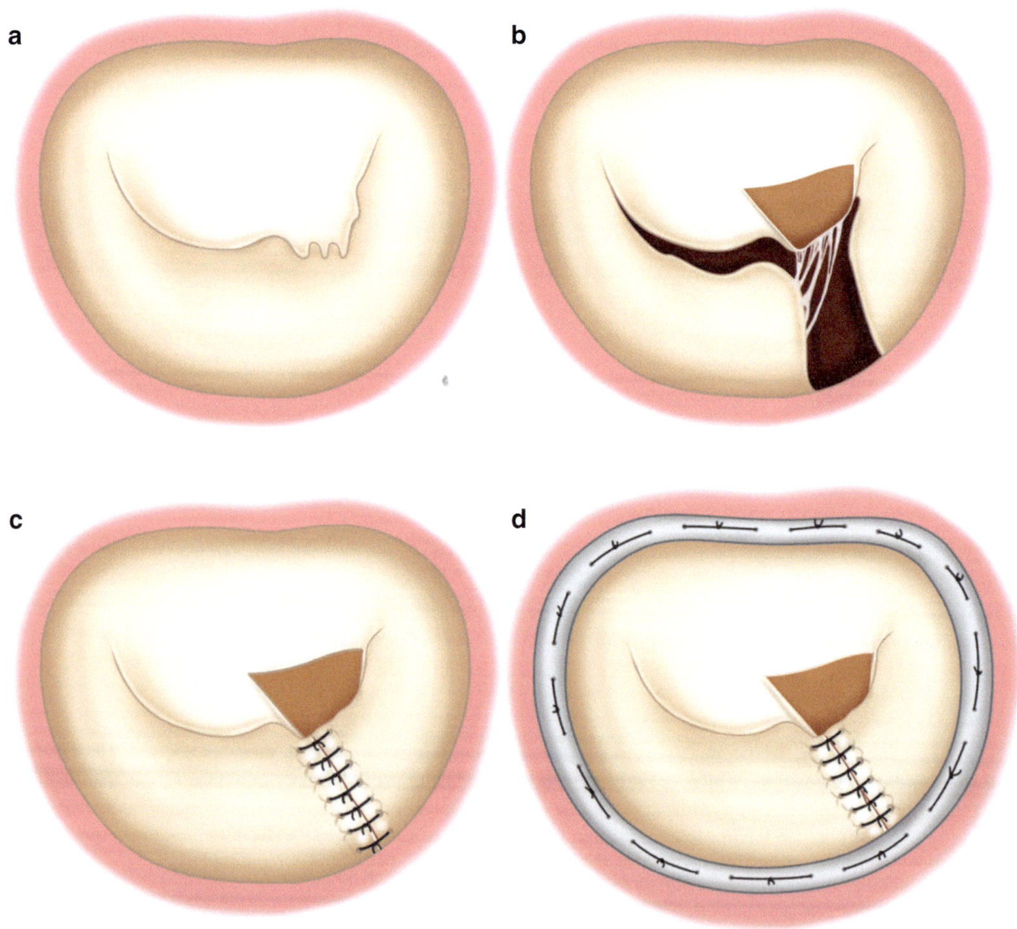

Fig. 8.5 Flip-over technique, which is performed by (**a**) detaching a quadrangular segment of the posterior leaflet from the annulus that lies directly opposite the prolapsing anterior leaflet segment, (**b**) flipping-over the segment with attached chordae, (**c**) suturing it to the atrial surface of the prolapsing anterior leaflet segment, whilst closing the defect in the posterior leaflet, followed by (**d**) ring annuloplasty

face of the prolapsing anterior leaflet segment. Any basal chordae that are attached to the ventricular surface of the posterior leaflet segment can be preserved. As with chordal transposition, the main advantage of this technique is that the transferred chords are of appropriate length. The resulting gap in the posterior leaflet is repaired using annular plication sutures and reconstruction of the residual segments of the posterior leaflet (as described in Chap. 7). Although patients with a very wide prolapsing segment can undergo a sliding annuloplasty in addition to the quadrangular resection, this is not recommended as it considerably reduces the orifice of the valve. Neo-chordae offer a better solution in these patients.

Chordal Shortening

Direct chordal shortening has been described and carried out in the past but the results are very poor with often early recurrence of regurgitation. Leaflet height reduction by reimplantation of the chords within the papillary muscle, however, allows a group of elongated chords to be shortened simultaneously. The technique involves performing a longitudinal incision, where the elongated chordae tendineae originate, from the tip of the papillary muscle, towards the base of the papillary muscle (Fig. 8.6). The elongated chordae can then be shortened by folding them into the deepest point of the incision and suturing them in position. Although this technique directly addresses the underly-

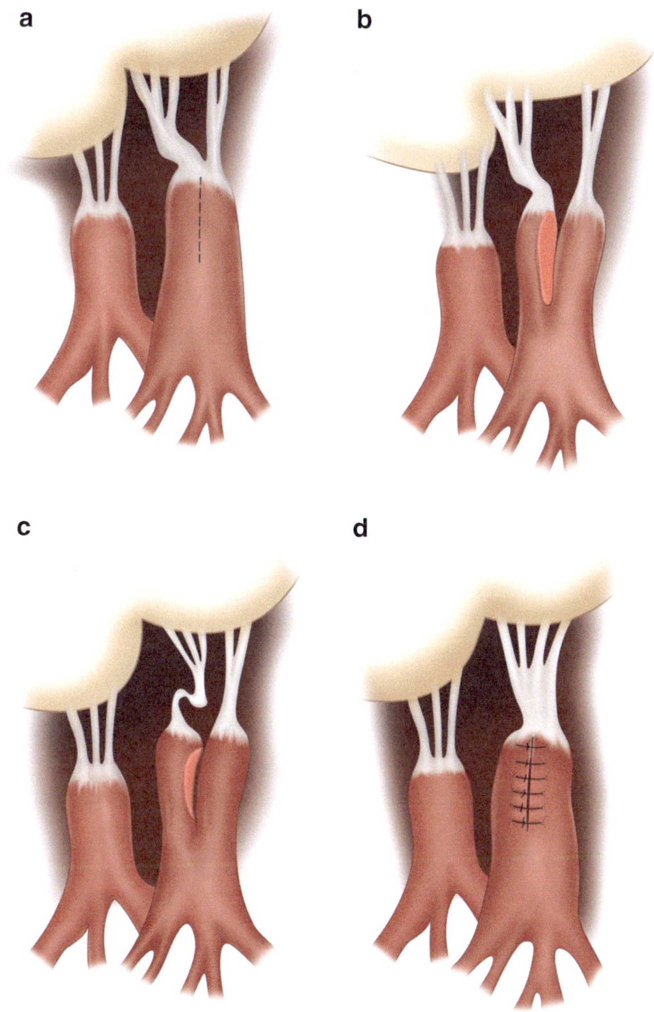

Fig. 8.6 Chordal shortening, which involves (**a**) identifying where the elongated chordae tendineae originate, (**b**) performing a longitudinal incision from the tip of the papillary muscle, towards the base of the papillary muscle. (**c**) The elongated chordae can then be shortened by folding them into the deepest point of the incision and (**d**) suturing them in position, to produce chordal length equal to the normal adjacent chordae

ing pathology, it also has unpredictable long-term results, with reports of chordal rupture and recurrent leaflet prolapse described.

Papillary Muscle Repositioning

In patients where all elongated chords arise from a single papillary muscle head, a wedge resection on the side of the papillary muscle can be used to reposition the tip of the papillary muscle thereby retensioning the elongated chordae (Fig. 8.7). The wedge resection is closed with interrupted non-pledgeted 4/0 Prolene sutures. The width of the resection will determine the degree of repositioning of the papillary muscle head and therefore the degree of retensioning.

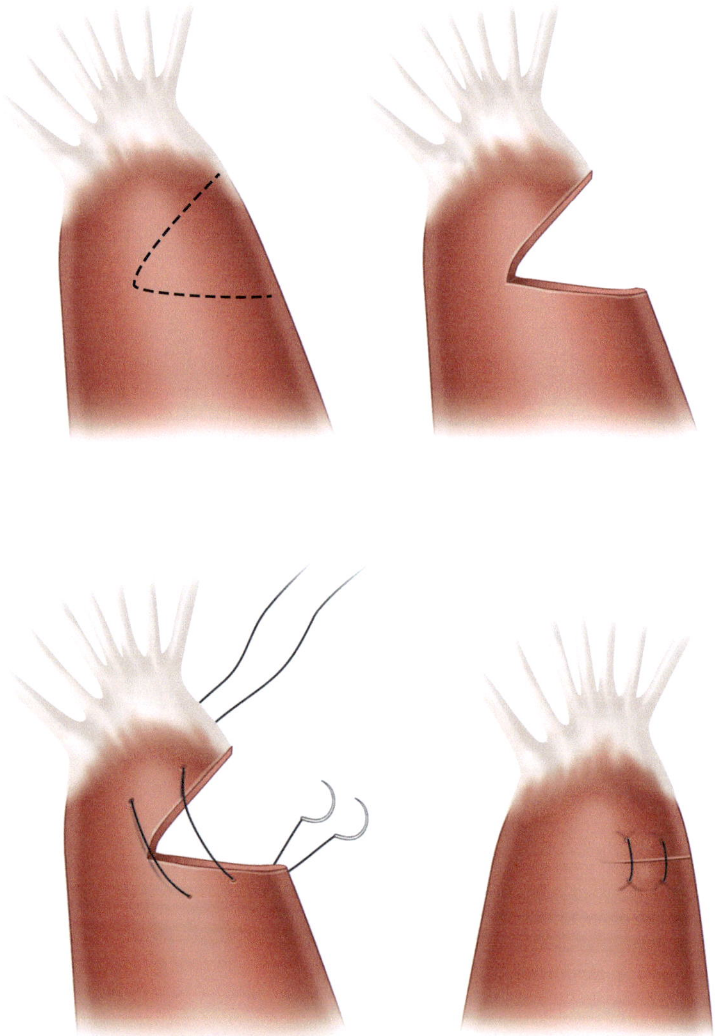

Fig. 8.7 Papillary muscle repositioning, which involves performing a wedge resection on the side of the papillary muscle to retension the elongated chordae. The wedge resection is closed with interrupted non-pledgeted 4/0 Prolene sutures

Leaflet Resection

As with techniques to treat posterior leaflet prolapse, excessive tissue in the prolapsing segments of the anterior leaflet can be excised. Triangular resection, not quadrangular resection, is performed following the radial lines drawn from the centre of the anterior annulus. Resection of the anterior leaflet is not very reliable with reports of early recurrence. In practise, this technique is usually only employed in patients with a large volume of the anterior leaflet billowing with chords of appropriate length. Patients with elongated or ruptured chordae tendineae will still need additional chordal support to complete the repair (Fig. 8.8).

Leaflet Plication

This is rarely indicated but can be used if there is a small cleft in the anterior leaflet, where the excess tissue can be tucked under the free edge of the leaflet.

Edge-to-Edge Technique

A primary indication for the Alfieri edge-to-edge technique is in the treatment of anterior leaflet prolapse. The free edge of the prolapsing leaflet is attached to the free edge of the corresponding segment on the opposing leaflet (Fig. 8.9). It is

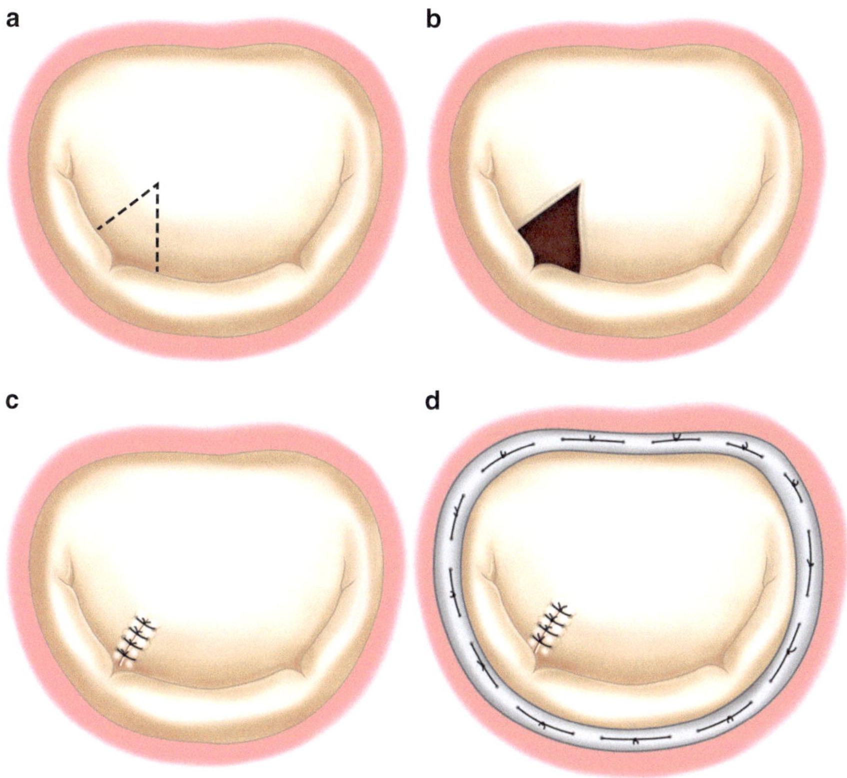

Fig. 8.8 Leaflet resection, which involves (**a**) identifying the area of prolapse, (**b**) performing a small triangular resection at the free edge of the anterior leaflet at the site of the prolapse, (**c**) closure using 5/0 polypropylene suture, followed by (**d**) ring annuloplasty

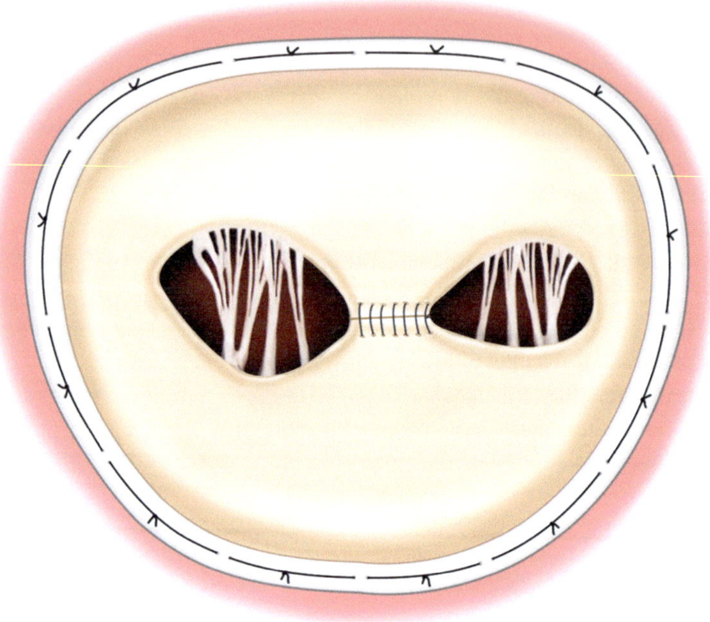

Fig. 8.9 Edge-to-edge repair of the mitral valve, resulting in a 'double-orifice' mitral valve

a functional rather than anatomical repair of the mitral valve. The crucial step of this technique is to accurately identify the origin of the regurgitant jet for optimal suture placement and to identify the exact point on the corresponding leaflet to avoid valve distortion and residual valve regurgitation. It results in a 'double-orifice' mitral valve, with openings that may or may not be of equal size and symmetrical. It is important that the sum of these two orifices is greater than 2.5 cm^2 to avoid post-operative mitral stenosis. Intraoperatively, the valve can be tested for stenosis using Hegar dilators and for competency by static testing with saline distension of the left ventricle. This relatively simple technique is reproducible and associated with relatively short ischaemic and cardiopulmonary bypass times. The name of the technique is somewhat misleading as the sutures are not placed at the "edge" of the leaflets but about 5–6 mm from the edge. It is more secure if it is done in two layers.

In addition to treating anterior leaflet prolapse, this technique can also be used as a rescue technique in patients with a heavily calcified mitral annulus. As with other procedures on the anterior leaflet, the edge-to-edge technique should usually be supported with a ring annuloplasty to avoid future annular dilatation. In particular, a minimum ring diameter of 30 mm should be used with the edge-to-edge technique to avoid the development of post-repair mitral stenosis.

Surgical Technique

Following placement of the annuloplasty sutures, which allowed much improved access and visualisation of the mitral valve leaflets and subvalvular apparatus, the mitral valve was assessed, using segmental analysis of the leaflets and the subvalvular apparatus, and correlated with the trans-oesophageal echocardiographical findings. In this patient, marked prolapse of the A2 segment of the anterior leaflet was observed, associated with ruptured chordae tendineae, which had originated from both the anterolateral and posteromedial papillary muscles (Fig. 8.10a).

Stay sutures (5/0 Prolene) were placed around the normal chordae tendineae attached on either side of the prolapsed area of the anterior leaflet and along the leading edge of the prolapsing segment. The exact number (usually

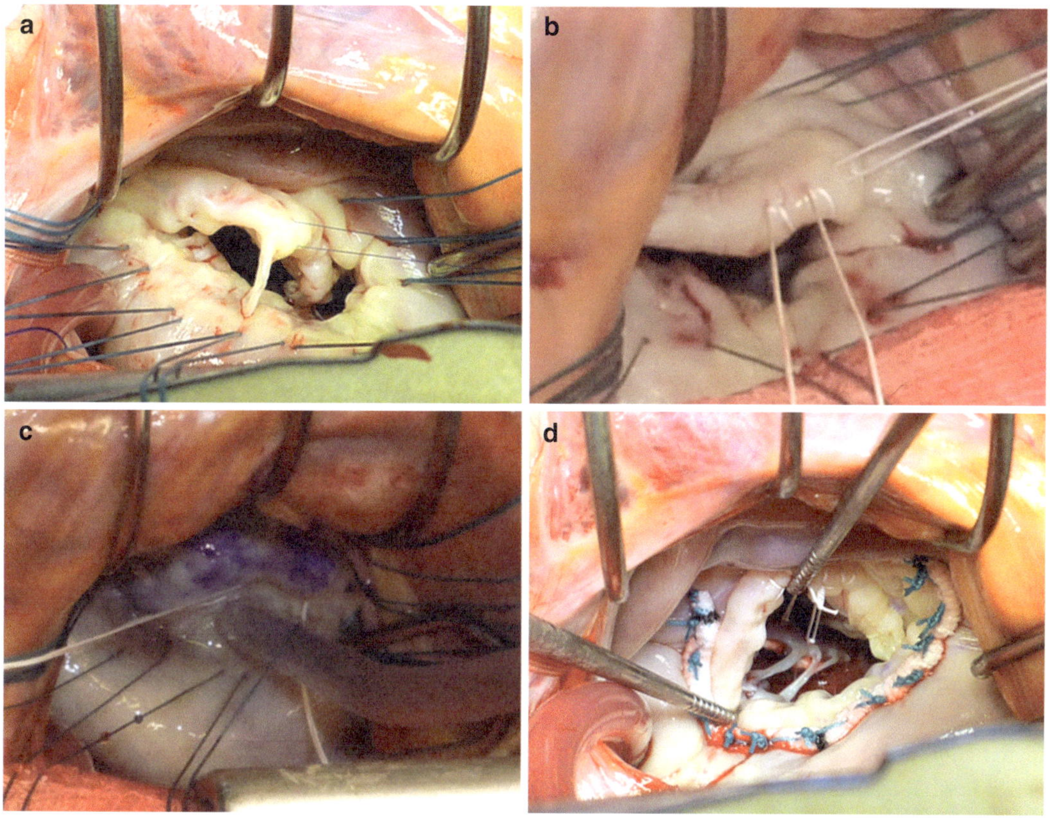

Fig. 8.10 Operative images illustrating (**a**) segmental analysis of the mitral valve, demonstrating isolated prolapse of the A2 segment of the anterior leaflet, secondary to a ruptured chord, (**b**) implantation of a Gore-Tex neo-chordae, (**c**) depth of coaptation assessed by the ink test and saline distension of the left ventricle, and (**d**) implantation of an annuloplasty band

2 or 3) is dependent upon the width of the prolapsing segment. Gentle traction on these stay sutures allowed the margins of prolapsed segment of the anterior leaflet to be clearly delineated, to assess the number of neo-chordae required and to identify the insertion point of the neo-chordae.

Access to papillary muscles can be sometimes be difficult but can be improved by mechanical retraction of the anterior leaflet using an additional retractor blade, leaflet retractor, large mechanical valve replacement sizer, Yankauer sucker tip or nerve hook. When choosing which papillary muscle head to insert the neo-chordae, it is useful though not an imperative, to respect anatomy and to use the origin of elongated or ruptured chordae as a guide to which papillary muscle head to use. The native chordae to A2 originate from both posteromedial and anterolateral papillary muscles and so if either papillary muscle head is small the most robust looking one may be chosen.

The neo-chordae were then placed by passing both limbs of a CV-4 Gore-Tex suture (W.L. Gore & Associates, Flagstaff, AZ, USA) through the fibrous part of the papillary muscle head, using a simple U-stich. Some surgeons feel it necessary to use pledgets on this suture but there is no evidence to support their use and if the suture needs to be replaced, the pledget needs to be retrieved to avoid the risk of subsequent embolization. It is not necessary to tie a knot in the Gore-Tex suture at the papillary muscle level. Not doing so allows an equal distribution of tension in both limbs of the suture, otherwise one limb may become tense and the other loose, if care is not taken to adjust

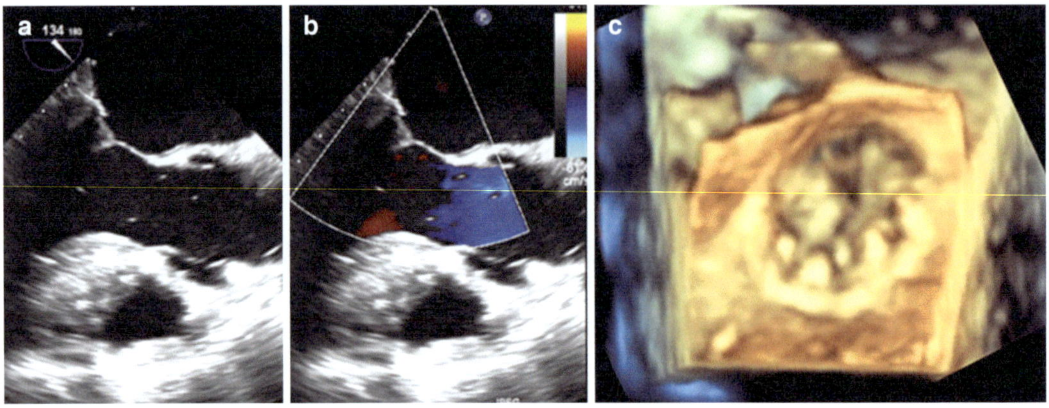

Fig. 8.11 Post-bypass intra-operative trans-oesophageal echocardiographical images, with (**a**) mid-oesophageal long-axis view demonstrating a good depth of coaptation between the anterior and posterior leaflets and no SAM, and (**b**) the corresponding image with colour flow Doppler showing a competent mitral valve with no residual mitral regurgitation. (**c**) Three-dimensional surgical view demonstrates the annuloplasty band in situ with the anterior leaflet below the annular plane and no longer prolapsing

their lengths appropriately. One of the limbs of the Gore-Tex suture was then passed through the prolapsing segment about 5 mm away from the leaflet edge and 2–3 mm away from the boundary of normal leaflet, from the ventricular side to the atrial side and then through a second time. This was then repeated for the second limb of the Gore-Tex neo-chord (Fig. 8.10b).

The provisional height of the Gore-Tex neochordae was then determined by using the posterior leaflet height and the level of the annulus as references to guide to the correct length and tension the implanted neo-chord. Competency of the mitral valve was then assessed with static testing, by injecting cold saline into the left ventricle, using a bulb syringe. With a left ventricle distended with saline, the depth of coaptation was assessed by marking the atrial surface of the mitral valve leaflets with a sterile marking pen (Fig. 8.10c). The depth of coaptation can be increased to achieve an optimal depth of at least 8 mm by adjusting the length of Gore-Tex beneath the leaflet. An appropriate sized annuloplasty band or ring was then chosen, according to the surface area of the whole mitral valve orifice (i.e. the surface area of the anterior and posterior leaflets together). The annuloplasty band was then implanted (Fig. 8.10d). Some surgeons feel the need to leave the fixation of the neo-chords until after ring implantation although this is not always necessary. Locking each end of the suture around the two lengths of suture beneath the valve prevents slipping of the knot and allows confident and firm tying.

A final saline test is performed to confirm the valve competency and positioning of the coaptation line. Should there be any residual regurgitation through clefts at the coaptation edge of the anterior or posterior leaflets, they may be closed using 5/0 Prolene.

Post-operative Echocardiogram

The post-repair trans-oesophageal echocardiogram (Fig. 8.11) confirmed:

1. Normal physiological functioning of the mitral valve complex with the absence of any residual prolapse or restriction of the anterior leaflet
2. No residual mitral regurgitation.
3. No systolic anterior motion of the mitral valve
4. The depth of leaflet coaptation was >8 mm.

Surgical Tips

1. Access to the papillary muscle heads is crucial when implanting Gore-Tex neo-chordae and can be augmented by mechanical retraction of the anterior leaflet
2. It is useful to respect anatomy and implant the Gore-Tex neo-chordae into the papillary muscle head from where the elongated or ruptured chordae originated but probably more important to choose a robust papillary muscle head to hold the neo-chordae
3. The anterior or posterior annulus can be used as a reference to guide the approximate length and tension of the implanted neo-chord, followed by fine tuning using a functional assessment with saline distension of the left ventricle

Comment

Anterior mitral valve leaflet prolapse has traditionally been considered a more challenging problem than posterior leaflet prolapse because of the geometry of the anterior leaflet, and is associated with less favourable long-term results. In view of this, contemporary repair techniques for the anterior leaflet tend to avoid resection and focus on the sub-valvular apparatus. Operative results of mitral valve surgery following chordal replacement for anterior leaflet prolapse have shown excellent outcomes, with an in-hospital mortality <1% and a low peri-operative complication rate. Long term outcome measures following chordal replacement for anterior mitral valve leaflet prolapse have also demonstrated excellent freedom from recurrent mitral regurgitation (85% with no or 1+ MR at 15 years) and freedom from reoperation (92% at 15 years). In this series of 608 patients, none of the repair failures were caused by failure of the Gore-Tex neo-chordae. In fact, at reoperation, the Gore-Tex neo-chordae were explanted and found to have maintained their flexibility, without evidence of any calcification.

Recommended Reading

Kasegawa H, Shimokawa T, Shibazaki I, Hayashi H, Koyanagi T, Ida T. Mitral valve repair for anterior leaflet prolapse with expanded polytetraflu- oroethylene sutures. Ann Thorac Surg. 2006;81:1625–31.

Morimoto H, Tsuchiya K, Nakajima M, Akashi O. Mitral valve repair for anterior leaflet prolapse: surgical techniques review and 16-year follow-up results. J Card Surg. 2008;23:426–30.

Pfannmüller B, Seeburger J, Davierwala P, Mohr FW. Repair of the anterior mitral leaflet prolapse. Expert Rev Med Devices. 2014;11(1):89–100.

Phillips MR, Daly RC, Schaff HV, Dearani JA, Mullany CJ, Orszulak TA. Repair of anterior leaflet mitral valve prolapse: chordal replacement versus chordal shortening. Ann Thorac Surg. 2000;69:25–9.

9 Bi-leaflet Prolapse

Keywords
Bi-leaflet prolapse · Systolic anterior motion (SAM) · Gore-Tex neo-chordae · Leaflet height reduction · Leaflet resection · Alfieri edge-to-edge technique · Barlow's disease · Myxomatous degeneration · Ring annuloplasty · Mitral regurgitation

Case History

A 40 year-old male presented with a long history of increasing dyspnoea on exertion, associated with a reduced exercise tolerance of 200 yards. He had no history of rheumatic fever or infective endocarditis. Clinical examination revealed a pan-systolic murmur (with late systolic accentuation) that radiated into the axilla.

Echocardiographical Findings

Trans-oesophageal 2-chamber and long-axis echocardiographic images revealed prolapse of the anterior and posterior mitral valve leaflets, where both leaflets can be seen to override the annular plane during systole (Fig. 9.1a, b). Colour flow Doppler across the mitral valve in these images demonstrated a complex severe regurgitant jet with several points of mitral regurgitation (MR) across the whole line of leaflet coaptation, consistent with bileaflet prolapse (Fig. 9.1a, b). This can also be seen on the 3D surgical view (Fig. 9.1c) and 3D reconstructions (Fig. 9.1d, e).

The left ventricular function was impaired with an ejection fraction of 47%. Quantification of the regurgitation, using the PISA method, revealed severe MR, with an effective orifice area of 56 mm^2 and regurgitant fraction of 67%, as well as a vena contracta of 0.85 cm. Associated with this, the left atrium and left ventricle were dilated (left atrial diameter 5.32 cm, left ventricular end-systolic diameter 4.6 cm and left ventricular end-diastolic diameter 6.2 cm).

Surgical Strategy

Mitral valve surgery for patients with Barlow's disease can prove challenging. These patients are usually young, often in the third or fourth decades of life, and it is common for the patient to have been notified much earlier in life that they had a cardiac murmur. Barlow's disease is characterised by excessively large leaflets, housed within a large valve orifice, usually greater than 40 mm and up to 50+ mm, in the inter-commissural plane. The posterior leaflet is commonly the same height as the anterior leaflet and sometimes taller. Depending upon the aorto-mitral angle, which can be seen in the long-axis view, there is an increased risk of systolic anterior motion (SAM) of the mitral valve in these patients. If the posterior leaflet is left too

N. Moorjani et al., *Operative Mitral and Tricuspid Valve Surgery*,
https://doi.org/10.1007/978-1-4471-4204-1_9

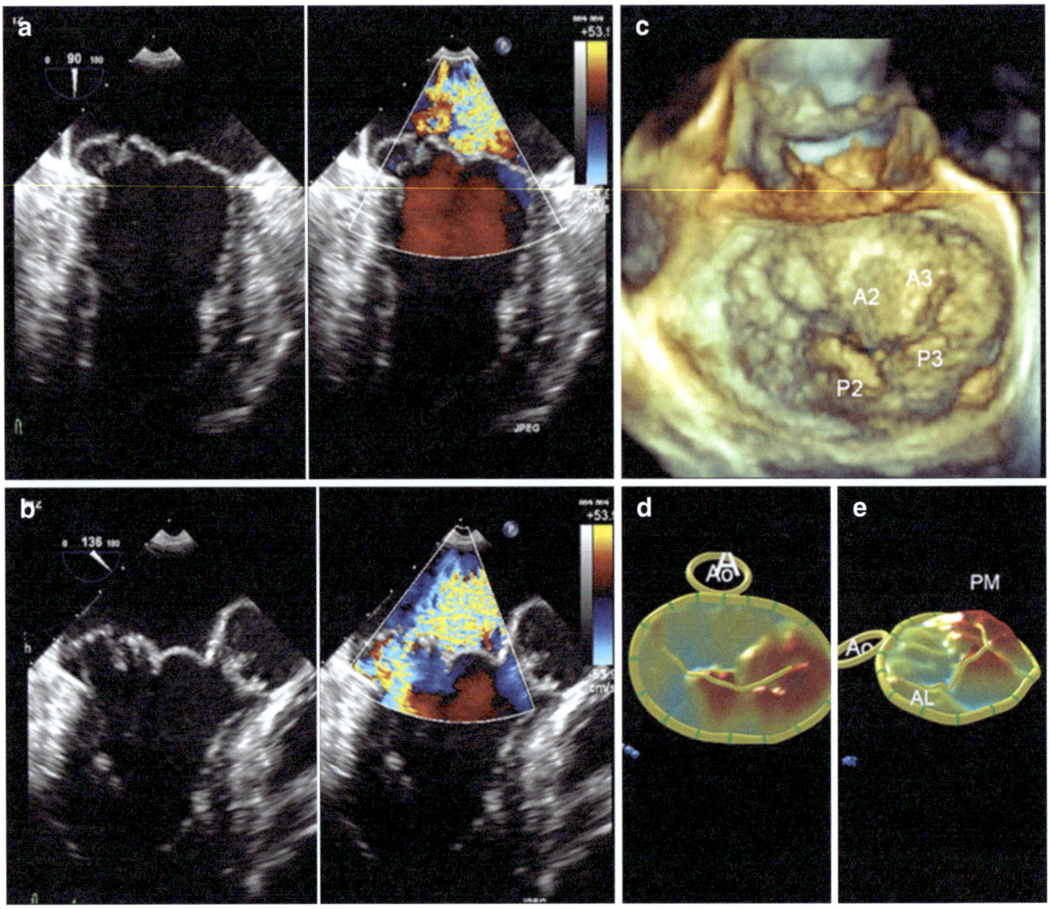

Fig. 9.1 Trans-oesophageal echocardiographical images demonstrating marked bi-leaflet prolapse, with both leaflets overriding the annular plane, on (**a**) mid-oesophageal 2-chamber and (**b**) long-axis views, causing a complex severe regurgitant jet with several points of regurgitation on the corresponding colour flow Doppler images. (**c**) Three-dimensional surgical view demonstrating prolapse of P2, P3, A2, A3 and the posteromedial commissure, as well as a flail P2 secondary to chordal rupture. (**d**, **e**) 3D reconstruction images illustrating the corresponding areas of prolapse (red)

high, then as it closes in systole, it is likely to collide with the anterior leaflet early, buckling it into the left ventricular outflow tract. The accelerating blood exiting the ventricle will then carry the leaflet into the outflow tract, meeting the septum and causing obstruction to flow and regurgitation through the mitral valve orifice.

There are usually significant abnormalities of the papillary muscles with multiple heads and often very high origin from the ventricular wall. The posteromedial commissural papillary muscle is often in multiple parts. These abnormalities lead to extreme variations in chordal length. The leaflets are commonly divided into multiple segments with deep indentations commonly reaching the annular margin. The leaflets billow and there is excessive motion of the leaflets at the annulus. This often leads to significant annular calcification, which may extend into the base of the leaflet tissue and into the papillary muscle heads. This calcification can extend from trigone to trigone along the posterior annulus but is only rarely seen in the septal portion. The excessive leaflet motion commonly gives rise to a grooved partial separation of the atrial endocardium and haemosiderin staining is commonly found (bluish green material along the annular groove). Although orifice dilatation (ventricular dilatation) occurs, the mitral orifice is naturally large in this setting.

Whilst the pre-operative echocardiogram images may suggest that both leaflets are prolapsing, quite often the anterior leaflet prolapse is as a result of lack of support from the posterior leaflet. Once the posterior leaflet prolapse has been corrected, proper leaflet coaptation will occur without anterior leaflet prolapse.

The key principles in repairing bi-leaflet prolapse include:

(a) Most importantly, identifying all of the components of prolapse of both leaflets.
(b) Deciding on whether the height of the posterior leaflet needs to be reduced to obviate the risk of SAM, as discussed above and elsewhere (see Chap. 15).
(c) Restoring normal leaflet excursion of the prolapsing segments with Gore-Tex neo-chordae.
(d) 'Fine-tuning' the repair by using cleft closure sutures, small triangular resections of the anterior leaflet, additional Gore-Tex neo-chordae or commissural closure sutures, if necessary.
(e) Implanting an annuloplasty band or ring to support the repair and prevent subsequent annular dilatation.

The first step in repairing these valves is to perform segmental analysis of the mitral valve both by trans-oesophageal echocardiography and intra-operative visualisation, using saline insufflation and nerve hook assessment. This will allow identification of which segments and commissures that will require repair, although it may involve all segments of both leaflets. Frequently the P1 segment is of more normal height and is not prolapsing. If that is the case, then it may be used as a reference point to judge the appropriate height of the rest of the leaflet. If all the segments are prolapsing, then, the annular plane is used as the 'point of reference' to determine the degree of prolapse of each of the segments and the height of the neo-chordae. It is also important to identify any annular or leaflet calcification, which will be very obvious. Any leaflet restriction through the calcification or any fibrous tissue must be identified and dealt with. Papillary muscle abnormalities, which are usually present, must also be identified. Ill-defined secondary and tertiary lesions are commonly missed on the echocardiogram and need to be addressed, as even if there is a degree of coaptation, they are likely to progress in later years. The presence of jet lesions on the posterior left atrial wall will identify the sites of prolapse.

Experience has shown that in cases of bi-leaflet prolapse, addressing the posterior leaflet problems first will allow the surgeon to decide whether or not the anterior leaflet will need any attention. As mentioned earlier, restoring the posterior leaflet to an even and normal coaptation plane will allow the operator to visualise any true anterior leaflet prolapse. The height of the posterior leaflet and the amount of prolapse first need to be assessed. Excessive height will increase the possibility of SAM and can be dealt with either through leaflet resection or neo-chordae shortened to the point where the leaflet is drawn down into the ventricle to achieve the correct coaptation point for the anterior leaflet. Whilst this latter method can give a good closure line, it can significantly restrict posterior leaflet motion. Appropriate adjustment of the leaflet height by resection can give a better-tailored result.

Leaflet resection techniques focus on the posterior leaflet and include resecting the base of the posterior leaflet subtending the tallest part of the leaflet anywhere from commissure to commissure, quadrangular resection with or without sliding plasty, targeted wedge resection, or multiple triangular resections. The choice between these resection techniques depends on the quantity of tissue in the posterior leaflet and specifically the height of the individual scallops, with the aim of the repair to produce a symmetrical (all scallops equal in height) posterior leaflet <1.5 cm tall.

To reduce the risk of SAM following valve repair, a commonly used technique to reduce the height of the posterior leaflet is to detach it from the posterior annulus and to resect an appropriate amount of basal leaflet (closest to the annulus) tissue, before reattaching the it (Fig. 9.2). The usually asymmetrical heights of the various segments of the posterior leaflet may require asymmetric excision of tissue to produce a

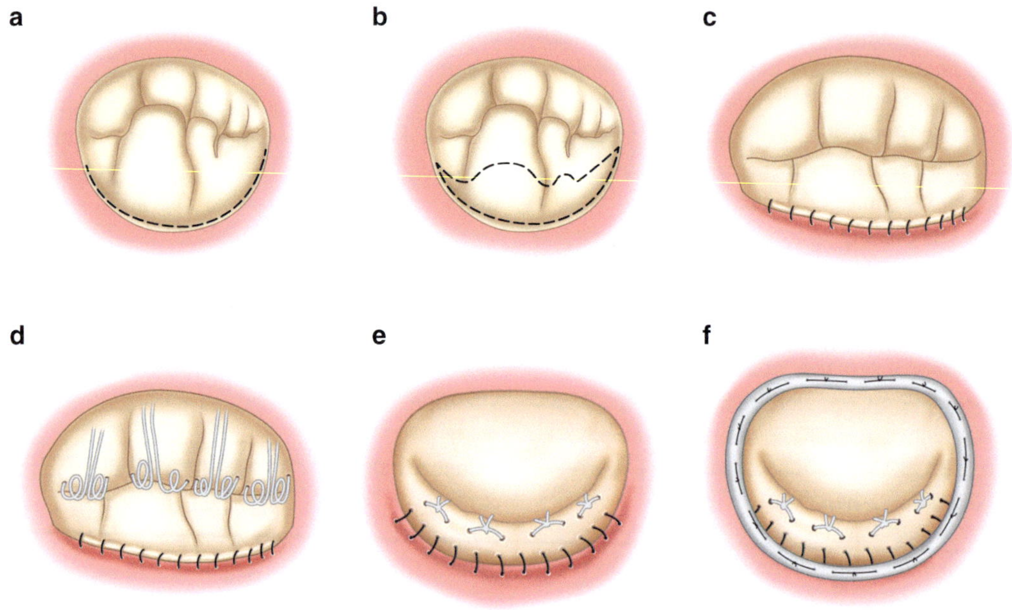

Fig. 9.2 Surgical repair of bi-leaflet prolapse by leaflet height reduction with (**a**) detachment of the posterior leaflet from the annulus, (**b**) resection of the basal portion of the posterior leaflet, (**c**) reattachment of the posterior leaflet to the annulus, (**d**) implantation of Gore-Tex neo-chordae to the markedly billowing and prolapsing posterior leaflet, (**e**) tying down the Gore-Tex neo-chordae, followed by (**f**) ring annuloplasty

symmetrical residual posterior leaflet following resection. Simply detaching and reattaching the posterior leaflet reduces the height of the leaflet by 3–6 mm, depending on the depth of suture placement from the leaflet edge during reattachment. This brings the line of coaptation towards the posterior annulus, thereby reducing the risk of anterior displacement of the mitral valve during systole into the left ventricular outflow tract. There may well be elongated or ruptured chordae along the free margin and this will need to be corrected by the insertion of neo-chordae. The choice of annuloplasty band or ring size is also important to prevent SAM.

Implanting Gore-Tex neo-chordae can also be used in these patients to achieve downward leaflet displacement, thereby preventing leaflet prolapse and significantly reducing the leaflet height. Neo-chordae used in this way transforms the prolapsing, billowing leaflet into a nearly vertical, buttress, which lies parallel to the posterior wall of the left ventricle and against which the anterior leaflet closes. Once posterior leaflet pathology has been repaired, the anterior leaflet can be assessed to identify whether the anterior leaflet prolapse is simply the result of a lack of support for the posterior leaflet or results from excessive chordal length. Ring or band annuloplasty is then performed to stabilize the repair, with sizing based on the area of the whole mitral valve orifice.

Once the primary lesions have been repaired, secondary lesions may become apparent. This happens because the dominant lesions overshadow lesser defects that lie in a different plane and are easily over-looked. It is important to correct leaflet bulges where the coaptation line is irregular. The aim of the repair is to achieve a competent valve that has no or minimal residual billowing of the leaflets, good depth of coaptation, a symmetrical closure line parallel to the posterior mitral valve annulus and is not at risk of SAM. This is evaluated with static testing, by injecting saline into the LV under enough pressure to distend the aortic root and marking the line of coaptation with methylene blue ink. The depth of coaptation is measured following saline evacuation from the LV and should be around 8–10 mm.

Another technique that is used for patients with bi-leaflet prolapse is the Alfieri edge-to-edge technique (Fig. 8.8), which can simplify the repair. Approximation of the central part of the valve on the P2 and A2 scallops of the mitral valve at the level of the annular plane can eliminate a significant amount of the myxomatous tissue from billowing and prolapsing, and hence abolish or significantly reduce the degree of regurgitation. Implantation of an annuloplasty ring is important to complete the repair. If regurgitation is not eliminated by this technique, however, its use is questionable, as valve insertion with complete subvalvar preservation will give a better long term result.

In some patients with mitral regurgitation caused by moderate bi-leaflet prolapse, in the absence of chordal elongation or rupture, simply placing an annuloplasty ring alone can block the outward movement of the posterior annulus (basal left ventricle), thereby eliminating the prolapse.

Surgical Technique

In this patient, horizontal mattress 2/0 Ethibond annuloplasty sutures were placed around the circumference of the posterior annulus, with a 5–10 mm width and approximately 1 mm apart. The mitral valve was assessed using segmental analysis of the leaflets and the subvalvular apparatus. This was correlated with the trans-oesophageal echocardiographical findings. Marked prolapse of all segments of the anterior and posterior leaflets was observed, associated with elongated chordae tendineae, originating from both the anterolateral and posteromedial papillary muscles. Stay sutures (5/0 Prolene) were placed on the anterior and posterior leaflets to provide better access to the subvalvular apparatus for subsequent Gore-Tex neo-chordae implantation (Fig. 9.3a).

Using gentle traction on the posterior leaflet stay sutures and posterior annuloplasty sutures, the heights of P1, P2 and P3 were assessed individually to determine whether any excess of tissue on the posterior leaflet would leave the valve at risk of SAM. The posterior leaflet was incised horizontally, at the mid-point of its insertion to the annulus, using a N°11 blade (Fig. 9.3b). The incision was then continued parallel to the posterior annulus, just short of both commissures, thereby detaching the posterior leaflet from the annulus (Fig. 9.3c). As the height of P2 was 28 mm, the base of the posterior leaflet was then resected (Fig. 9.3d), to reduce its height. This moved the line of coaptation posteriorly, thereby reducing the risk of SAM and subsequent left ventricular outflow tract obstruction. The extent of resection depends on the degree of excess tissue of the posterior leaflet, ensuring that height of the posterior leaflet is <15 mm throughout its circumference. Any annular calcification was then debrided.

The posterior leaflet was then reattached to the annulus, using 4/0 Prolene (Fig. 9.3e) and the degree of prolapse of the anterior and posterior leaflets was then reassessed with a reduced posterior leaflet height. In this patient, it was apparent that Gore-Tex neo-chordae were only required for the posterior leaflet. Using gentle traction on the anterior and posterior leaflet stay sutures, both the anterolateral and posteromedial papillary muscles could be accessed. Pledgeted CV-4 Gore-Tex neo-chordae were passed through the fibrous part of the papillary muscles using a horizontal mattress technique (Fig. 9.3f). Gore-Tex neo-chordae placed to the right of the midline on the posterior leaflet were anchored to the posteromedial papillary muscle, whilst those placed to the left of the midline were anchored to the anterolateral papillary muscle. The native chordae were also used as a guide to determine which head of the papillary muscles to insert the neo-chordae. The free ends of the neo-chordae were then placed through the leaflets approximately 5 mm from the free edge using a single-loop technique.

Competency of the mitral valve was then assessed with static testing, by injecting cold saline into the left ventricle using a bulb syringe. The free ends of the Gore-Tex neo-chordae were then tied with the leaflets at, or just below the annular plane and when competency of the mitral valve had been achieved. Each neo-chord was tied with a total of 12 knots (6 in each direction) to ensure that the Gore-Tex knots did not loosen.

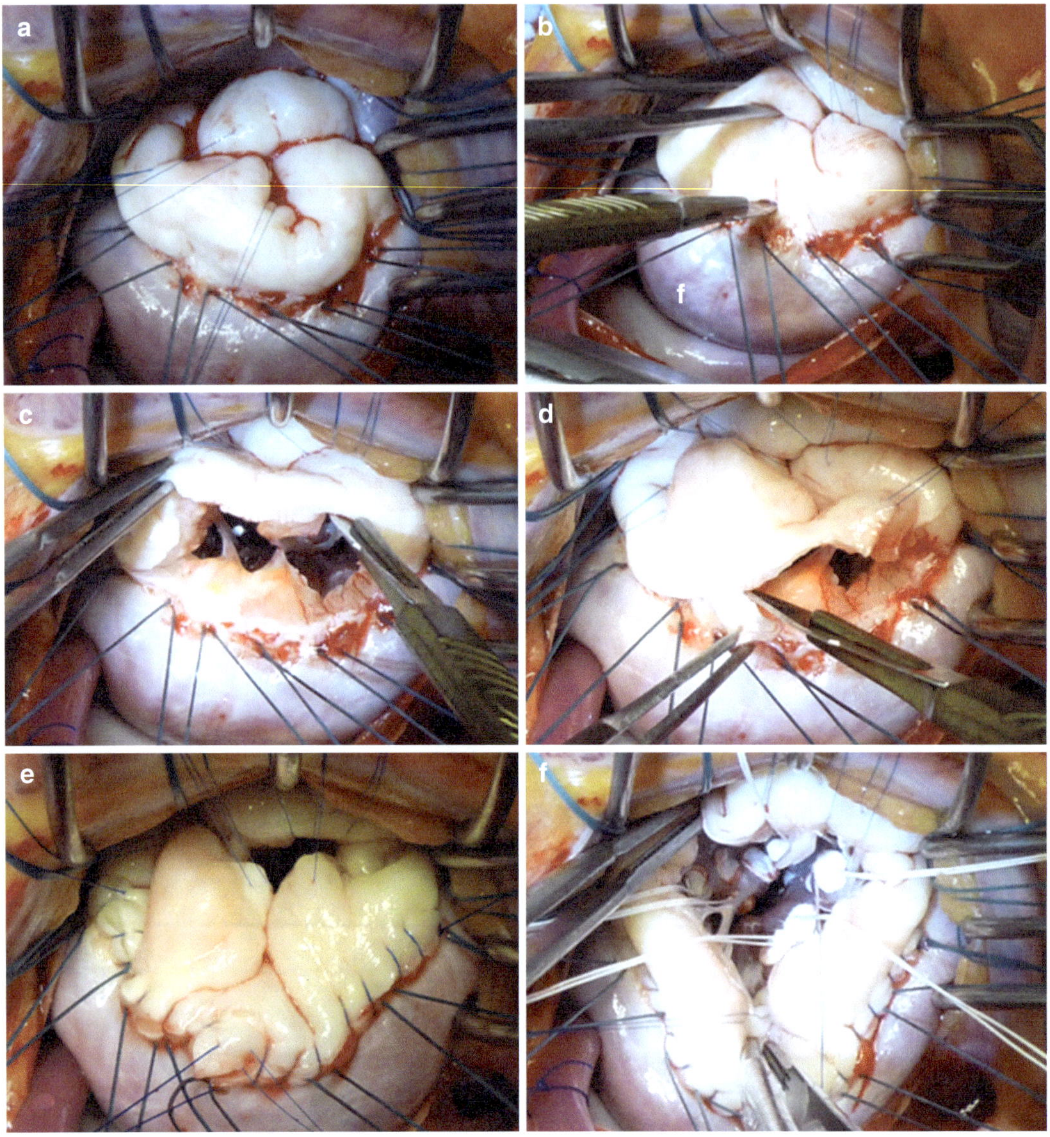

Fig. 9.3 Operative images illustrating (**a**) segmental analysis of the mitral valve, demonstrating marked bi-leaflet prolapse, (**b**) incision at the centre of the annular attachment of the posterior leaflet, (**c**) extension of the incision just short of the anterolateral and posteromedial commissures, (**d**) excision of the basal portion of the posterior leaflet to reduce its height, (**e**) reattachment of the posterior leaflet to the annulus using 4/0 Prolene and (**f**) implantation of Gore-Tex neo-chordae to the anterolateral and posteromedial papillary muscles

With the left ventricle distended with saline, marking the atrial surface of the mitral valve leaflets with a sterile pen allowed assessment of the depth of coaptation, which ought to achieve an optimal depth of least 8–10 mm. An appropriately sized annuloplasty band was then chosen, according to the surface area of the whole mitral valve orifice (i.e. the surface area of the anterior and posterior leaflets together), and inserted using the already placed annuloplasty sutures. Following implantation of the annuloplasty band, injecting cold saline again allowed the mitral valve to be assessed for competency, adequate depth of coaptation,

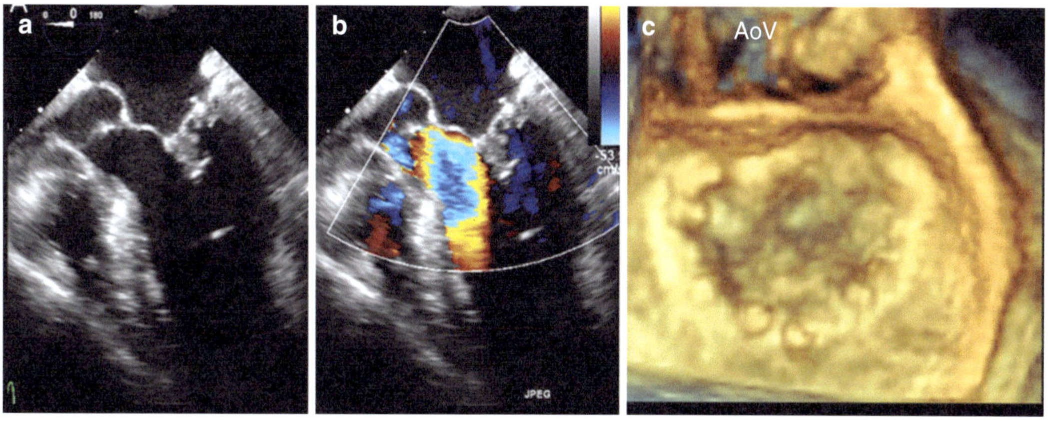

Fig. 9.4 Post-bypass intra-operative trans-oesophageal echocardiographical images demonstrating a good depth of coaptation between the anterior and posterior leaflets and no SAM on (**a**) mid-oesophageal 5-chamber view and a competent mitral valve with no residual mitral regurgitation on (**b**) the corresponding view with colour flow Doppler. (**c**) Three-dimensional surgical view in systole demonstrates the annuloplasty band in situ and no residual prolapse. AoV aortic valve

that the coaptation line runs parallel to the posterior annulus and that the height of the posterior leaflet was ~15 mm. Although unlikely with this technique, any residual regurgitation through the clefts at the coaptation edge were closed using 5/0 Prolene.

It is important to note in this patient that no additional work was needed for the anterior leaflet once the posterior leaflet prolapse was addressed. This pseudo-prolapse of the anterior leaflet seen preoperatively resolved once the posterior leaflet was repaired.

Post-operative Echocardiogram

The post-repair trans-oesophageal echocardiogram (Fig. 9.4) confirmed:

1. Normal physiological functioning of the mitral valve complex with no residual mitral regurgitation.
2. The depth of leaflet coaptation was >8 mm.
3. The height of the posterior mitral valve leaflet was <15 mm.
4. No systolic anterior movement of the mitral valve leaflets into the left ventricular outflow tract or left ventricular outflow obstruction.

Surgical Tips

1. Repair is usually feasible in patients with bi-leaflet prolapse.
2. Segmental analysis of the mitral valve is crucial to clearly identify which segments require repair.
3. The use of multiple Gore-Tex neochordae allows preservation of the mitral valve leaflet tissue to increase the surface area of coaptation.
4. Often, reduction of the height of the posterior leaflet is important to reduce the risk of SAM.
5. The use of an annuloplasty band or ring will stabilise the posterior portion of the mitral annulus preventing subsequent annular dilation.
6. Obtaining an adequate and even depth of coaptation (8–10 mm) is important for the long-term durability of the repair.

Comment

Results of mitral valve surgery for bileaflet prolapse have shown excellent outcomes, with an in-hospital mortality <1% and a low peri-operative complication rate. Although somewhat inferior to those for isolated posterior leaflet prolapse, most published results of mid to long term outcome measures have demonstrated excellent freedom from recurrent mitral regurgitation (90% with <2+ MR at 8 years), freedom from reoperation (95% at 8 years) and survival (89% at 8 years).

Recommended Reading

Bellitti R, Petrone G, Buonocore M, Nappi G, Santé P. Anatomic reconstruction in degenerative mitral valve bileaflet prolapse: long-term results. Ann Thorac Surg. 2014;97(2):563–8.

David TE, Ivanov J, Armstrong S, Christie D, Rakowski H. A comparison of outcomes of mitral valve repair for degenerative disease with posterior, anterior, and bileaflet prolapse. J Thorac Cardiovasc Surg. 2005;130:1242–9.

Jouan J, Berrebi A, Chauvaud S, Menasché P, Carpentier A, Fabiani JN. Mitral valve reconstruction in Barlow disease: long-term echographic results and implications for surgical management. J Thorac Cardiovasc Surg. 2012;143(4 Suppl):S17–20.

Miura T, Ariyoshi T, Tanigawa K, Matsukuma S, Yokose S, Sumi M, Hisatomi K, Tsuneto A, Hashizume K, Eishi K. Technical aspects of mitral valve repair in Barlow's valve with prolapse of both leaflets: triangular resection for excess tissue, sophisticated chordal replacement, and their combination (the restoration technique). Gen Thorac Cardiovasc Surg. 2015;63(2):61–70.

Okada Y, Nasu M, Koyama T, Shomura Y, Yuzaki M, Murashita T, Fukunaga N, Konishi Y. Outcomes of mitral valve repair for bileaflet prolapse. J Thorac Cardiovasc Surg. 2012;143(4 Suppl):S21–3.

Commissural Prolapse

10

Keywords
Commissural prolapse · Papillary muscle · Commissural closure · Gore-Tex neo-chordae · Papillary muscle shortening · Commissural resection and reconstruction · Commissuroplasty · Mitral regurgitation · Ring annuloplasty

Case History

A 62 year-old female presented with a prolonged history of increasing exertional dyspnoea associated with lethargy. There was no history of rheumatic fever or infective endocarditis. She had previously been diagnosed with mitral regurgitation, which had been monitored with serial echocardiography for several years.

Echocardiographical Findings

Trans-oesophageal mid-oesophageal 4-chamber echocardiographic images revealed prolapse of the posteromedial commissure, secondary to ruptured chordae tendineae (Fig. 10.1a). Doppler flow across the mitral valve in this view demonstrated a very eccentric jet of mitral regurgitation (MR) (Fig. 10.1b). Quantification of the regurgitation, using the PISA method, revealed severe MR, with an effective regurgitant orifice area of 62 mm^2 and a regurgitant fraction of 54%, associated with a vena contracta of 0.73 cm. The left atrium (diameter 4.84 cm) and left ventricle (end-systolic diameter 4.5 cm and end-diastolic diameter 6.8 cm) were dilated. Left ventricular systolic function was impaired with an ejection fraction of 52%. Isolated prolapse of the posteromedial commissure was confirmed on the mid-oesophageal 2-chamber (Fig. 10.1c) and three dimensional (3D) 'surgical' views (Fig. 10.1d).

Surgical Strategy

Commissural prolapse may be limited to either the anterior or the posterior leaflet but often involves both. The posteromedial commissure is the most frequent site. Echocardiographic diagnosis of commissural prolapse can be difficult and may be missed, being overshadowed by more prominent lesions especially in the setting of Barlow's disease. Therefore, careful intra-operative inspection is essential.

The anatomical support of the commissural leaflet tissue is normally provided by a characteristic 'fan' of chordae tendineae arising from 'horse-shoe' shaped papillary muscles (Fig. 1.10). It is, however, common to find significant congenital anatomical variation of the posteromedial papillary muscle and its associated chords. This diminishes the required mechanical

N. Moorjani et al., *Operative Mitral and Tricuspid Valve Surgery*,
https://doi.org/10.1007/978-1-4471-4204-1_10

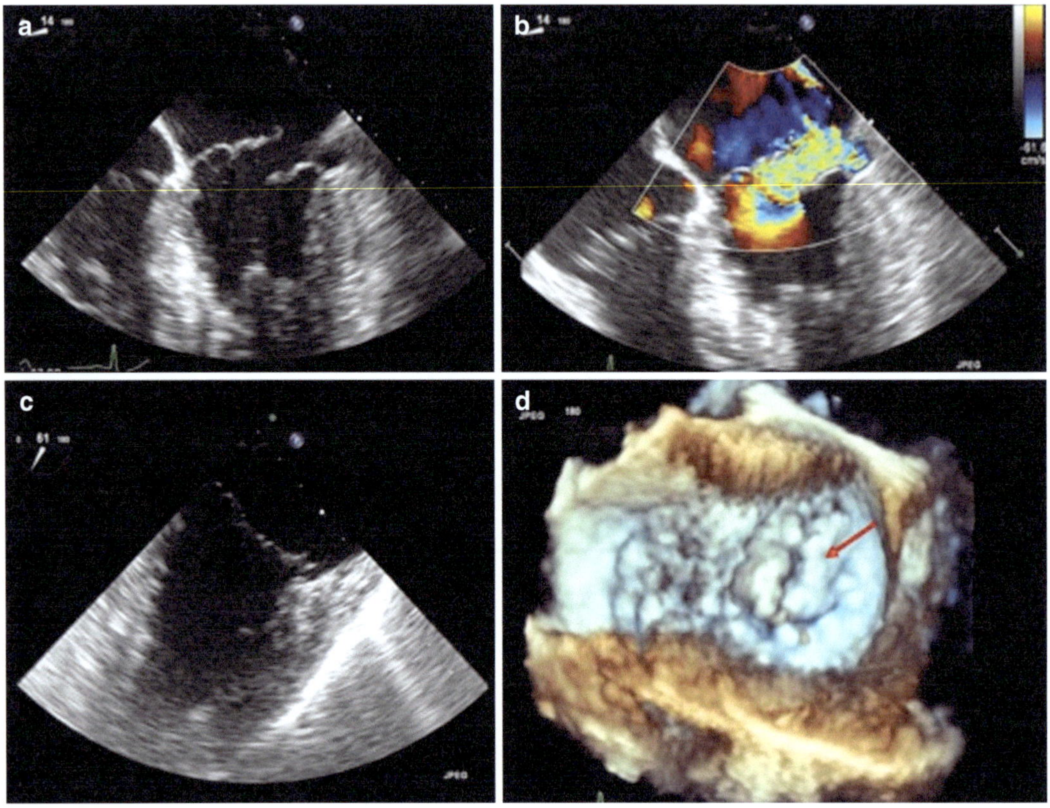

Fig. 10.1 Trans-oesophageal echocardiographical images demonstrating prolapse of the posteromedial commissure, secondary to ruptured chordae tendineae on (**a**) mid-oesophageal 4-chamber view, with corresponding (**b**) colour flow Doppler revealing a very eccentric regurgitant jet sweeping horizontally across the anterior leaflet, and (**c**) mid-oesophageal 2-chamber view. (**d**) Three-dimensional surgical view demonstrating posteromedial commissural prolapse (red arrow)

support in this critical region. The established lesion may involve one or both of the leaflets, their chordae tendineae and associated papillary muscles, with chordal elongation or rupture being the most easily visible manifestations. Even though the chordal lesion is the obvious one, it is always accompanied by some malformation of the valve components, such as high rising papillary muscles, often with multiple heads, several of which may be very small. There may be a complete lack of chordal support (Fig. 10.2).

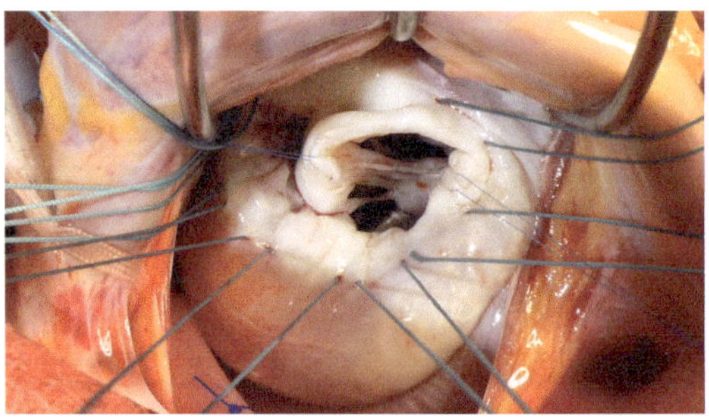

Fig. 10.2 Absence of chordae at the posteromedial commissure

Tissue destruction from endocarditis may also present with commissural prolapse. This lesion is usually associated with a pre-existing anatomical lesion of the kind described above.

Whilst commissural prolapse is often regarded as a difficult lesion to repair satisfactorily, there are a variety of techniques described to restore competence with excellent long-term clinical and echocardiographic results. The choice between these techniques is determined by the underlying aetiology and the nature of the resulting anatomical lesion.

For limited lesions, commissural closure with inverting sutures may give a satisfactory result. Carpentier referred to a variant of this technique as the 'Magic' stitch. The implantation of Gore-Tex neo-chordae to either or both leaflet margins works well with more extensive lesions where there is a paucity or absence of natural chordae. In some cases, limited resection, which is usually confined to the posterior leaflet portion of the commissure, with or without sliding plasty or annular plication will give good results. Papillary muscle translocation or shortening has regained popularity with some surgeons, although the originally described chordal shortening, as proposed by Carpentier, has been shown to be unstable with time. The setting of bi-leaflet commissural prolapse with elongated fan chords or short chords associated with high rising papillary muscles within the ventricle is the ideal lesion for this technique. Sometimes the distance between the tips of the papillary muscles and the leaflet margin is so small that the use of neo-chords is impossible.

Commissural Closure

This technique, which is also known as a para-commissural edge-to-edge repair or modified 'Magic' suture, provides a simple functional (rather than anatomical) method for managing a patient with limited commissural prolapse, especially in patients with a large mitral valve orifice area. It involves using a 5/0 polypropylene suture placed 5 mm from the leaflet edges to imbricate the leaflet edges at the site of the commissural prolapse, restoring competency (Fig. 10.3). More than one suture may be necessary. When using this technique, it is important to consider the resultant effective valve orifice area to avoid producing mitral stenosis.

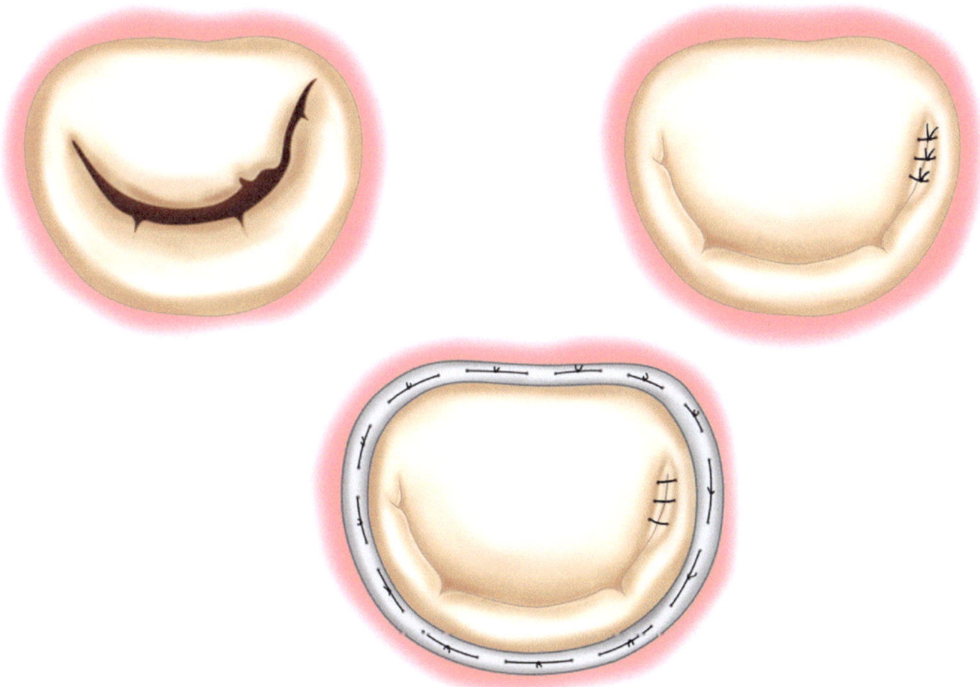

Fig. 10.3 Chordal prolapse treated by commissural closure using a 5/0 polypropylene suture, followed by placement of an annuloplasty ring

Chordal Replacement

As with anterior or posterior mitral valve leaflet prolapse, neo-chordal implantation aims to restore normal leaflet coaptation height and normal planar closure. Elongated or ruptured chordae tendineae are supplanted with Gore-Tex polytetrafluoroethylene (PTFE) sutures (W.L. Gore & Associates, Flagstaff, AZ, USA). The major advantage of this technique is that it does not require the excision of valve tissue, thereby preserving leaflet morphology, mobility and the maximal possible orifice area of the mitral valve. Chordal replacement is performed by passing both limbs of pledgeted or non-pledgeted CV-4 Gore-Tex sutures through the fibro-muscular part of the papillary muscle head that was providing chordal support to the prolapsing segment of the commissure and then through the leaflet tissue (Fig. 8.2), using the previously described single loop technique (see Chap. 8). The height of the Gore-Tex neo-chordae are adjusted by raising or lowering the leaflet height on the suture. The result can then be assessed with saline distention of the left ventricle. With the ventricle tensioned, the height and evenness of the coaptation margin is marked using a sterile pen. When a satisfactory position has been obtained, the Gore-Tex sutures are locked with twelve secure knots as previously described.

Leaflet Resection

Localised leaflet resection of unsupported leaflet tissue at the commissure with subsequent recon-

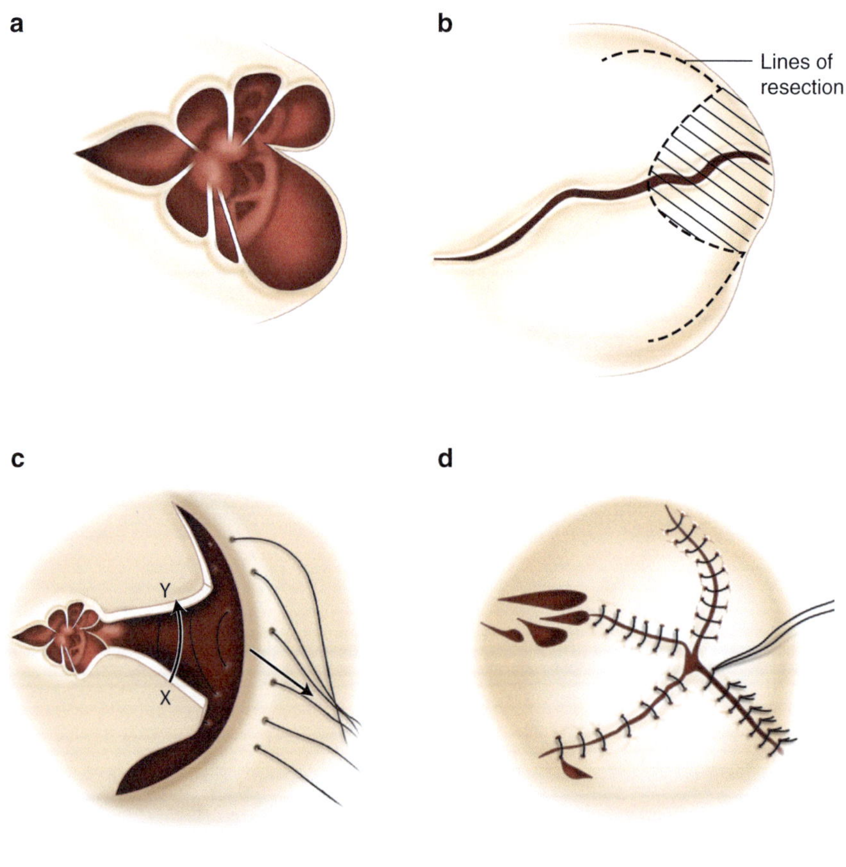

Fig. 10.4 Commissural resection and reconstruction. (**a**) Posteromedial commisural prolapse, (**b**) quadrangular resection of the commissure with sliding plasty of both the anterior and posterior leaflets, (**c**) compression annuloplasty sutures followed by (**d**) commissural reconstruction

struction can be also used and is very useful when there is a significant excess of leaflet tissue, for example in Barlow's disease (Fig. 10.4). This may involve a limited wedge or quadrangular resection, with the annular distance being greater than the marginal distance to prevent tension on the reunited leaflet edges. Simple annular plication or a sliding plasty is almost invariably required (see Chap. 7). An additional commissural closure suture may also be required to support the newly created commissure.

Papillary Muscle Shortening

This technique is useful for commissural prolapse caused by elongation of multiple chordae arising from the same papillary muscle head. Downward displacement of the papillary muscle head can be achieved by a small triangular wedge resection at the base of the head, using the prolapsing distance as a guide to the size of the wedge of tissue to be resected (Fig. 8.6). The papillary muscle head is then secured within the trench using a pledgeted 4/0 Prolene suture. An alternative technique is to make a longitudinal split in the papillary muscle and then resuturing the head to a lower point on the papillary muscle. This technique seems to work better than the original chordal shortening method described by Carpentier because the displaced muscle will heal into the rest of the papillary muscle whereas the imbricated chords do not.

The rationale for choosing between these different techniques depends upon the type and extent of commissural prolapse, the degree of excess leaflet tissue present and the size of the mitral valve area. Although, commissural closure is a simple, reproducible technique that is the most common method employed to repair short lengths of commissural prolapse, it is a non-physiological technique that reduces the effective mitral valve orifice area. In an attempt to achieve a more physiological repair, patients with limited commissural prolapse can be treated with limited leaflet resection alone provided that the residual leaflet tissue is supported by chords that produce good coaptation. Neo-chordal implantation is an excellent option for patients with extensive commissural prolapse. In isolated posterior leaflet commissural prolapse, leaflet resection, combined with annular plication or sliding plasty may be indicated. In patients with elongation of multiple chordae originating from a single papillary muscle head, especially in the presence of very short chords associated with a high origin of the papillary muscle from the ventricular wall, shortening may be the ideal technique to treat the prolapse and restore competency at the commissural area. In patients with extensive tissue destruction following endocarditis causing commissural prolapse, the defect can be repaired with autologous pericardium, bovine pericardium, autologous tricuspid valve posterior leaflet or a mitral homograft. It is important to assess the remainder of the mitral valve scallops, as commissural prolapse often occurs in conjunction with prolapse of other parts of the anterior or posterior leaflets. After repair of the commissural prolapse, the procedure is completed with implantation of an annuloplasty ring or band.

Surgical Technique

The mitral valve was assessed, using segmental analysis of the leaflets and the subvalvular apparatus, and correlated with the trans-oesophageal echocardiographical findings. Marked prolapse of the posteromedial commissure was observed, associated with ruptured chordae tendineae, which originated from the multiple heads of the posteromedial papillary muscle. In addition, there was an excess of leaflet tissue.

Horizontal mattress annuloplasty sutures (2/0 Ethibond) were placed around the circumference of the mitral valve, with a 5 mm width and approximately 1 mm apart, to provide much improved access and visualisation of the mitral valve leaflets and subvalvular apparatus for subsequent repair. Stay sutures (5/0 Prolene) were placed around the normal chordae tendineae attached on either side of the prolapsed area of the posteromedial commissure. Gentle traction on these stay sutures allowed the margins of prolapsed commissure to be clearly delineated and to assess the subvalvular apparatus. This revealed that the ruptured chordae

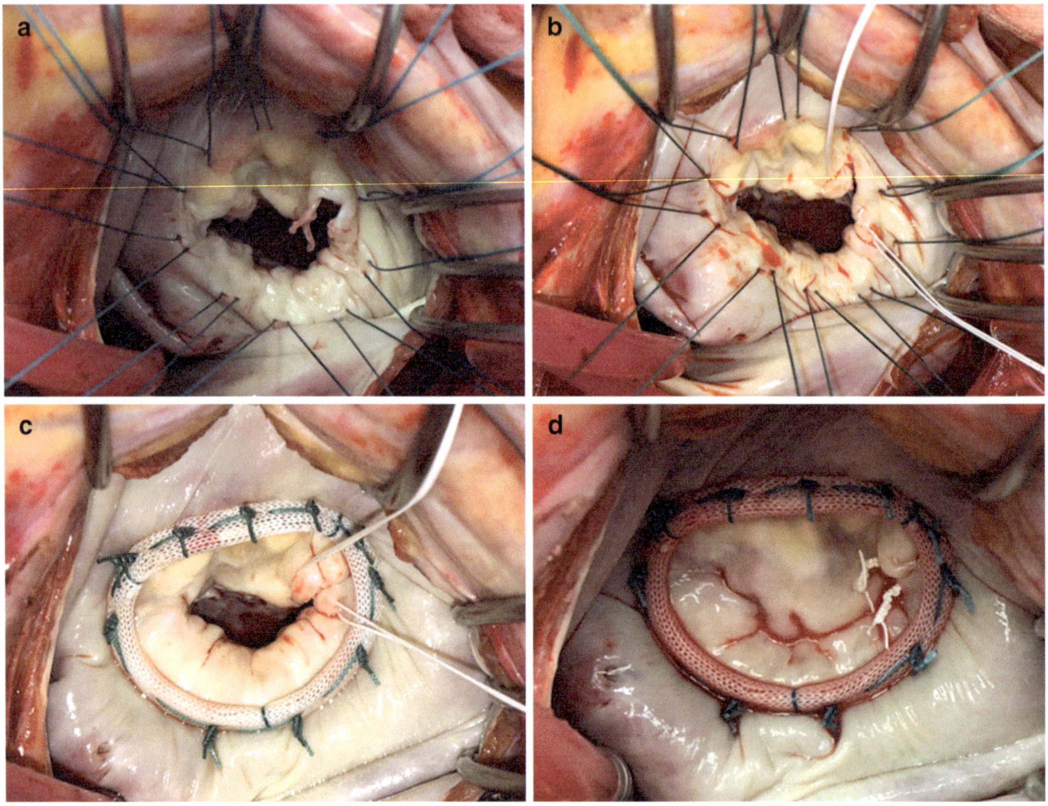

Fig. 10.5 Operative images illustrating (**a**) segmental analysis of the mitral valve, demonstrating isolated prolapse of the posteromedial commissure, secondary to chordal rupture, (**b**) implantation of two Gore-Tex neo-chordae at the posteromedial commissure, (**c**) implantation of an annuloplasty ring, and (**d**) following tying the Gore-Tex neo-chordae, saline distension of the left ventricle demonstrating a competent mitral valve

originated from the different heads of the posteromedial papillary muscle (Fig. 10.5a).

In view of this, the commissural prolapse was repaired using chordal replacement. A neo-chord was placed by passing both limbs of a CV-4 Gore-Tex suture (W.L. Gore & Associates, Flagstaff, AZ, USA) through the fibrous part of the anterior head of the posteromedial papillary muscle, using a simple U-stich. One of the limbs of the Gore-Tex suture was then passed through the prolapsing commissural segment of the anterior leaflet about 5 mm away from the leaflet edge and 2–3 mm away from the boundary of normal leaflet, from the ventricular side to the atrial side and then through a second time. This was then repeated for the second limb of the Gore-Tex neo-chord (Fig. 10.5b). A second CV-4 Gore-Tex neo-chord was placed through the fibrous part of the posterior head of the posteromedial papillary muscle and in a similar fashion through the prolapsing commissural segment of the posterior leaflet.

The provisional height of the Gore-Tex neo-chordae was then determined by using the level of the annulus as a reference to guide to the correct length and tension of the implanted neo-chord. Competency of the mitral valve was then assessed with static testing, by injecting cold saline into the left ventricle, using a bulb syringe. With a left ventricle distended with saline, the depth of coaptation was assessed by marking the atrial surface of the mitral valve leaflets with a sterile pen. The depth of coaptation can be increased to achieve an optimal depth of at least 8 mm by adjusting the length of Gore-Tex suture beneath the leaflet.

A 34 mm Physio II annuloplasty ring (Edwards Lifesciences, Irvine, CA) was then chosen, according to the surface area of the whole mitral valve orifice, and tied down in situ (Fig. 10.5c).

Following tying of the neo-chordae, distension of the left ventricle with cold saline allowed the mitral valve to be assessed to demonstrate an adequate depth of coaptation, symmetrical coaptation line and the absence of residual prolapse at the posteromedial commissure (Fig. 10.5d).

Post-operative Echocardiogram

The post-repair trans-oesophageal echocardiogram (Fig. 10.6) confirmed:

1. Normal physiological functioning of the mitral valve complex with no residual mitral regurgitation at the posteromedial commissure or any degree of mitral stenosis
2. No residual prolapse at the posteromedial commissure
3. The depth of leaflet coaptation was >8 mm.

Surgical Tips

1. A number of different operative techniques exist for treating commissural prolapse and the rationale for choosing between them depends upon the type and extent of commissural prolapse, the proximity of the papillary muscles to the leaflet, the degree of excess leaflet tissue present and the size of the mitral valve area.
2. If commissural prolapse is caused by elongated chordae tendineae, without abnormally high papillary muscles, chordal replacement can provide an excellent repair technique
3. Chordal replacement for commissural prolapse should be supported by implantation of an annuloplasty ring

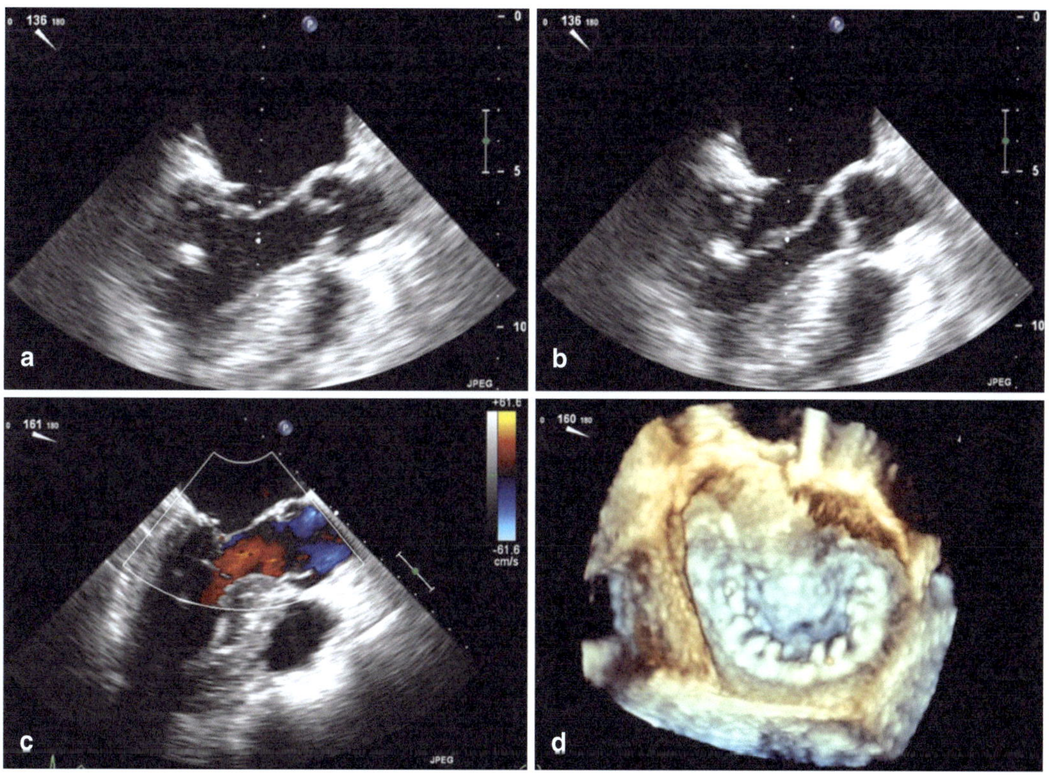

Fig. 10.6 Post-bypass intra-operative trans-oesophageal echocardiographical long-axis images demonstrating no SAM and a 9 mm depth of coaptation between the anterior and posterior leaflets in (**a**) systole and (**b**) diastole, and a competent mitral valve with no residual mitral regurgitation on (**c**) the colour flow Doppler. (**d**) Three-dimensional image demonstrating a competent mitral valve with no prolapse of the posteromedial commissure

Comment

Results of mitral valve surgery following repair of commissural prolapse using a variety of techniques have shown excellent outcomes, with an in-hospital mortality <2% and a low peri-operative complication rate. Long-term outcome measures have also demonstrated excellent freedom from recurrent mitral regurgitation (91.4% with < moderate MR at 10 years), freedom from reoperation on the mitral valve (92.5% at 10 years) and survival (96.7% at 10 years).

Recommended Reading

Aubert S, Barreda T, Acar C, Leprince P, Bonnet N, Ecochard R, Pavie A, Gandjbakhch I. Mitral valve repair for commissural prolapse: surgical techniques and long term results. Eur J Cardiothorac Surg. 2005;28(3):443–7.

De Bonis M, Lapenna E, Taramasso M, Pozzoli A, La Canna G, Calabrese MC, Alfieri O. Is commissural closure associated with mitral annuloplasty a durable technique for the treatment of mitral regurgitation? A long-term (≤15 years) clinical and echocardiographic study. J Thorac Cardiovasc Surg. 2014;147(6):1900–6.

Shimizu A, Kasegawa H, Tabata M, Fukui T, Takanashi S. Long-term outcomes of mitral valve repair for isolated commissural prolapse: up to 17-year experience. Ann Thorac Surg. 2015;99(1):43–7.

Ischaemic Mitral Regurgitation

11

Keywords
Ischaemic mitral regurgitation · Coronary artery disease · Myocardial infarction · Coronary artery bypass grafting · Reduction annuloplasty · Restricted leaflet motion · Papillary muscle displacement · Leaflet augmentation · Mitral valve replacement · Papillary muscle relocation

Case History

A 67 year-old man presented with a history of increasing dyspnoea on exertion, associated with a reduced exercise tolerance of 400 yards. He had previously sustained an inferior myocardial infarction resulting in impaired left ventricular function. Clinical examination revealed a pan-systolic murmur, radiating into the axilla and a laterally displaced apex beat. Moderate bilateral peripheral oedema was also present. Coronary angiography revealed severe three vessel coronary artery disease, with an occluded right coronary artery.

Echocardiographical Findings

Trans-thoracic parasternal long-axis and apical 3-chamber echocardiographic images revealed restriction of the both the anterior and posterior mitral valve leaflets, associated with dilatation of the mitral valve annulus (Fig. 11.1a, b). This tenting effect resulted in the characteristic 'seagull' sign of the anterior leaflet in ischaemic mitral regurgitation, with a bending angle >45°. Doppler flow across the mitral valve demonstrated a posteriorly directed jet of mitral regurgitation (MR), consistent with posterior leaflet restriction, caused by ischaemic fibrosis in the wall of the left ventricle following myocardial infarction (Fig. 11.1c, d). This was also observed on the 3D images, where tethering of both leaflets can be seen, especially in the P2-P3 region (Fig. 11.1e, f).

Quantification of the regurgitation, using the PISA method, revealed severe MR, with an effective orifice area of 43 mm^2 and regurgitant volume of 63 mL, associated with a vena contracta of 0.72 cm. The left atrium (diameter 6.1 cm) and left ventricle (end-systolic diameter 5.1 cm and end-diastolic diameter 6.7 cm) were dilated, associated with impaired left ventricular function, with an ejection fraction of 39%. Peak MR velocity, a measure of closing forces on the MV, was obtained by continuous-wave Doppler.

It is important to note that the Doppler echocardiographic thresholds that are used to define the severity of ischaemic mitral regurgitation previously differed from those used for degenerative mitral valve disease, where severe ischaemic MR was characterized by an effective regurgitant orifice area $\geq$20 mm^2, regurgitant volume (RV) >30 mL/beat and vena contracta width $\geq$4 mm.

N. Moorjani et al., *Operative Mitral and Tricuspid Valve Surgery*,
https://doi.org/10.1007/978-1-4471-4204-1_11

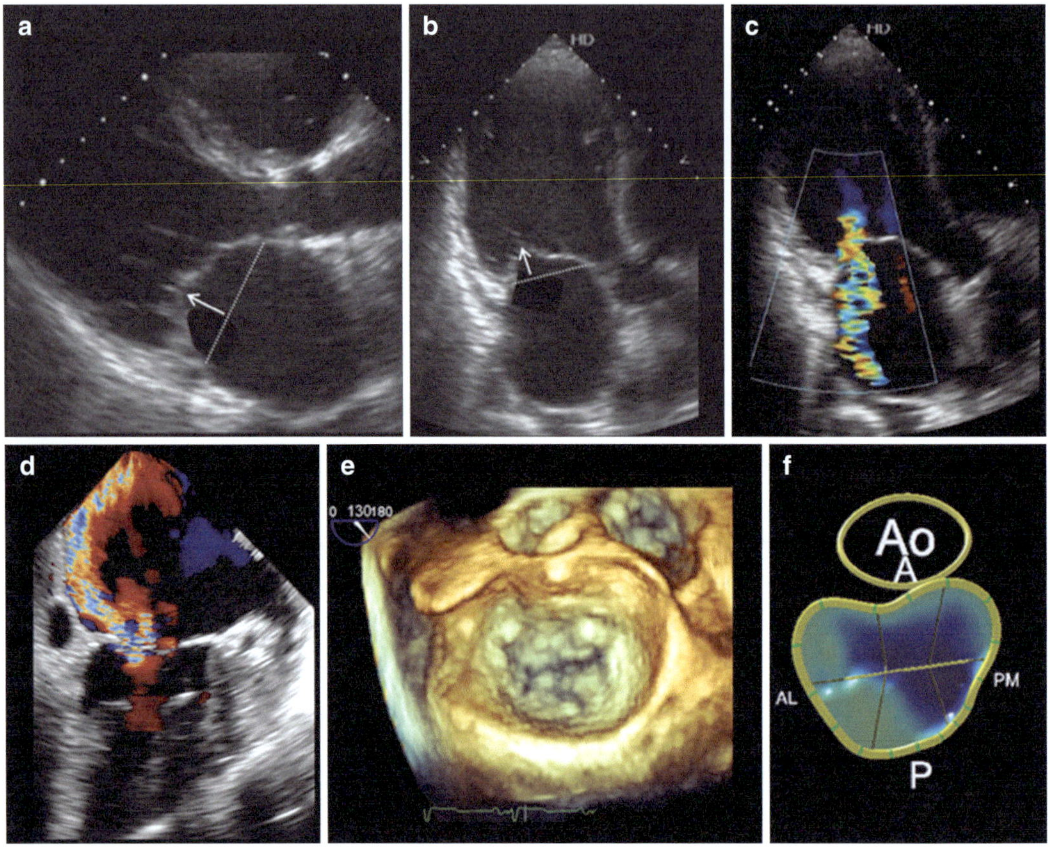

Fig. 11.1 Trans-thoracic echocardiographical images demonstrating tethering and restricted movement of both the anterior and posterior leaflets, increased tenting height (white arrow), measured from the annular plane (dotted line), with thinning of the basal inferior wall on (**a**) parasternal long-axis view and (**b**) apical 3-chamber views, causing (**c**) severe posteriorly directed mitral regurgitation on the corresponding apical 3-chamber colour flow Doppler image. Trans-oesophageal images confirming the eccentric posteriorly directed regurgitation on the (**d**) mid-oesophageal 2-chamber view and leaflet restriction and thickening on the (**e**) 3D surgical view. (**f**) Three-dimensional reconstruction demonstrates the leaflet coaptation plane is pulled into left ventricle due to tethering primarily of P3 but also involves A3, A2 and P2 (dark blue regions). A anterior, P posterior, Ao aorta, AL anterolateral papillary muscle, PM posteromedial papillary muscle

In the 2017 update to the AHA guidelines, these values have been brought into line with the values used to define degenerative mitral regurgitation, with severe ischaemic MR now characterized by an effective regurgitant orifice area ≥ 40 mm^2, regurgitant volume >60 mL/beat and vena contracta width ≥ 7 mm.

Pathophysiology

Chronic ischaemic mitral regurgitation (IMR) is a disease of the myocardium. Abnormalities of the infarcted left ventricular wall and the papillary muscle distort leaflet function. The leaflets and chords are normal. It is important to distinguish these patients from those in whom non-ischemic mitral valve disease co-exists with coronary artery disease (CAD), where there is no causal relationship between the MR and CAD. Similarly, although mitral regurgitation associated with dilated cardiomyopathy has some pathophysiological similarities with ischaemic mitral regurgitation, it should be considered aetiologically distinct. In addition, acute ischaemic mitral regurgitation may occur secondary to isolated papillary muscle ischaemia and rupture.

Chronic IMR is usually produced by a complex interaction of pathophysiological processes involved in the global and regional remodelling processes that follow myocardial infarction, including an increase in the end-diastolic LV volume, sphericity and wall stress, and subsequent ventricular dilatation.

In combination with fibrosis and atrophy of the infarcted papillary muscle, regional remodelling results in posterolateral displacement of the papillary muscles from the annular plane, producing tethering of the chordae tendineae, restricted leaflet movement and subsequent impaired coaptation and apposition of the leaflets during systole (Fig. 11.2).

Although both papillary muscles are usually displaced during the ventricular remodelling process, IMR is more commonly associated with transmural infarction of the posteroinferior LV wall, which affects the posteromedial papillary muscle. Although the posteromedial papillary muscle is attached to the medial half of both the anterior (A2/A3) and posterior (P2/P3) mitral valve leaflets, the displacement is more marked on the posterior leaflet (P2/3), as the anterior annulus is relatively fixed (Fig. 11.3).

More diffuse ventricular ischaemia produces global left ventricular dilatation resulting in annular dilatation and apical displacement of the papillary muscles, producing apical tethering of both mitral valve leaflets. The annular dilatation usually occurs with an increase in the septal-lateral diameter greater than that of the commissure-commissure diameter, thereby altering the mitral annulus to a more circular shape. This is associated with flattening of the normal, non-planar, saddle-shaped mitral annulus. This three-dimensional shape of the normal annulus involves significant peaks at the mid-septal annulus with nadirs at the commissures and is important for stress distribution across the leaflet. Although most of the dilatation is in the posterior annulus, the anterior annulus also dilates but to a lesser extent.

The regional and global LV remodelling result in different patterns of leaflet tethering

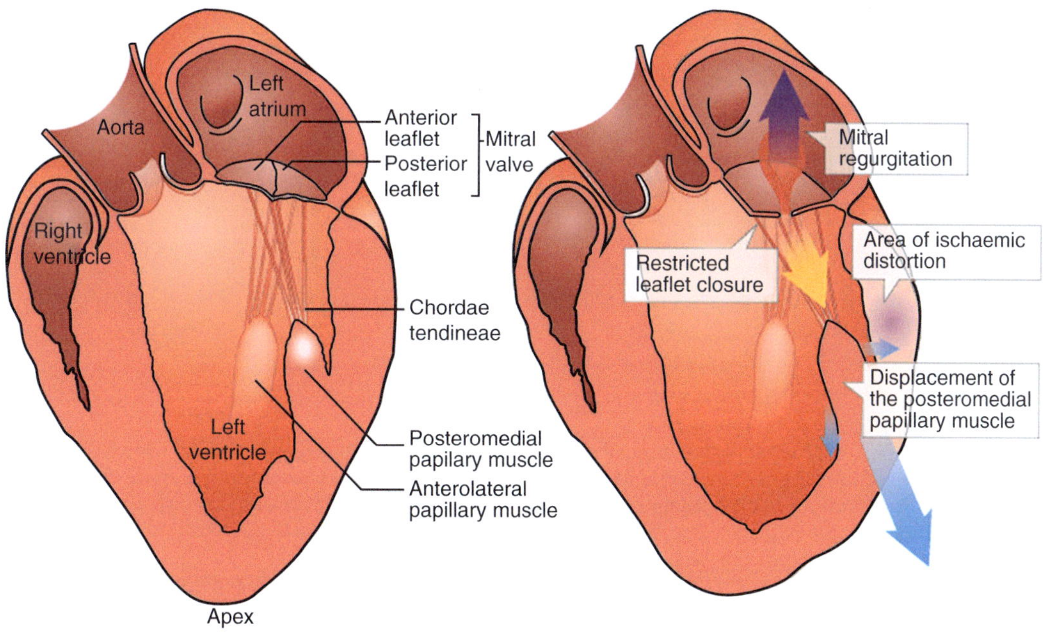

Fig. 11.2 Papillary muscle displacement following myocardial infarction resulting in leaflet tethering, impaired leaflet coaptation and subsequent ischemic mitral regurgitation. (Reproduced with permission from Taramasso M, et al. Valvular disease: Functional mitral regurgitation: should all valves be replaced? *Nat Rev Cardiol.* 2016;13(2):65–6.)

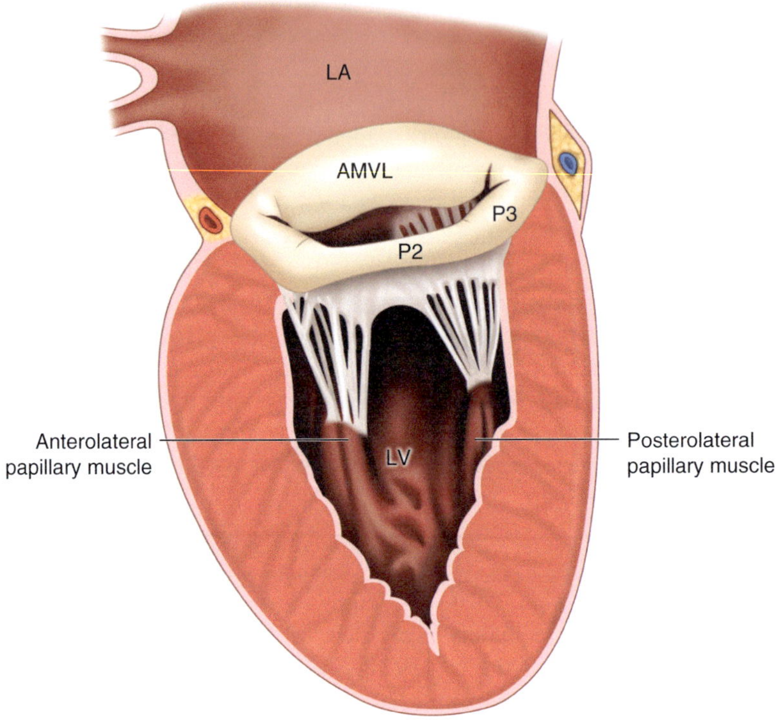

Fig. 11.3 Ischaemic mitral regurgitation caused by tethering of the leaflets, which is more prominent in the region of the P2 and P3 scallops of the mitral valve. LA left atrium, AMVL anterior mitral valve leaflet, LV left ventricle

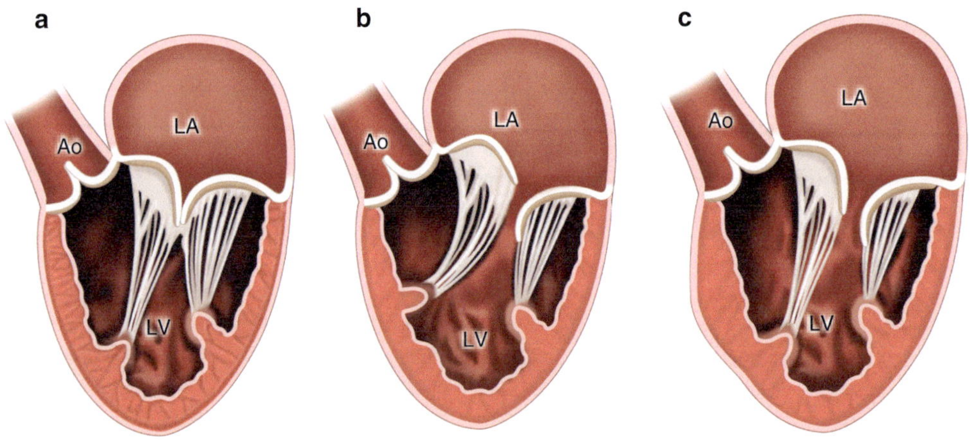

Fig. 11.4 (**a**) Normal LV shape and size producing a good depth of mitral valve leaflet coaptation and no mitral regurgitation. (**b**) Regional LV remodelling resulting in lateral displacement of the posteromedial papillary muscle, asymmetrical leaflet tethering and a posteriorly directed jet of mitral regurgitation. (**c**) Global LV remodelling resulting in annular dilatation, apical displacement of both papillary muscles, symmetrical leaflet tethering and a central jet of mitral regurgitation. LA left atrium, LV left ventricle, Ao aorta

(Fig. 11.4). Asymmetric tethering is characterized by regional LV remodelling with displacement of the posteromedial papillary muscle causing posterior leaflet restriction and a posteriorly directed jet of eccentric MR. Symmetric tethering generally results from global LV remodelling with apical displacement of both papillary muscles and annular dilatation, resulting typically in a central MR jet. Asymmetric tethering is often related to inferior or posterior myocardial infarction, whereas symmetric tethering is related to anterior myocardial infarction or to both anterior and posterior myocardial infarction.

Decreased closing forces of the mitral valve, secondary to systolic dysfunction, also contribute to the regurgitation. The mitral regurgitation becomes self-perpetuating with increased volume overload, further left ventricular remodelling, producing further papillary muscle displacement and annular dilatation, which induces further mitral regurgitation. Although the mitral valve is an innocent bystander in the pathological process of ventricular ischaemia, histological analysis of leaflet tissue in these patients has shown structural changes in the leaflet architecture caused by abnormal stretching.

Surgical Strategy

Chronic IMR may complicate up to 50% of patients with myocardial infarction, with moderate or severe regurgitation occurring in more than 10% of patients. It is associated with a poor prognosis, where mortality increases with increasing severity of the mitral regurgitation. The 5-year survival is 47% in patients with mild IMR and 29% in those with moderate or severe IMR. Despite advances in mitral valve surgery, the optimal approach to the management of ischaemic mitral regurgitation remains controversial. The homogeneity of pathophysiological mechanisms that produce ischaemic mitral regurgitation mean that a single strategy cannot be applied equally to all patients with ischaemic mitral regurgitation. The different surgical options in the management of IMR include coronary artery bypass alone, or in combination with repair techniques, such as reduction annuloplasty, sub-valvular chordal or papillary muscle techniques, leaflet augmentation and ventricular reshaping, or valve replacement. It is important to note, however, that mitral regurgitation is only partly responsible for the final clinical outcome of these patients, with progressive ventricular remodelling and deteriorating ventricular contractility meaning that some patients, ultimately, will not benefit from any surgical procedure on the mitral valve.

Coronary Artery Bypass Grafting

Although the current American College of Cardiology/American Heart Association guidelines recommend intervention on the mitral valve at the time of CABG for severe ischemic MR, the indication for moderate MR is less clearly defined. In patients with recruitable myocardium through revascularisation, CABG alone has the potential to reverse the IMR by restoring regional wall motion. This is especially true if the regurgitation is less than moderate. In patients with moderate or severe regurgitation, the regurgitation is likely to persist and indeed to worsen as the ventricle continues to dilate as the fibrous tissue within the ventricular muscle stretches. These results were confirmed by a large prospective randomised study, where the presence of mitral regurgitation was increased in patients with moderate IMR undergoing CABG alone as compared to CABG with reduction annuloplasty.

Complete coronary artery bypass grafting, especially of viable ischemic LV segments, is important to restore ventricular contractility as progression of IMR has been reported after incomplete coronary artery revascularisation. The pre-operative assessment of left ventricular viability is also important in establishing whether non-viable scarred myocardium is present to determine the type of intervention on the mitral valve. Severe or moderate to severe mitral regurgitation associated with irreversible ischaemic structural damage will be best managed by insertion of a prosthetic valve (usually tissue), with complete sub-valvar preservation by re-implantation of the chords to the annulus.

Reduction Annuloplasty

Patients with mild/moderate mitral regurgitation with evidence of recruitable myocardium can be managed either by CABG alone or in the presence of more than mild MR by the insertion of an annuloplasty ring. The goal is to restore a good coaptation height between the leaflets. This is achieved with the use of a relatively smaller mitral annuloplasty ring than would be used in degenerative valve lesions. The literature describes the use of rings of one to two sizes smaller. Sizing is based on the surface area of the aortic leaflet and the inter-trigonal distance. Traditionally, complete, rigid or semi-rigid annuloplasty rings are used, rather than a flexible ring or band, to reduce the anteroposterior (septal-lateral) diameter of the mitral valve orifice, thereby restoring mitral annular geometry and increasing the surface area of coaptation.

This technique, however, only deals with annular dilatation and does not address the other main pathophysiological mechanism of IMR, namely leaflet tethering. In fact, reduction annuloplasty may make posterior leaflet tethering worse, by shifting the mobile posterior annulus anteriorly. Reduction annuloplasty requires the tethered anterior leaflet to coapt with an essentially fixed posterior leaflet to maintain valve competency. Unsurprisingly, a significant number of these patients develop recurrent moderate or severe mitral regurgitation in the medium-term (up to 30–50% at 5 years) because of progressive left ventricular dilatation. Consistent with this, MV repair with reduction annuloplasty for ischemic mitral regurgitation has not been shown to confer any survival advantage. In addition, there have been reports of mitral stenosis in patients with marked downsizing annuloplasty.

Several risk factors (Fig. 11.5) have been identified to be associated with recurrent mitral regurgitation following reduction annuloplasty, in whom additional surgical procedures for preventing MR recurrence may be warranted (Table 11.1).

In addition, it is thought that flat annuloplasty rings atrialise the commissures, which increases the distance between the posterior leaflet and the papillary muscles, thereby potentially increas-

Table 11.1 Risk factors associated with recurrence of mitral regurgitation following reduction annuloplasty

Anterior and posterior tethering angle	>45°
Anterior excursion angle	<35°
Anterior leaflet bending angle	>25°
Coaptation length	<4 mm
Tenting height/coaptation depth	>10 mm
Tenting area	>2.5 cm^2
Systolic inter-papillary muscle distance	>20 mm
Mitral annular diameter	>3.7 cm
Left ventricular end-systolic volume	>145 mL
Left ventricular end-systolic diameter	>65 mm
Left ventricular sphericity index	>0.7
Left ventricular end-diastolic index	>3.5 cm/m^2
Wall motion score	>1.5
Myocardial performance index	>0.9

Anterior and posterior tethering angles represent the angle between the mitral valve annulus and the anterior or posterior mitral valve leaflets
Anterior excursion angle is the angle between the leaflet during systole and diastole and represents the degree of leaflet restriction
Coaptation length is the distance that the mitral leaflets are in contact during systole and normally is >8 mm
Tenting height/coaptation depth is the distance from the mitral annulus to the line of leaflet coaptation during systole and normally is <6 mm
Tenting area is the mid-systolic area between the mitral annulus and the leaflets
Left ventricular sphericity index is the ratio of the long-axis length to the short-axis length and is used as a surrogate for increased MV tethering due to adverse LV remodelling
Left ventricular end-diastolic index is the left ventricular end-systolic diameter divided by body surface area

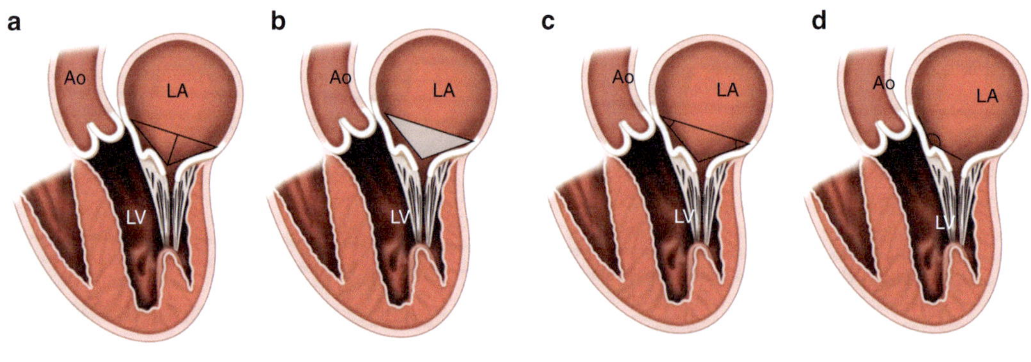

Fig. 11.5 Markers of leaflet tethering, quantified on echocardiographical assessment, including (**a**) tenting height, (**b**) tenting area, (**c**) anterior and posterior leaflet tethering angles, and (**d**) anterior leaflet bending angle. LA left atrium, LV left ventricle, Ao aorta

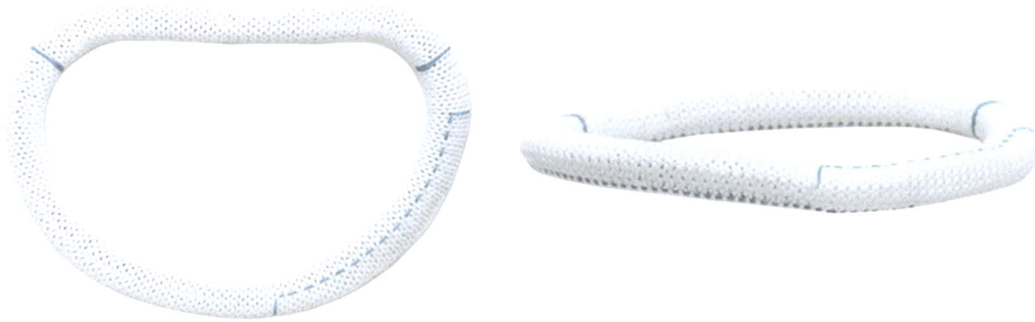

Fig. 11.6 Carpentier-McCarthy-Adams IMR ETlogix annuloplasty ring, with reduced anteroposterior diameter and an asymmetric design with a reduced P2-P3 curvature. (Reproduced with permission from Edwards Lifesciences, Irvine, CA, USA)

ing tethering of the posterior leaflet. Newer, specifically designed ischaemic mitral regurgitation annuloplasty rings have been introduced, which incorporate septal-lateral diameter reduction and have a saddle-shape to compensate for the tethered P2/P3 scallops of the posterior leaflets, thereby restoring the 3D shape of the annulus to normalise leaflet stress, and can be true-sized to the inter-commissural distance and anterior leaflet (Fig. 11.6). Long term results of these are awaited.

A comprehensive approach to the repair of the ischemic mitral valve, however, must consider all aspects of the pathophysiological process. In view of this, newer adjunctive techniques have been developed that focus on the subvalvular apparatus, including the chordae tendineae, papillary muscles and left ventricular free wall, in an attempt to address the underlying pathophysiological mechanisms of IMR and achieve better long-term results. Identifying which patients will benefit from sub-valvular repair, however, remains a challenge. The addition of technically complex repair techniques needs to be considered in the context of prolonged bypass times in a patient undergoing coronary artery bypass grafting with an already impaired left ventricle.

Leaflet Extension

Augmentation of the posterior leaflet has been suggested as an adjunct to address the leaflet tethering, increase leaflet curvature (a surrogate for reduced valve stress) and increase the depth of coaptation of the mitral leaflets. It is important that both leaflets are pliable, and that there is no leaflet or annular calcification. The posterior leaflet is detached at its annular margin, from the middle of the P2 scallop up to the posteromedial commissure, allowing a long ovo-rectangular shaped pericardial patch (approximately 1 × 4 cm) to be implanted, using a continuous locking 4/0 or 5/0 Prolene suture (Fig. 11.7). This allows a true-sized annuloplasty ring to be implanted, measured against the intercommissural distance and the anterior leaflet, thereby significantly increasing the depth of coaptation in the region most affected by leaflet tethering. Extending the P2 and P3 scallops by approximately 1 cm allows a safety margin to compensate for any further ventricular enlargement and papillary muscle displacement. Long-term follow-up is required to establish whether the bovine patch remains pliable to maintain adequate leaflet motion.

Chordal Cutting

The secondary mitral chords are the strong load bearing chords and in IMR are responsible for tethering of the leaflets, as a result of their size and strength. This tethering of the body of the leaflet produces the 'seagull sign' seen on echocardiography.

Cutting of secondary chords is advocated by some surgeons to correct the altered subvalvular

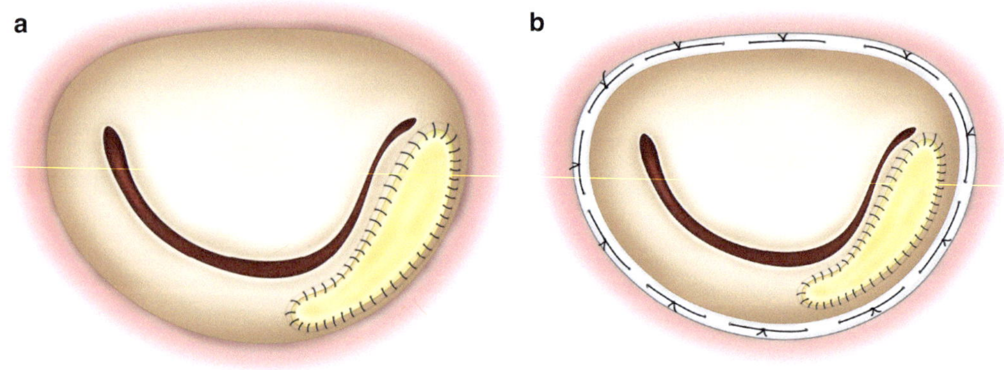

Fig. 11.7 (**a**) Implantation of a bovine pericardial patch to augment the tethered P2/P3 scallops of the posterior mitral valve leaflet, followed by (**b**) implantation of an annuloplasty ring

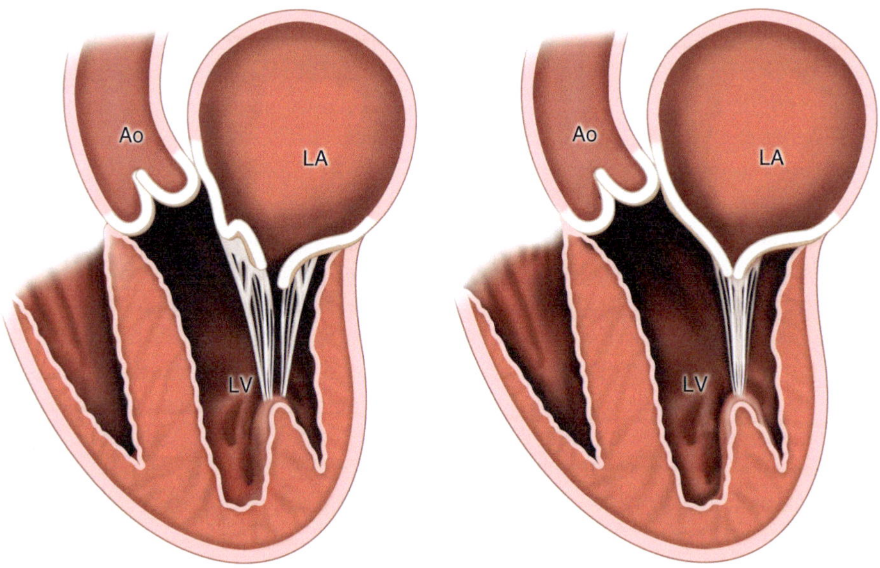

Fig. 11.8 Translocation of secondary chordae of the anterior mitral valve leaflet from the body to the free edge, thereby reducing leaflet tethering in ischaemic mitral regurgitation

geometry associated with IMR. Secondary chords to the anterior leaflet, posterior leaflet and commissure, arising from the affected papillary muscle are cut, whereas those arising from the normal papillary muscle are not divided. This reduces tethering of the chordae tendineae on the leaflets, improves leaflet movement and increases the depth of coaptation. There are concerns about the effects of secondary chord cutting. Reduced structural support for the leaflets and reduced support for the left ventricle through disruption of valvular-ventricular continuity may lead to progressive left ventricular distension and leaflet prolapse. In view of this, the secondary chords can be translocated to the free edge of the leaflet (Fig. 11.8), which may be further strengthened by inserting Gore-Tex neochordae. The primary and tertiary chordae are left in situ to preserve valvular-ventricular continuity.

Papillary Muscle Relocation

This technique is based on the concept that the distance between the mitral annulus and the

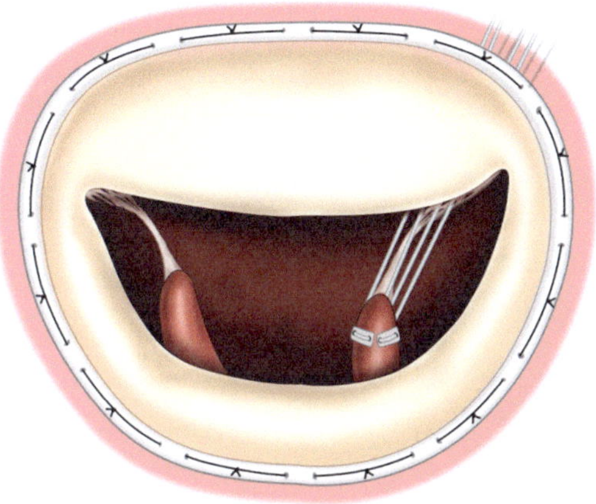

Fig. 11.9 Papillary muscle relocation using a CV4 Gore-Tex trans-ventricular suture to approximate the posteromedial papillary muscle towards the mitral valve annulus at the level of the posteromedial commissure

posterior papillary muscle is an important determinant of the leaflet tethering. The displaced posterior papillary muscle can be relocated using a trans-ventricular suture to approximate it towards the mitral annulus and counteract the altered subvalvular geometry involved in ischaemic mitral regurgitation. Through an atriotomy, the papillary muscle can be approximated to the mitral annulus at the level of the posteromedial commissure (Fig. 11.9).

An alternative technique is to access the head of the posterior papillary muscle via an aortotomy and then pass the pledgeted CV4 Gore-Tex suture through the mid-point of the anterior annulus, which lies beneath the commissure between the non-coronary and left coronary aortic cusps, and exteriorise it through the aortic wall (Fig. 11.10). The suture can then be tied under echocardiographical guidance in the loaded beating heart to reposition the displaced posterior papillary muscle toward the mid-point of the anterior annulus. This technique is supported with implantation of an annuloplasty ring.

Papillary Muscle Sling

This technique involves placing a 4 mm Gore-Tex tube around the base of both papillary muscles.

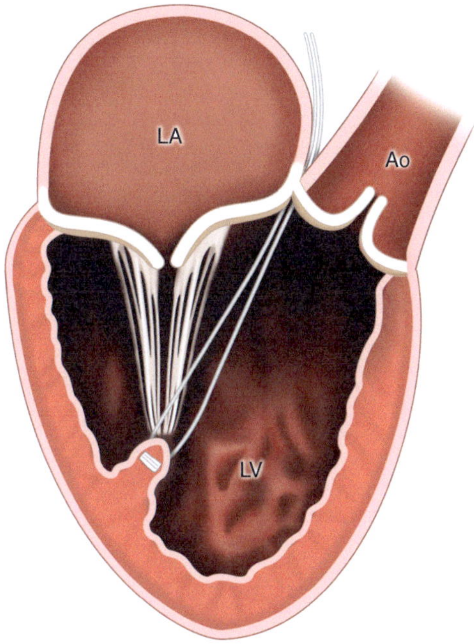

Fig. 11.10 Papillary muscle relocation using a CV4 Gore-Tex trans-ventricular suture to approximate the posteromedial papillary muscle towards the mitral valve annulus. The suture is exteriorised through the aortic wall and can be tied on a loaded beating heart

The sling is then tightened to decrease the distance between both papillary muscles, thereby realigning the papillary muscles and reducing the tension on the chordae tendineae. A moderately undersized (30 mm) annuloplasty ring is also placed. An alternative to this technique involves simply suturing the heads of the papillary muscles together to reduce papillary muscle displacement and leaflet tethering (Fig. 11.11).

Ventricular Techniques

In an attempt to address the ventricular remodelling process that is responsible for ischaemic mitral regurgitation, several 'ventricular' techniques have been proposed. These include surgical ventricular restoration (Fig. 11.12), which uses an endoventricular patch to exclude an infarcted anterior ventricular wall, thereby restoring the ventricular elliptical shape, and reducing left ventricular volume, papillary muscle

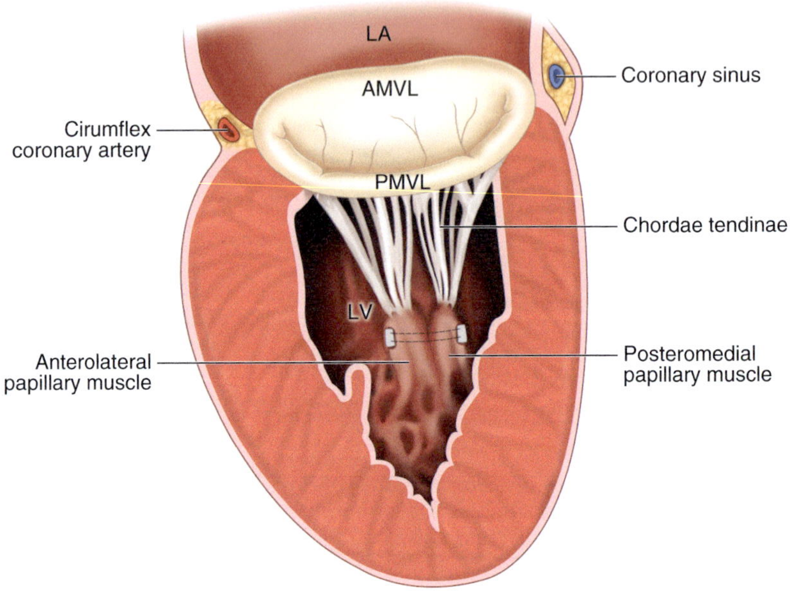

Fig. 11.11 Papillary muscle approximation using a pledgeted 4/0 Prolene suture. LA left atrium, LV left ventricle, AMVL anterior mitral valve leaflet, PMVL posterior mitral valve leaflet

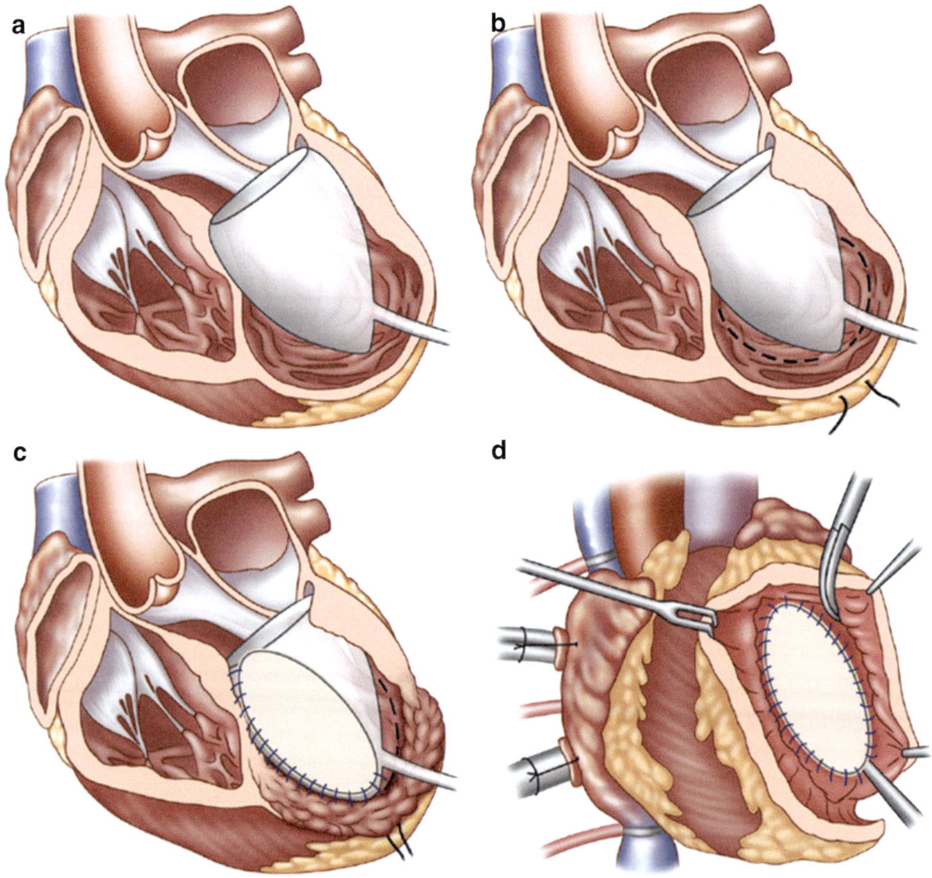

Fig. 11.12 Surgical ventricular restoration, with (**a**) insertion of an endoventricular balloon that is used to define the post-procedural left ventricular volume (50 mL/m^2), (**b**) placement of an endoventricular purse-string suture (Fontan stich) at the boundary between scarred fibrotic myocardium and normal contractile myocardium, (**c**) implantation of a bovine pericardial patch to close the residual defect in the ventricular wall and (**d**) closure of the ventriculotomy

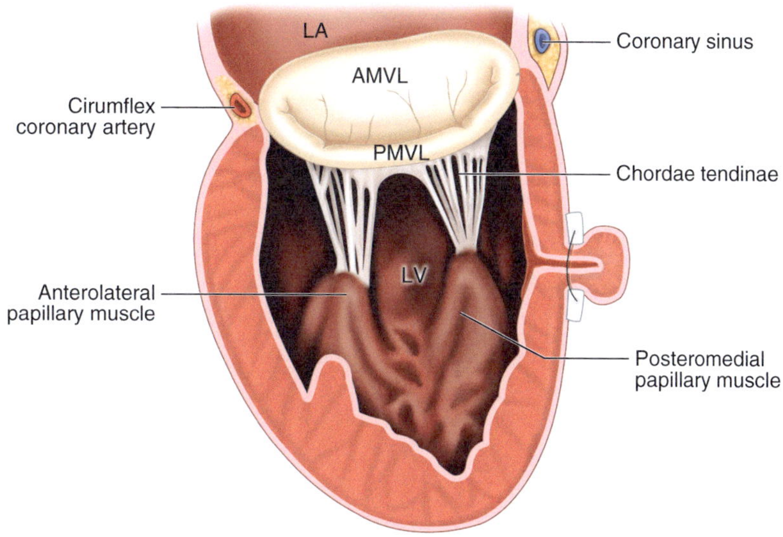

Fig. 11.13 Infarct plication used to reduce papillary muscle displacement. LA left atrium, LV left ventricle, AMVL anterior mitral valve leaflet, PMVL posterior mitral valve leaflet

displacement and subsequent MR; infarct plication (Fig. 11.13), where the infarcted inferolateral wall of the left ventricle is plicated using Teflon buttressed mattress sutures to help approximate the displaced papillary muscle towards the mitral annulus; and external compression devices, such as the Acorn Corcap (Fig. 11.14a) and Coapsys device (Fig. 11.14b), which again reduce wall stress and restore a more elliptical LV shape, thereby reducing papillary muscle displacement.

Mitral Valve Replacement

Historically, patients with IMR were treated by mitral valve replacement without preservation of the sub-valvular apparatus. This was associated with very poor long-term outcomes as a result of disruption of the valvular-ventricular continuity and subsequent left ventricular enlargement and impaired contractility. More recently, mitral valve replacement with sub-valvular preservation has been compared to mitral valve repair with reduction annuloplasty in a large multi-centre prospective randomised controlled trial of patients with severe ischaemic mitral regurgitation. It demonstrated that there was no significant difference between the groups for major adverse cardiac or cerebrovascular events or survival at 12 months but that replacement produced a significantly more durable correction of the mitral regurgitation, associated with reduced recurrence of heart failure symptoms and hospital readmissions.

Sub-valvular preservation involves restoring normal ventricular geometry by maintaining ventricular-annular continuity and thereby supporting the ventricular wall. The anterior leaflet is detached from the annulus (Fig. 11.15a) and divided between the chordal insertion from each papillary muscle head (Fig. 11.15b). The triangular portion of leaflet tissue without chordal insertion is resected (Fig. 11.15c) and the prosthetic valve sutures are placed through the remaining tissue and passed through the annulus in preparation for valve insertion (Fig. 11.15d).

If the posterior leaflet is shallow, it may be left in situ and sutures passed through the leaflet and the annulus. If necessary, it is possible to maximise the size of replacement valve by detaching the posterior leaflet for its entire length and dividing it in the middle, as for the anterior leaflet, and then reattaching it. This allows full development of the posterior leaflet circumference. If the native chordae tendineae cannot be preserved, which is unusual in the setting of ischaemic mitral regurgitation, Gore-Tex neo-chordae can be used to reattach the papillary muscles to the mitral annulus. Preservation of all the chordae results in the maintenance of more normal ventricular volumes and better systolic function compared with partial preservation.

Fig. 11.14 External compression of the left ventricle, to reduce ventricular dilatation and displacment of the papillary muscles in ischaemic cardiomyopathy, using (**a**) Acorn CorCap and (**b**) Coapsys devices. AMVL anterior mitral valve leaflet, PMVL posterior mitral valve leaflet, LA left atrium, LV left ventricle

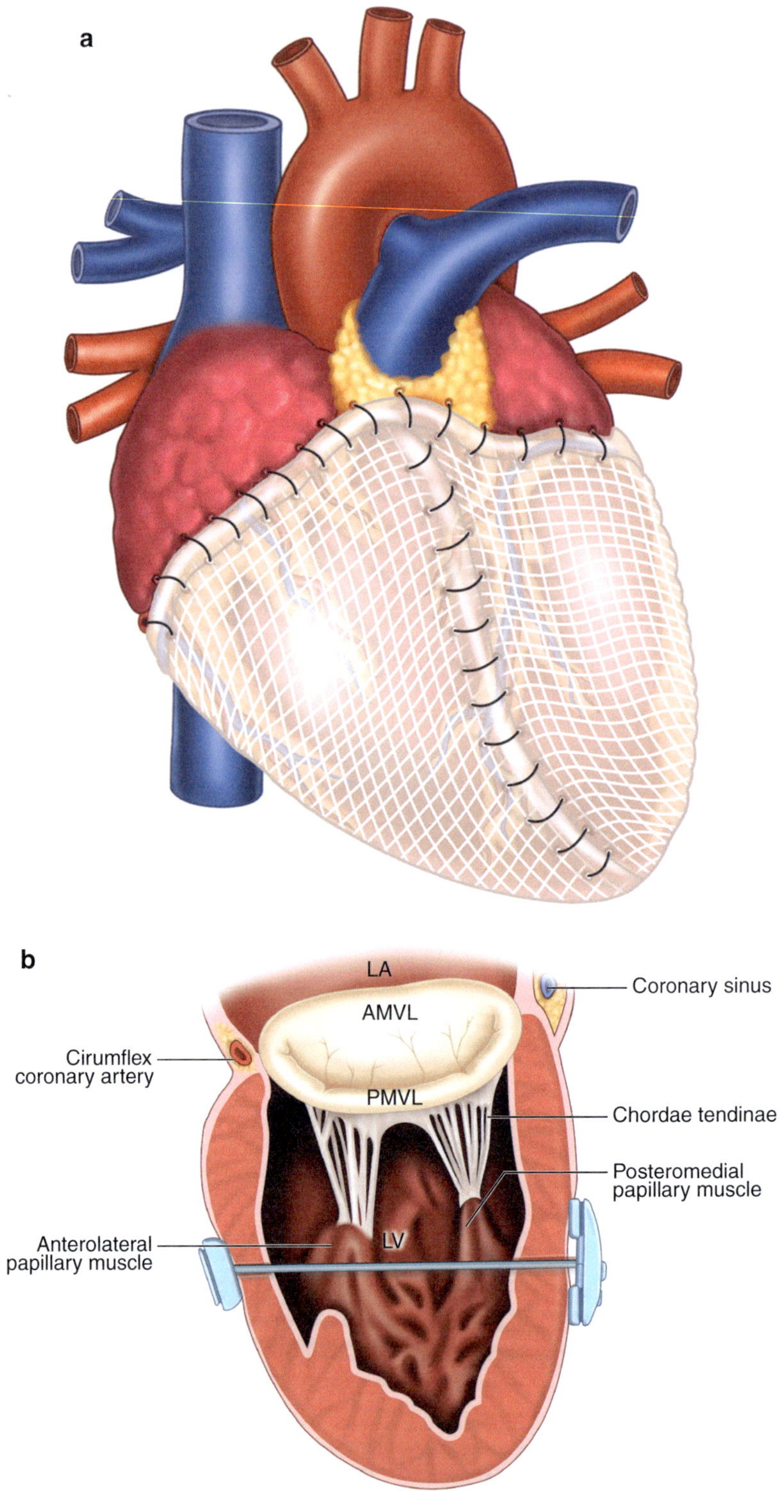

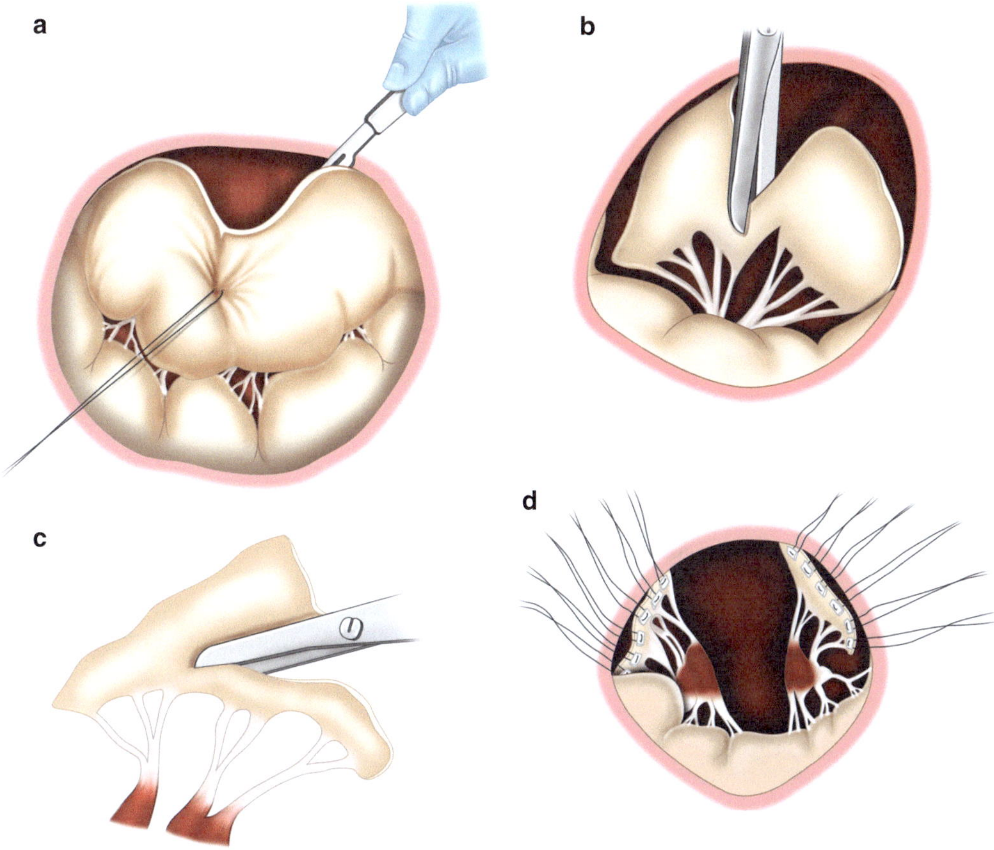

Fig. 11.15 Chordal-sparing mitral valve replacement with (**a**) detachment of the anterior leaflet from the annulus, (**b**) division of the anterior leaflet between the chordal insertion from each papillary muscle head, (**c**) resection of the triangular portion of leaflet tissue without chordal insertion, and (**d**) implantation of the prosthetic valve sutures through the residual leaflet tissue

Often a bioprosthesis is implanted, irrespective of age, as the median survival for patients with ischaemic mitral regurgitation is 5 years, thereby avoiding anticoagulation-related adverse events. Common sense dictates that prosthetic mitral valve insertion with preservation of the subvalvular apparatus is preferable to a repair procedure, especially if a sub-optimal result is obtained, as a prosthetic valve will provide a more durable correction of the mitral regurgitation. For patients with multiple comorbidities, complex regurgitant jets (more than one jet), or severe tethering of both mitral leaflets, mitral valve replacement is a better option

The decision to intervene in ischaemic mitral regurgitation, and if so, whether to repair or replace, can be challenging. A number of factors need to be considered including the severity of mitral regurgitation, the aetiology of mitral regurgitation (annular dilation, restricted leaflet motion or a combination), severity of LV impairment, age of the patient and presence of significant co-morbidities. It is important to appreciate that mitral valve repair in the context of IMR does not treat the underlying primary cause of the regurgitation and that progressive left ventricular dilatation after the repair may cause further

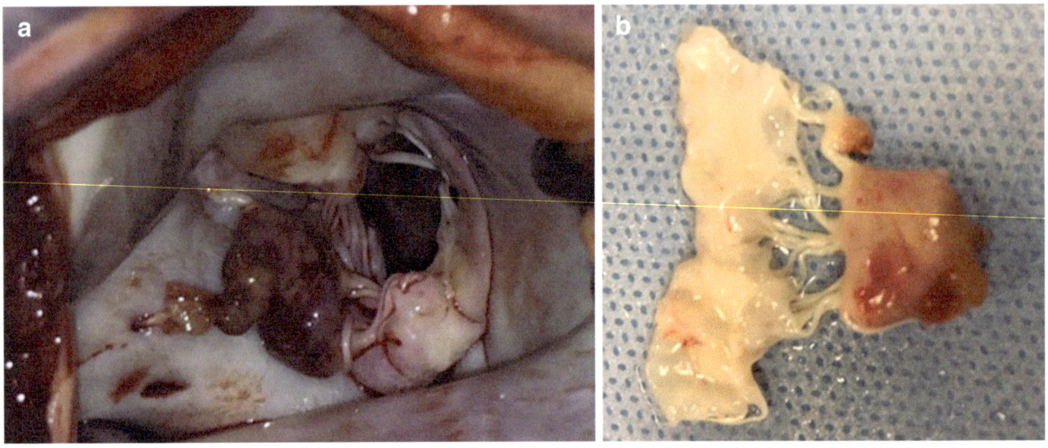

Fig. 11.16 (**a**) Ruptured posteromedial papillary muscle following acute inferior myocardial infarction and (**b**) resected papillary muscle with attached chordae tendineae and P2 scallop of posterior mitral valve leaflet

displacement of the papillary muscles and recurrence of the MR.

1. CABG alone is used for patients with mild-moderate IMR but with significant myocardial viability, suggesting that they will experience reverse remodelling and an improvement in LV contractility following revascularisation.
2. Annular and sub-valvular mitral valve repair with CABG can be considered for patients with moderate IMR and symptoms of heart failure or scarred and non-viable inferolateral LV wall, who are unlikely to improve with CABG alone. When performing mitral repair for IMR, it is important to identify the exact mechanisms responsible for IMR in order to perform the appropriate surgical procedure to restore valve competency.
3. Chordal preserving mitral valve insertion plus CABG is used for patients with severe IMR, moderate IMR with high risk of recurrence with repair (such as complex IMR jets, tethering of both leaflets) and patients with multiple co-morbidities. Further research is on-going to more clearly define the subset of patients with severe IMR where repair can be considered. These patients include those without significant risk factors for recurrence (Table 11.1), such as increased left ventricular end-systolic volume, tethering angle and tenting height.

In patients with severe acute ischaemic mitral regurgitation secondary to papillary muscle rupture (Fig. 11.16), mitral valve replacement may also be required, again preserving as much sub-valvular apparatus as possible.

Surgical Technique

The lesion set in patients with ischaemic mitral regurgitation is best assessed pre-operatively with trans-oesophageal echocardiography because of the functional nature of the lesion. Whilst segmental analysis of the mitral valve using saline insufflation and nerve hook assessment converts the ultrasound data into direct visualisation of the problem, it cannot replace accurate close scrutiny of the pre-operative trans-oesophageal assessment with an expert investigational cardiologist. This allows the best assessment of the morbid anatomy and planning of the operative procedure.

The annular plane is used as the 'point of reference' to determine the degree of tethering of each of the segments. It is also important to identify any valvular calcification, sub-valvular pathology or annular dilatation, which may be contributing to the incompetence of the valve. The presence of a jet lesion may help to identify the direction of the regurgitant blood.

In this case, marked restriction of the P2-P3 segments of the posterior leaflet was observed, secondary to tethering of the chordae from the

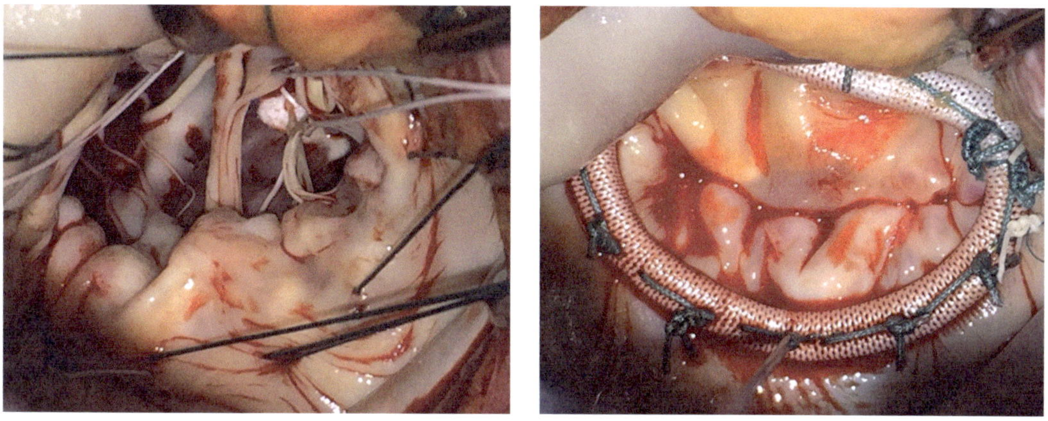

Fig. 11.17 Operative images illustrating (**a**) restriction of the P2-P3 segment of the posterior leaflet, placement of the annuloplasty sutures, and insertion of the CV4 Gore-Tex suture for papillary muscle relocation, and (**b**) implantation of a Carpentier-McCarthy-Adams IMR ETlogix annuloplasty ring (Edwards Lifesciences, Irvine, CA) and fixing of the papillary muscle relocation sutures on the atrial side of the annulus at the level of the posteromedial commissure and P3

posterolateral papillary muscle, as well as dilatation of the mitral valve annulus. Horizontal mattress ring annuloplasty sutures (2/0 Ethibond) had been placed around the circumference of the mitral valve, with a 5–10 mm width and approximately 1 mm apart to improve visualisation of the valve. The sutures placed in the region of the P2-P3 segment of the posterior mitral valve annulus need to be very secure with good depth into the ventricular muscle to deal with the tension in this area produced by the ventricular distortion.

The secondary chordae originating from the posteromedial papillary muscle and attaching to the anterior leaflet, posterior leaflet and posteromedial commissure, were then cut immediately below their attachment to the ventricular side of the leaflets and reattached to the leaflet free edge, using 5/0 Prolene. To relocate the posteromedial papillary muscle, 2 Teflon-pledgeted CV4 Gore-Tex sutures were then placed from the fibrous head of the posteromedial papillary muscle through the mitral annulus at the level of the posteromedial commissure and P3 (Fig. 11.17a).

The mitral valve annulus was then sized according to the intercommisural distance and height of the anterior leaflet, which resulted in moderate under-sizing of the whole valve area. A 30 mm Carpentier-McCarthy-Adams IMR ETlogix annuloplasty ring (Edwards Lifesciences, Irvine, CA) was chosen, as it is a semi-rigid complete ring, and has an asymmetric three-dimensional design, with reduced P2-P3 curvature to compensate for a tethered P2-P3 segment and a decreased the anteroposterior distance to compensate for annular dilatation, thereby increasing the depth of leaflet coaptation.

The ring was then tied in situ and competency of the mitral valve assessed with static testing, by injecting cold saline into the left ventricle, using a bulb syringe. The correct length of the papillary muscle relocation sutures can then be determined and tied on the atrial side of the annulus (Fig. 11.17b).

Post-operative Echocardiogram

The post-repair trans-thoracic echocardiogram (Fig. 11.18) confirmed:

1. Restoration of physiological functioning of the mitral valve complex with excellent bileaflet motion, reduced annular dimension and absence of leaflet tethering.
2. Excellent depth of coaptation (8 mm) with no residual mitral regurgitation
3. Significantly reduced tenting height (4 mm) and tenting area (1.1 cm^2)
4. No evidence of mitral stenosis, systolic anterior motion of the mitral valve (SAM) or left ventricular outflow obstruction (LVOTO).

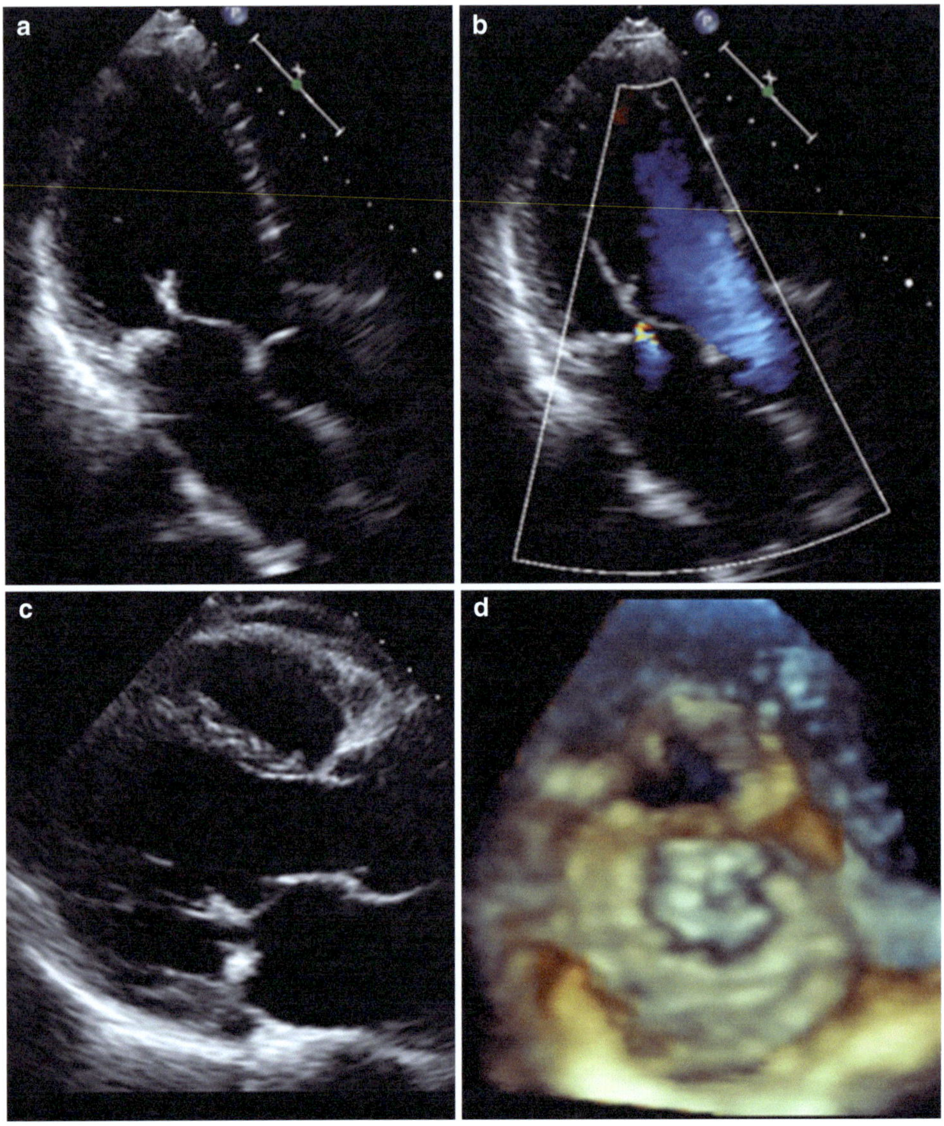

Fig. 11.18 Post-operative trans-thoracic echocardiographical images demonstrating the annuloplasty ring in situ, with a competent mitral valve, no residual mitral regurgitation, excellent bi-leaflet motion and reduced leaflet tethering on (**a**) apical 3-chamber view with (**b**) corresponding colour flow Doppler image, (**c**) parasternal long-axis view and (**d**) 3D surgical short-axis view

Surgical Tips

1. Reduction annuloplasty with a specifically designed complete rigid or semi-rigid ring will address the annular dilatation component of ischaemic mitral regurgitation
2. Excessive downsizing may worsen leaflet tethering and result in recurrent mitral regurgitation
3. Adjunctive measures of secondary chord cutting and papillary muscle relocation may be required to address leaflet tethering
4. It is important to identify the preoperative risk factors for recurrent mitral regurgitation and use sub-valvular techniques to restore the valve to a physiological configuration

Comment

The Cardiothoracic Surgical Trials Network (CTSN) have recently published the results of two prospective randomised trials to help guide the management of patients with ischaemic mitral regurgitation. The first compared chordal preserving mitral valve replacement with reduction annuloplasty mitral valve repair in 251 patients with severe ischemic MR. At 24 months, both groups showed evidence of reverse remodelling but no significant difference for left ventricular systolic volume index (primary outcome measure) or survival between the groups. There was, however, a 58.8% incidence of at least moderate regurgitation in the repair group, as compared to 3.8% in the replacement group. Further studies are being carried out from pre-operative echocardiographic data to determine a subgroup of patients that would benefit from repair in the setting of severe IMR.

The second trial compared coronary artery bypass grafting alone versus CABG plus reduction annuloplasty mitral valve repair in 301 patients with moderate ischaemic MR. Unlike previous prospective randomised controlled trials assessing this cohort of patients, there was no significant difference in the left ventricular end-systolic volume index (a surrogate for reverse remodelling) at 12 months. As expected, however, patients undergoing CABG alone had a 31.1% incidence of moderate or severe regurgitation, as compared to 11.2% in the repair group. There was no significant difference in peri-operative mortality (2.7% in CABG group versus 1.3% in the CABG plus repair group) or major adverse cardiac and cerebrovascular events between the groups. Similarly, further studies are being performed pertaining to myocardial viability to determine which patients with moderate IMR will benefit from CABG alone.

Longer term results of these studies are awaited to determine the effect of recurrence of significant regurgitation and use of contemporary surgical techniques on survival and functional status.

Recommended Reading

Acker MA, Parides MK, Perrault LP, Moskowitz AJ, Gelijns AC, Voisine P, Smith PK, Hung JW, Blackstone EH, Puskas JD, Argenziano M, Gammie JS, Mack M, Ascheim DD, Bagiella E, Moquete EG, Ferguson TB, Horvath KA, Geller NL, Miller MA, Woo YJ, D'Alessandro DA, Ailawadi G, Dagenais F, Gardner TJ, O'Gara PT, Michler RE, Kron IL, CTSN Investigators. Mitral-valve repair versus replacement for severe ischemic mitral regurgitation. N Engl J Med. 2014;370(1):23–32.

Chan KM, Punjabi PP, Flather M, Wage R, Symmonds K, Roussin I, Rahman-Haley S, Pennell DJ, Kilner PJ, Dreyfus GD, Pepper JR, for the RIME Investigators. Coronary artery bypass surgery with or without mitral valve annuloplasty in moderate functional ischemic mitral regurgitation: final results of the randomized ischemic mitral evaluation (RIME) trial. Circulation. 2011;116(21):2502–10.

Fattouch K, Guccione F, Sampognaro R, Panzarella G, Corrado E, Navarra E, Calvaruso D, Ruvolo G. Efficacy of adding mitral valve restrictive annuloplasty to coronary artery bypass grafting in patients with moderate ischemic mitral valve regurgitation: a randomized trial. J Thorac Cardiovasc Surg. 2009;138(2):278–85.

Goldstein D, Moskowitz AJ, Gelijns AC, Ailawadi G, Parides MK, Perrault LP, Hung JW, Voisine P, Dagenais F, Gillinov AM, Thourani V, Argenziano M, Gammie JS, Mack M, Demers P, Atluri P, Rose EA, O'Sullivan K, Williams DL, Bagiella E, Michler RE, Weisel RD, Miller MA, Geller NL, Taddei-Peters WC, Smith PK, Moquete E, Overbey JR, Kron IL, O'Gara PT, Acker MA, CTSN Investigators. Two-year outcomes of surgical treatment of severe ischemic mitral regurgitation. N Engl J Med. 2016;374(4):344–53.

Kron IL, Hung J, Overbey JR, Bouchard D, Gelijns AC, Moskowitz AJ, Voisine P, O'Gara PT, Argenziano M, Michler RE, Gillinov M, Puskas JD, Gammie JS, Mack MJ, Smith PK, Sai-Sudhakar C, Gardner TJ, Ailawadi G, Zeng X, O'Sullivan K, Parides MK, Swayze R, Thourani V, Rose EA, Perrault LP, Acker MA, CTSN Investigators. Predicting recurrent mitral regurgitation after mitral valve repair for severe ischemic mitral regurgitation. J Thorac Cardiovasc Surg. 2015;149(3):752–61.

Lorusso R, Gelsomino S, Vizzardi E, D'Aloia A, De Cicco G, Lucà F, Parise O, Gensini GF, Stefàno P, Livi U, Vendramin I, Pacini D, Di Bartolomeo R, Miceli A, Varone E, Glauber M, Parolari A, Giuseppe Arlati F, Alamanni F, Serraino F, Renzulli A, Messina A, Troise G, Mariscalco G, Cottini M, Beghi C, Nicolini F, Gherli T, Borghetti V, Pardini A, Caimmi PP, Micalizzi E, Fino C, Ferrazzi P, Di Mauro M, Calafiore AM, ISTIMIR Investigators. Mitral valve repair or replacement for ischemic mitral regurgitation? The Italian Study on the Treatment of Ischemic

Mitral Regurgitation (ISTIMIR). J Thorac Cardiovasc Surg. 2013;145(1):118–39.

Smith PK, Puskas JD, Ascheim DD, Voisine P, Gelijns AC, Moskowitz AJ, Hung JW, Parides MK, Ailawadi G, Perrault LP, Acker MA, Argenziano M, Thourani V, Gammie JS, Miller MA, Pagé P, Overbey JR, Bagiella E, Dagenais F, Blackstone EH, Kron IL, Goldstein DJ, Rose EA, Moquete EG, Jeffries N, Gardner TJ, O'Gara PT, Alexander JH, Michler RE, Cardiothoracic Surgical Trials Network Investigators. Surgical treatment of moderate ischemic mitral regurgitation. N Engl J Med. 2014;371(23):2178–88.

Taramasso M, Maisano F. Valvular disease: functional mitral regurgitation: should all valves be replaced? Nat Rev Cardiol. 2016;13(2):65–6.

Vassileva CM, Boley T, Markwell S, Hazelrigg S. Meta-analysis of short-term and long-term survival following repair versus replacement for ischemic mitral regurgitation. Eur J Cardiothorac Surg. 2011;39(3):295–303.

Mitral Valve Infective Endocarditis 12

Keywords
Infective endocarditis · Annular abscess · Vegetation · Leaflet reconstruction · Autologous pericardium · Bovine pericardium · Mitral regurgitation · Mitral valve replacement · Bacteraemia · Embolisation

Case History

A 63 year-old gentleman presented with a 4-week history of fever, night sweats and increasing dyspnoea on exertion, associated with lethargy. He had no previous history of rheumatic fever but had recently undergone a dental extraction. Clinical examination revealed a pyrexia (38.2 °C) and a pansystolic murmur. Blood cultures revealed streptococcus sanguinis, associated with a raised white blood cell count (15,600/μL) and C-reactive protein (238 mg/dL).

Echocardiographical Findings

Trans-thoracic apical 4-chamber echocardiographic image revealed the presence of a 0.7 cm vegetation on the anterior mitral valve leaflet, associated with normal movement of both the anterior and posterior leaflets (Fig. 12.1a). This was also observed on the parasternal long-axis view (Fig. 12.1b), where the vegetation can be seen as a mobile mass attached to the atrial surface of the anterior leaflet. Doppler flow across the mitral valve demonstrated a jet of mitral regurgitation (MR), through a perforation in the anterior leaflet (Fig. 12.1c).

Trans-oesophageal echocardiographic images confirmed the presence of the vegetation on the atrial surface of the anterior leaflet, associated with normal movement of both the anterior and posterior leaflets on mid-oesophageal long-axis and 4-chamber views (Fig. 12.2a, b), associated with a jet of mitral regurgitation (MR) through the perforation seen on the corresponding colour flow Doppler image (Fig. 12.2c).

Quantification of the regurgitation, using the PISA method, revealed severe MR, with a regurgitant volume of 67 mL and regurgitant fraction of 53%, associated with a vena contracta of 0.76 cm. The left atrium was not dilated (3.9 cm) and the left ventricular size and function were preserved, with a left ventricular end-systolic diameter of 3.7 cm, left ventricular end-diastolic diameter of 5.2 cm and ejection fraction of 67%. The three-dimensional short-axis surgical view clearly demonstrates the perforation in the body of the anterior leaflet (Fig. 12.2d).

N. Moorjani et al., *Operative Mitral and Tricuspid Valve Surgery*,
https://doi.org/10.1007/978-1-4471-4204-1_12

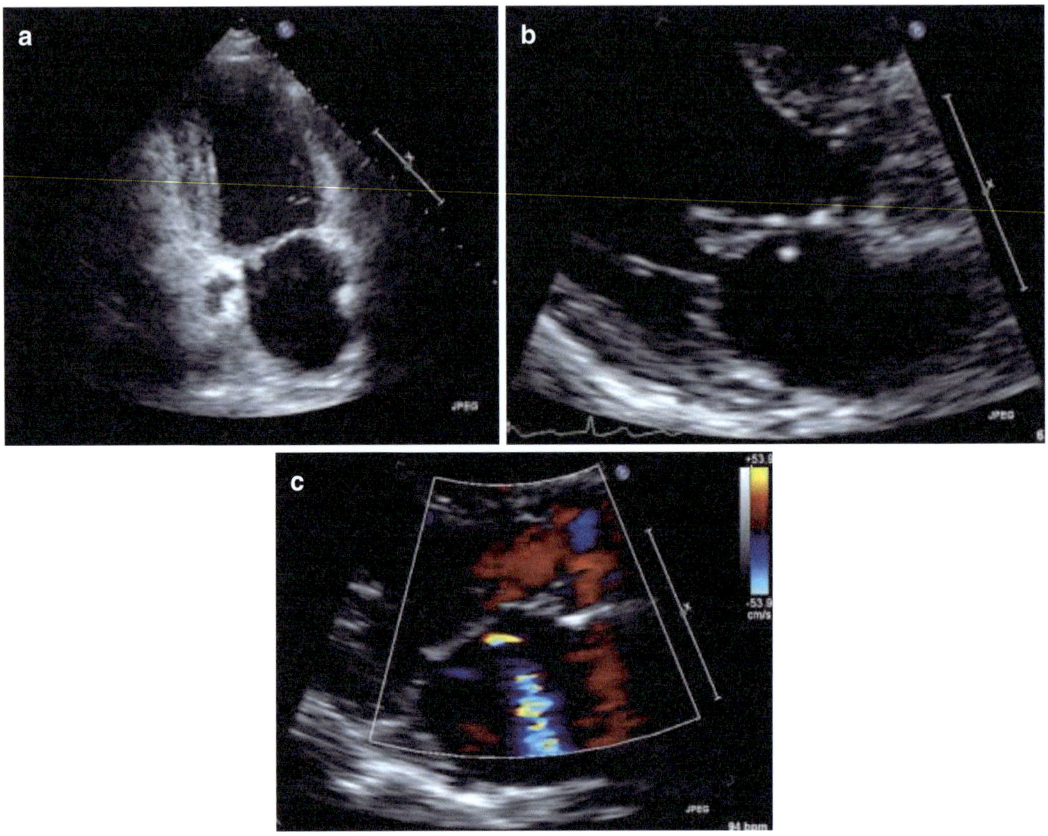

Fig. 12.1 Trans-thoracic echocardiographical images demonstrating a 0.7 cm vegetation lying on the atrial side of the anterior mitral valve leaflet on (**a**) apical 4-chamber and (**b**) parasternal long-axis views, associated with a jet of severe mitral regurgitation through the perforation on (**c**) the corresponding parasternal long-axis colour flow Doppler image

Pathophysiology

Normal cardiac endothelium is resistant to infection and even with transient bacteremia, endogenous immune mechanisms, including thrombocidins (microbicidal proteins released by platelets), help to prevent endocarditis. Patients with endothelial disruption or non-laminar blood flow, such as those with some degree of valve dysfunction (stenosis or regurgitation) are at risk of sterile platelet-fibrin thrombus formation. The Venturi effect usually causes the thrombus to form on the low-pressure side of the turbulent blood flow, such as with mitral regurgitation on the atrial side of the valve in patients with mitral regurgitation.

Subsequent bacteraemia allows colonisation of the pre-existing thrombus, resulting in vegetation formation. The bacteraemia can be induced by an invasive procedure, such as dental extraction, endoscopy or surgery in the presence of infection. The organisms are able to multiply within the platelet-fibrin thrombus and are 'protected' from the body's immune system. The most common organisms associated with native valve endocarditis include *Streptococcus viridans, Staphylococcus aureus, Staphylococccus epidermidis* and the enterococcus *Streptococcus faecalis*. Amongst their properties, these organisms are able to induce platelet aggregation, bind to the surface of the fibrin-platelet thrombus, as they possess fibronectin receptors, and resist the bactericidal action of complement and certain platelet proteins.

The pathological effects of infective endocarditis are secondary to spread into the surrounding

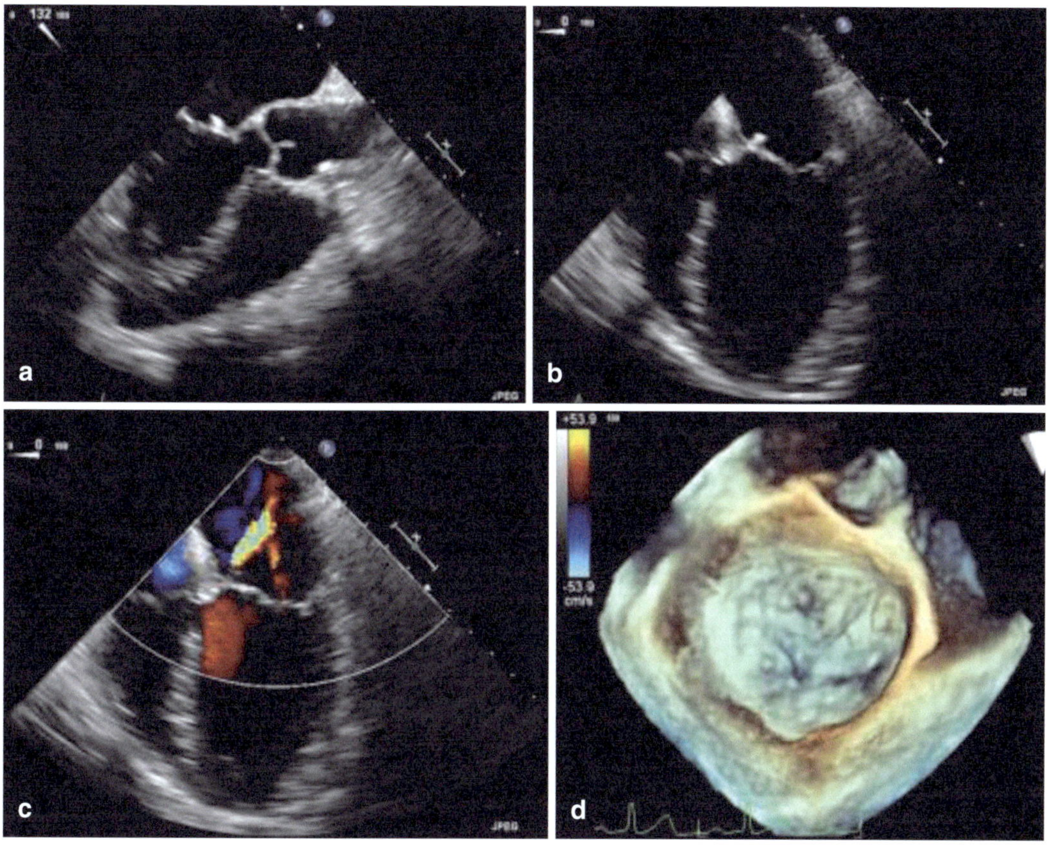

Fig. 12.2 Trans-oesophageal echocardiographical images demonstrating a 0.7 cm vegetation of the atrial surface of the anterior mitral valve leaflet on mid-oesophageal (**a**) long-axis and (**b**) 4-chamber views, associated with a jet of severe mitral regurgitation through the perforation on the corresponding colour flow Doppler image, and (**d**) a perforation visible in the body of the anterior leaflet on a 3D short-axis view

tissues causing local tissue destruction, such as leaflet perforation or peri-annular abscess formation. In addition, embolisation of the vegetation can result in peripheral abscesses, such as cerebral, renal or splenic. Peripheral effects of the infective endocarditic process can also occur secondary to immune complex deposition, such as vasculitis or glomerulonephritis.

Surgical Strategy

Although a proportion of patients with mitral valve infective endocarditis can be treated medically with antibiotics, surgical intervention is often required and should be initiated early to reduce the risk of on-going valve destruction or embolisation. When operating on these patients, it is important to first determine whether repair is feasible or replacement is necessary. Although mitral valve repair in this setting may prolong the ischaemia time, there is evidence of both short and long-term advantages of repair over replacement, including a lower incidence of recurrent endocarditis, improved freedom from reoperation and long-term survival advantage in this patient cohort.

Indications for Surgery

1. Uncontrollable sepsis despite appropriate antibiotics for an adequate time (7 days)
2. Abscess formation in the annulus or leaflets

3. Uncontrollable heart failure (although this is unusual these days)
4. Significant embolisation from large vegetations on the leading edge of the leaflets
5. Any of the above in association with *staphylococcus aureus* infection

The timing of surgery needs to be carefully considered, especially as early surgery in the presence of significant on-going infection runs the risk of recurrence of infection, particularly in the presence of an artificial valve.

During the operation, it is important to avoid excessive manipulation of the heart before the aortic cross-clamp has been applied, to avoid systemic embolisation of infected tissue. The key principle in determining the feasibility of valve repair in patients with mitral valve infective endocarditis is to identify the lesions caused by the infective process and the extent of tissue destruction. There are several patterns of destruction encountered in these patients, including perforation of the anterior leaflet, destruction of the posterior leaflet, commissural prolapse and annular abscess. It is quite common to find anterior leaflet perforation in patients with concomitant endocarditis of the aortic valve, due to jet lesions onto the aorto-mitral curtain and anterior leaflet.

Leaflet Reconstruction

In patients where the regurgitation is caused by leaflet perforation, it is important to assess whether it is possible to resect the infected tissue with a clear margin, whilst leaving enough native tissue to form a competent valve. If the valve is deemed repairable, all macroscopically infected and inflamed tissue is excised to ensure that the residual native tissue is free from infection, with a 2 mm margin. The residual tissue must be strong enough to hold suture material.

Repair of a defect in the anterior leaflet is usually possible, even if up to 50% of the leaflet body is involved, so long as the leading edge of the anterior leaflet, along the coaptation line, is intact. The defect in the leaflet body may be repaired with fresh autologous pericardium, glutaraldehyde-treated autologous pericardium or bovine pericardium. Bovine pericardium is used if autologous pericardium is not available, such as in patients undergoing reoperation. Bovine pericardium, as well as glutaraldehyde-treated autologous pericardium, also have the advantage of being easier to handle and are used for more complex reconstructions. Although deceullarised porcine intestinal submucosa (CorMatrix©) has also been used for leaflet patch augmentation, there have been reports of patch dehiscence or tearing using this material.

The pericardium is implanted using a continuous locking 5/0 Prolene suture, to avoid purse-stringing the patch (Fig. 12.3). It is important to oversize the patch to ensure that there is no tension on the leaflet causing restricted leaflet motion. In some patients, additional Gore-Tex neo-chordae are required to support the free edge of the anterior leaflet.

Infective lesions of the posterior leaflet can usually be treated by resection, using the standard principles of triangular or quadrangular resection, with or without annular plication and sliding plasty. In addition, some patients will require patch augmentation or Gore-Tex neo-chordae to support the leaflet body and free edge, respectively (Fig. 12.4).

Infective destruction of the anterolateral or posteromedial commissure, however, can be more difficult to treat. Following resection of the infected adjacent segments, sliding plasty is often required to advance posterior leaflet tissue to reconstruct the commissure (Fig. 12.5). Again additional patch augmentation, Gore-Tex neo-chordae or annular plication may also be required to support the commissural reconstruction.

The vegetation and any resected tissue should be sent for microbiological analysis. Any

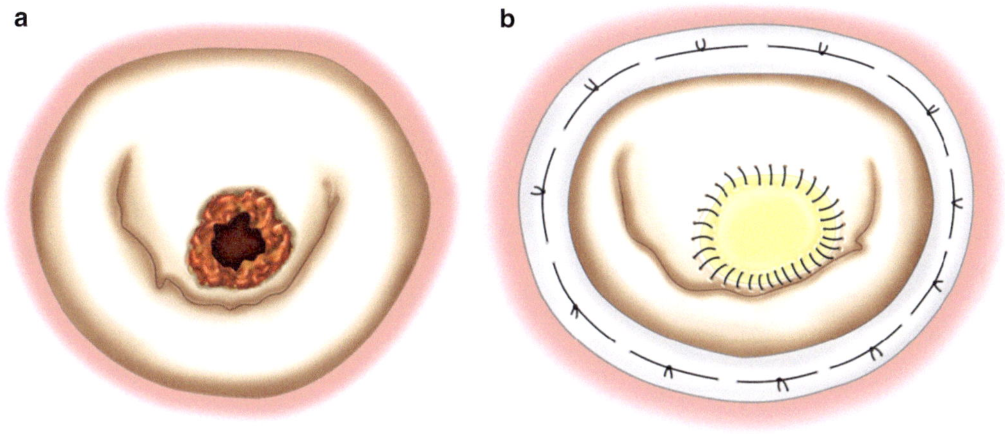

Fig. 12.3 (**a**) Perforation of the anterior mitral valve leaflet caused by the presence of a vegetation and infective destruction of the native tissue, and (**b**) repair with bovine pericardial patch augmentation of the anterior leaflet and ring annuloplasty

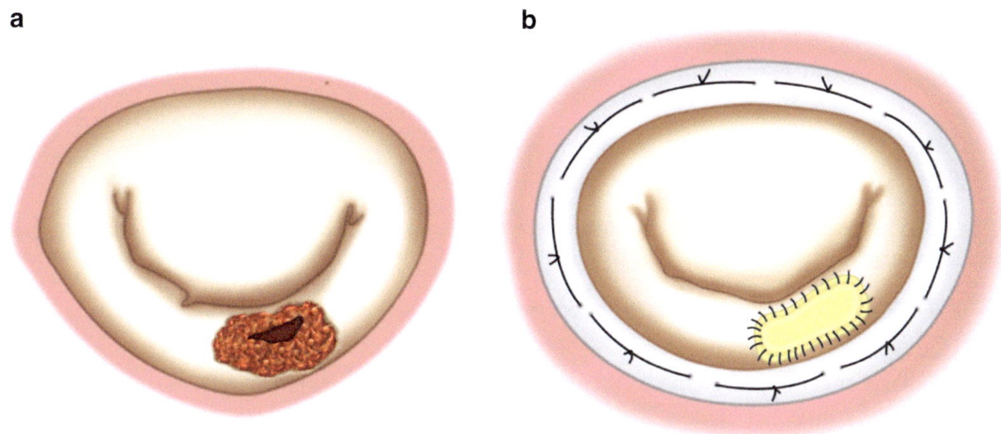

Fig. 12.4 (**a**) Perforation of the posterior leaflet caused by the presence of a vegetation and infective destruction of the native tissue, and (**b**) repair with bovine pericardial patch augmentation of the posterior leaflet and ring annuloplasty

underlying mitral valve pathology, which may have contributed to the development of the infective endocarditis, should also be treated during the repair procedure using standard techniques. Degenerative mitral valve prolapse is the most common underlying cardiac lesion that predisposes to mitral valve infective endocarditis.

Once the repair procedure has been completed, it is important to stabilise the mitral valve annulus with an annuloplasty band or ring, thereby relieving the tension on the leaflets by optimising the coaptation zone. Although some advocate avoidance of using prosthetic material in these patients, there is no evidence that using

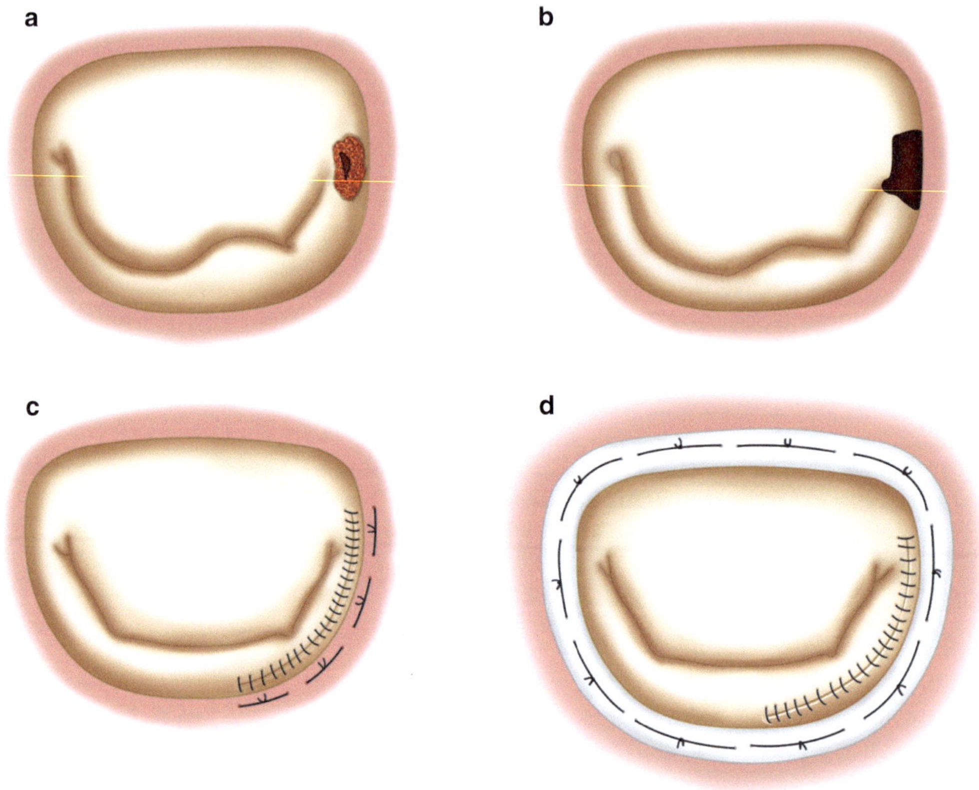

Fig. 12.5 (**a**) Prolapse of the posteromedial commissure caused by the presence of a vegetation and infective destruction of the underlying native tissue, (**b**) debridement of the infected tissue by quadrangular resection, (**c**) repair with sliding plasty advancement of the medial half of the posterior leaflet and commissuroplasty, followed by (**d**) ring annuloplasty

an annuloplasty ring or band increases the risk of recurrent endocarditis but it does increase the longevity of the repair.

Annular Reconstruction

In patients with infective endocarditis of the mitral valve, it is important to explore the surrounding tissues to assess for the presence of any peri-annular abscess or spread onto the aorto-mitral curtain. If present, extension of the infective process into the posterior annulus with resulting peri-annular abscess formation will require extensive debridement of the annulus and the abscess cavity, followed by reconstruction of the posterior annulus and atrioventricular groove (Fig. 12.6). An oversized fresh autologous or bovine pericardial patch is used to cover the defect in the atrioventricular groove and attached to the adjacent posterior walls of the left ventricle and left atrium using a continuous 4/0 Prolene suture. It is important to place the sutures in the ventricle distant from the edges of the resected material to ensure a strong suture line. Left atrial and ventricular pressures help to maintain

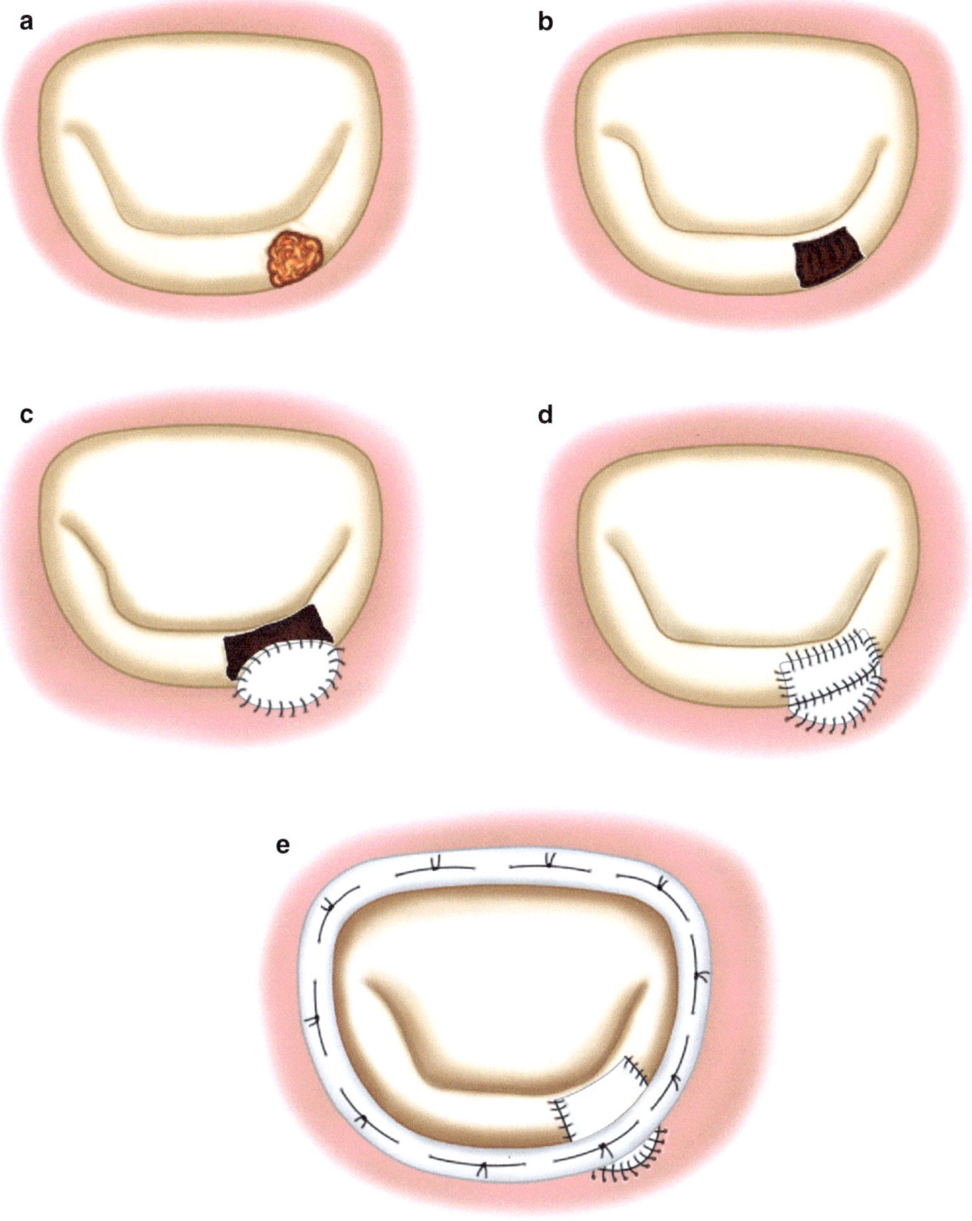

Fig. 12.6 (**a**) Abscess of the posterior mitral valve annulus, (**b**) debridement of infected tissue extending into the atrioventricular groove, (**c**) bovine pericardial patch reconstruction of the atrioventricular groove, extending onto the posterior wall of the left ventricle and left atrium, (**d**) bovine pericardial patch reconstruction of the posterior leaflet and (**e**) ring annuloplasty to support the repair

apposition of the patch against the posterior wall of the heart. The reconstructed posterior annulus with pericardial patch can then be used to receive the interrupted valve annuloplasty or replacement sutures, which will additionally help to secure the patch in situ.

If repair is not possible and replacement is necessary, the choice between a mechanical or biological valve should be made with the usual considerations, as there is no difference in recurrent endocarditis rates between the two valve choices.

Following all surgery for mitral valve endocarditis (repair or replacement), organism-specific intravenous antibiotics should be continued as dictated by current international recommendations, usually for 4–6 weeks. If organisms are grown from the resected material, it is the authors recommendation that antibiotic treatment should continue for 6 weeks with a full endocarditis screen two weeks after the completion of the treatment.

Surgical Technique

The mitral valve was assessed, using segmental analysis of the leaflets and the subvalvular apparatus, and correlated with the trans-oesophageal echocardiographical findings. A 0.7 cm vegetation was identified on the atrial surface of the anterior leaflet, with associated perforation (Fig. 12.7a). The infective process had spread into adjacent areas of the anterior leaflet but was not involving the chordae tendinae or posterior leaflet. The aortic valve was also free from any visible infection.

Stay sutures (5/0 Prolene) were placed around the chordae tendineae attached on either side of the perforated area of the anterior leaflet. Gentle traction on these stay sutures gave better access and visualisation of the anterior leaflet. The vegetation and any residual infected leaflet surrounding the perforation were excised and sent for microbiological analysis (Fig. 12.7b). At this stage, it was important to assess the degree of destruction to the surrounding tissues and whether

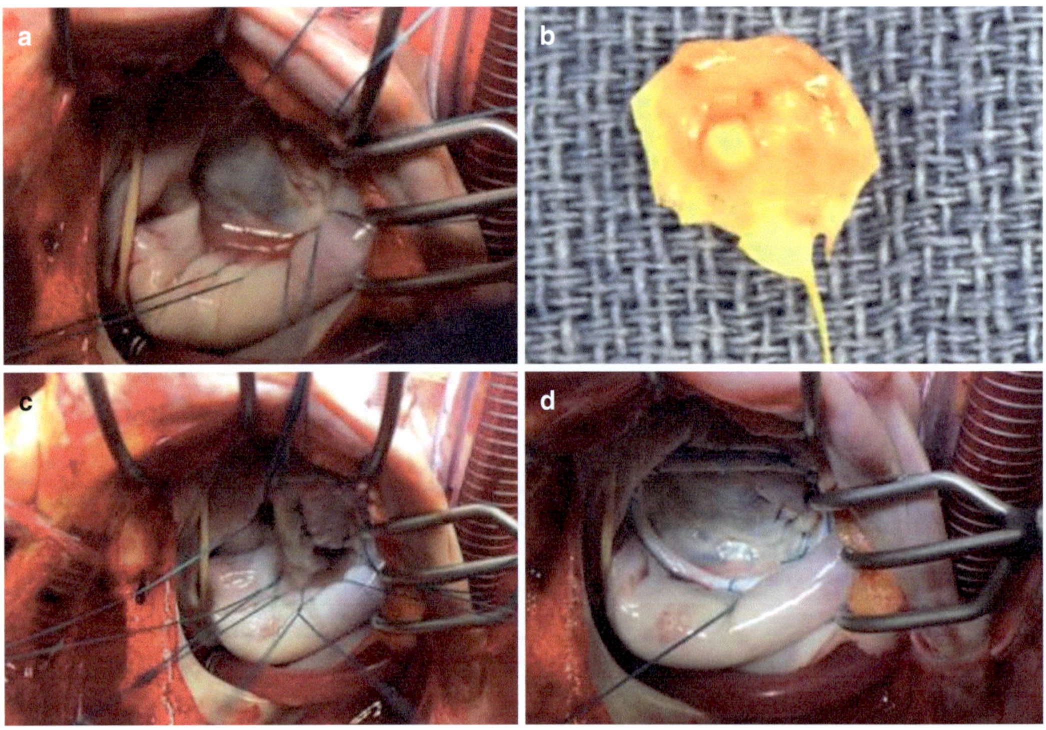

Fig. 12.7 Operative images illustrating (**a**) 0.7 cm vegetation lying on the atrial surface of the A3 scallop of the anterior leaflet, (**b**) resected vegetation and surrounding infected tissue, (**c**) closure of the defect in the A3 segment of the leaflet with a bovine pericardial patch and (**d**) implantation of an annuloplasty ring to support the repair

enough of the valvular and subvalvular structures remained intact and free from the infective process to produce a competent valve by repair.

A bovine pericardial patch was then used to close the defect in the anterior leaflet using continuous locking 5/0 Prolene with a tension-free anastomosis (Fig. 12.7c). Competency of the mitral valve was assessed with static testing, by injecting cold saline into the left ventricle, using a bulb syringe. Horizontal mattress band annuloplasty sutures (2/0 Ethibond) were placed around the circumference of the mitral valve, with a 5 mm width and approximately 1 mm apart. The appropriate sized annuloplasty ring was then chosen, according to the surface area of the whole mitral valve orifice, and tied down in situ.

Following implantation of the annuloplasty ring, injecting cold saline again allowed the mitral valve to be assessed for competency, adequate depth of coaptation (>8 mm) and that the coaptation line runs parallel to the posterior annulus (Fig. 12.7d).

Post-operative Echocardiogram

The post-repair trans-oesophageal echocardiogram (Fig. 12.8) confirmed:

1. No residual vegetation
2. Competency of the mitral valve with no residual mitral regurgitation.
3. The depth of leaflet coaptation was >8 mm.

Surgical Tips

1. Complete debridement of the vegetation and adjacent infected and inflamed tissue is necessary to reduce the risk of recurrence
2. Assess that there is enough residual tissue after resection to allow for repair
3. Augment any defects in the leaflet tissue or annulus with bovine or fresh autologous pericardium
4. Support the leaflet repair procedure with an annuloplasty ring.

Comment

For endocarditis patients who have limited valve destruction, the results of mitral valve repair have shown excellent outcomes, with an in-hospital mortality of 3% and a low peri-operative complication rate. In general, however, patients with acute mitral valve endocarditis have an operative mortality of 10–20%. Long term outcome measures at 10 years of patients who have undergone repair have also demonstrated excellent freedom from recurrent mitral regurgitation (91% with no or 1+ MR), freedom from reoperation (91%) and survival (80%). Meta-analyses and large series comparing repair versus replacement in patients with mitral valve infective endocarditis have

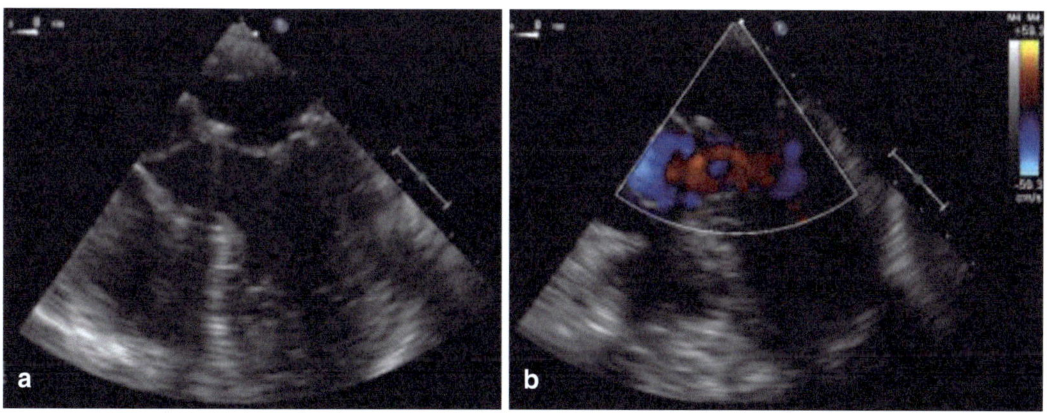

Fig. 12.8 Post-bypass intra-operative trans-oesophageal echocardiographical images demonstrating a competent mitral valve, with no residual mitral regurgitation, no residual vegetation and 9 mm depth of coaptation between the anterior and posterior leaflets

shown better short and long-term outcome measures, with a lower operative mortality, increased long-term survival, reduced risk of recurrent endocarditis and reduced need for a reoperation in patients undergoing repair. The increased incidence of reoperation in patients undergoing replacement for mitral valve endocarditis is related to paravalvular leaks, structural valve deterioration and prosthetic valve endocarditis.

Recommended Reading

AATS Surgical Treatment of Infective Endocarditis Consensus Guidelines Writing Committee Chairs, Pettersson GB, Coselli JS, Writing Committee, Pettersson GB, Coselli JS, Hussain ST, Griffin B, Blackstone EH, Gordon SM, SA LM, Woc-Colburn LE. The American Association for Thoracic Surgery (AATS) consensus guidelines: surgical treatment of infective endocarditis. J Thorac Cardiovasc Surg 2017. 2016;153(6):1241–58.

de Kerchove L, Price J, Tamer S, Glineur D, Momeni M, Noirhomme P, ElKhoury G. Extending the scope of mitral valve repair in active endocarditis. J Thorac Cardiovasc Surg. 2012;123(4 Suppl):S91–5.

Evans CF, Gammie JS. Surgical management of mitral valve infective endocarditis. Semin Thorac Cardiovasc Surg. 2011;23(3):232–40.

Feringa HH, Shaw LJ, Poldermans D, Hoeks S, van der Wall EE, Dion RA, Bax JJ. Mitral valve repair and replacement in endocarditis: a systematic review of literature. Ann Thorac Surg. 2007;83(2): 564–70.

Sareyyupoglu B, Schaff HV, Suri RM, Connolly HM, Daly RC, Orszulak TA. Safety and durability of mitral valve repair for anterior leaflet perforation. J Thorac Cardiovasc Surg. 2010;139(6):1288–93.

Shimokawa T, Kasegawa H, Matsuyama S, Seki H, Manabe S, Fukui T, Morita S, Takanashi S. Long-term outcome of mitral valve repair for infective endocarditis. Ann Thorac Surg. 2009;88(3):733–9.

Zegdi R, Debièche M, Latrémouille C, Lebied D, Chardigny C, Grinda JM, Chauvaud S, Deloche A, Carpentier A, Fabiani JN. Long-term results of mitral valve repair in active endocarditis. Circulation. 2005;111(19):2532–6.

Zhao D, Zhang B. Are valve repairs associated with better outcomes than replacements in patients with native active valve endocarditis? Interact Cardiovasc Thorac Surg. 2014;19(6):1036–9.

13 Extensive Mitral Annular Calcification

Keywords
Mitral annular calcification · Degenerative mitral valve disease · En bloc resection · Annular reconstruction · Pericardial patch reconstruction · Decalcification · Mitral valve replacement · Atrioventricular disruption · Circumflex coronary artery

Case History

A 78 year-old lady presented with a prolonged history of increasing exertional dyspnoea associated with lethargy. She had no history of rheumatic fever or infective endocarditis and had been followed up with serial echocardiography over several years with known mitral regurgitation. A chest radiograph demonstrated a C-shaped calcific outline of the mitral annulus with the open part lying adjacent to the left ventricular outflow tract (Fig. 13.1a). Coronary angiography demonstrated no flow limiting coronary artery lesions but marked calcification of the mitral annulus could clearly be visualised during fluoroscopy (Fig. 13.1b).

Echocardiographical Findings

Trans-thoracic parasternal long-axis echocardiographic images revealed prolapse of the posterior mitral valve leaflet (Fig. 13.2a). This was also observed on the apical 4-chamber and 3-chamber views (Fig. 13.2b, c), where the posterior leaflet can be seen to override the annular plane during systole. In both of these images, an irregular, echo-dense mass was observed at the angle between the left ventricular wall and the posterior leaflet. This was further visualised on a parasternal short-axis view of the mitral valve, demonstrating extensive posterior mitral annular calcification at the junction of the atrioventricular groove and posterior leaflet (Fig. 13.2d). The mitral annular calcification was graded as severe as it extended along the entire posterior annulus, from trigone to trigone, with the maximum width of the calcification 7 mm. The septal part of annulus was spared.

Images derived from a trans-oesophageal probe allowed segmental analysis of the posterior leaflet dysfunction and showed isolated prolapse of a tall P2 segment with associated chordal rupture, in the mid-oesophageal long-axis view (Fig. 13.3a). Colour flow Doppler across the mitral valve demonstrated an anterior directed jet of mitral regurgitation (MR), confirming posterior leaflet prolapse as the dominant lesion (Fig. 13.3b). Quantification of the regurgitation, using the PISA method revealed severe MR with an effective regurgitant orifice area of 51 mm^2, regurgitant volume of 65 mL and regurgitant fraction of 56%, associated with a vena contracta of 0.81 cm. The left atrium was dilated at 5.17 cm but the left ventricular size was preserved. The

N. Moorjani et al., *Operative Mitral and Tricuspid Valve Surgery*,
https://doi.org/10.1007/978-1-4471-4204-1_13

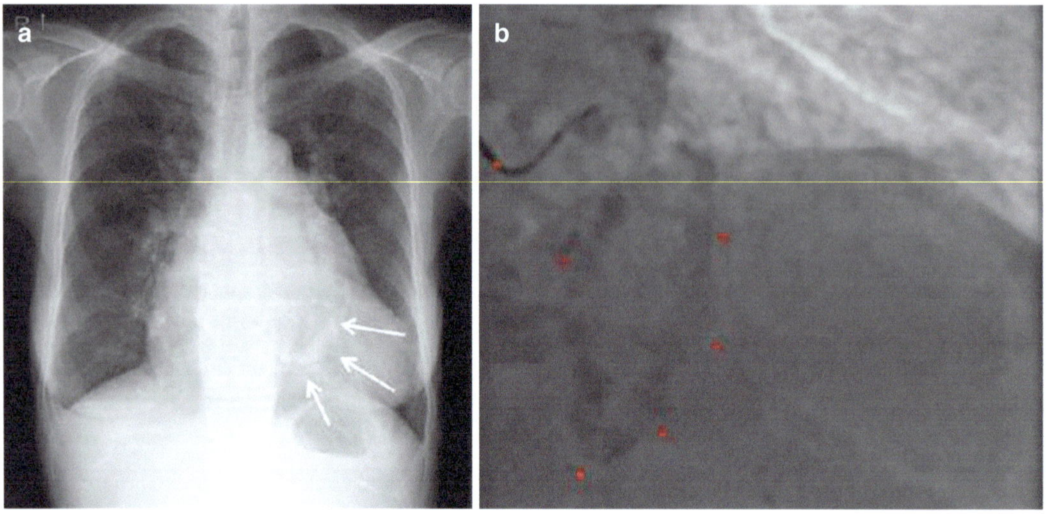

Fig. 13.1 (**a**) Chest radiograph and (**b**) fluoroscopic image demonstrating extensive mitral annular calcification (arrows)

left ventricular end-systolic diameter was 3.7 cm and left ventricular end-diastolic diameter 5.2 cm, with an ejection fraction of 67%. In addition, calcification of the posterior mitral valve annulus can clearly be seen on mid-oesophageal 2-chamber (Fig. 13.3c) and long-axis (Fig. 13.3d) views. Three-dimensional (3D) short-axis images also demonstrate the prolapsing P2 segment of the posterior leaflet and extensive calcification of the posterior mitral annulus in diastole (Fig. 13.3e) and systole (Fig. 13.3f).

In view of this, a multi-slice spiral computed tomography scan (Fig. 13.4) was performed to further delineate the exact location and extent of the annular calcification, which demonstrated the calcification extending into the left ventricular muscle postero-inferiorly.

Pathophysiology

Mitral annular calcification (MAC) represents a chronic degenerative calcific process that begins in the atrio-ventricular junction of the mitral valve and affects the posterior annulus to varying degrees. It seems to occur at the point of maximum flexion of the posterior leaflet on the annulus and exaggerated motion might be a stimulus for this. It has been suggested that the underlying pathological process of MAC is similar to atherosclerosis, and hence an association of MAC with hypertension, diabetes mellitus, smoking, hyperlipidaemia and cardiovascular atheromatous disease but there is no evidence for this. Increased stress on the mitral valve is a more likely risk factor for MAC, as it is so often found in patients with mitral valve prolapse of probable life long duration. Hypertension or aortic stenosis, which result in increased mitral valve closing pressure, have also been suggested as potential risk factors producing excess annular tension and subsequent annular degeneration but, again, there is no more than circumstantial evidence for this. In patients with degenerative mitral valve disease, extensive MAC has a bimodal distribution, occurring either in younger patients with Barlow's disease or in the elderly patients with fibroelastic deficiency. MAC has a reported prevalence of 8–15% and whilst it is more commonly found in the elderly, it can occur in significantly younger patients. Patients with chronic kidney disease, especially if undergoing dialysis may have a higher incidence. Several patients with significant and long-standing mitral regurgitation are found to have a white creamy material in the annular reflection of the posterior leaflet, which can extend into the left ventricular muscle at the

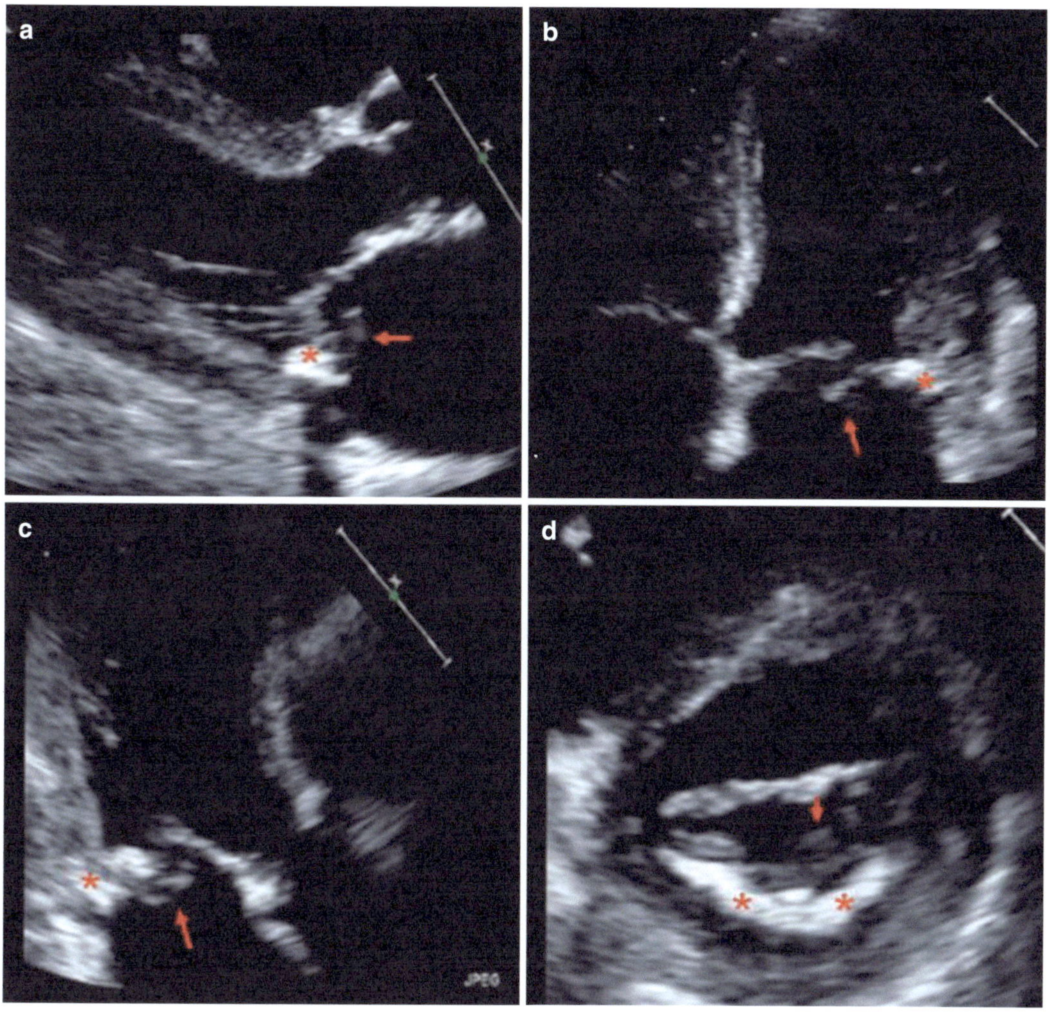

Fig. 13.2 Trans-thoracic echocardiographical images demonstrating prolapse of the P2 segment of the posterior mitral valve leaflet (red arrow), secondary to ruptured chordae tendineae and extensive posterior mitral annular calcification (red star) on (**a**) parasternal long-axis, (**b**) apical 4-chamber, (**c**) apical 3-chamber and (**d**) parasternal short-axis views

base of the heart. This may be a precursor of the calcification.

The severity of MAC can be qualitatively categorised on a trans-thoracic parasternal short-axis image as mild (focal, limited echodensity of the mitral annulus), moderate (marked echodensity involving between 1/3 and 1/2 of the annular circumference) or severe (marked echodensity involving >1/2 of the annular circumference or with intrusion into the left ventricular inflow tract, Fig. 13.5). A maximal width of the calcification from the anterior to the posterior edge >4 mm can also be used to define severe MAC.

The presence of extensive MAC destroys the normal dynamic changes of the mitral annulus that occur during the cardiac cycle. Systolic contraction of the base of the left ventricle at the annulus that is important in valve closure and competency is lost. Extension of the calcification process from the annulus onto the base of the mitral valve tissue causes restricted basal leaflet motion contributing to the development of mitral valve dysfunction. In addition, traction on the

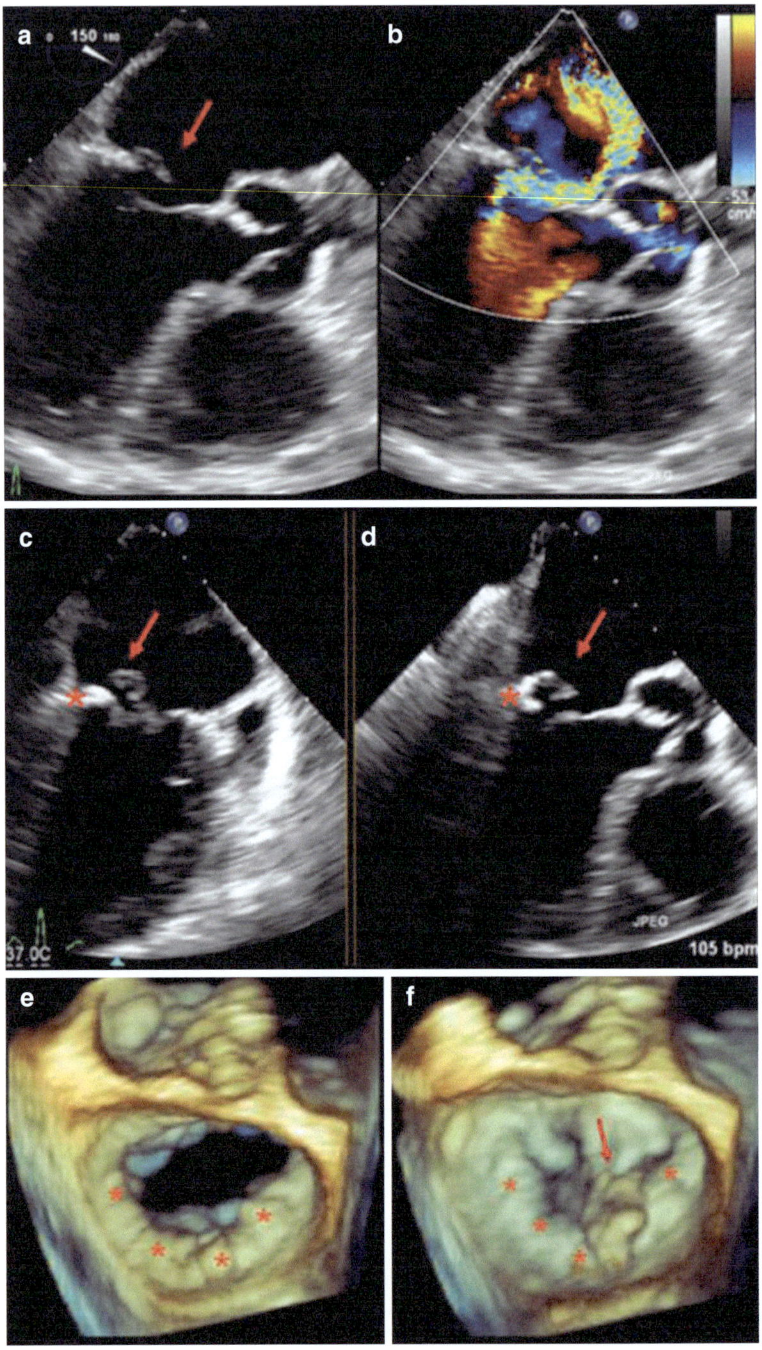

Fig. 13.3 Trans-oesophageal echocardiographical images demonstrating P2 prolapse (red arrow), secondary to a ruptured chordae tendineae, on (**a**) the long-axis view, resulting in severe eccentric anteriorly directed mitral regurgitation on (**b**) the corresponding colour flow Doppler image. In addition, the extensive posterior mitral annular calcification (red star) can be seen on (**c**) the mid-oesophageal 2-chamber, (**d**) mid-oesophageal long-axis, (**e**) diastolic 3D surgical and (**f**) systolic 3D surgical views

leaflets by MAC increases the tension on the attached chordae and the risk of subsequent chordal elongation or rupture. The leaflet hinge point progresses away from the annulus into the body of the leaflet.

The presence of MAC is associated with conduction delays and heart block, which is thought to be secondary to direct extension of calcific deposits into conducting tissue or diffuse degenerative disease of the conduction tissue.

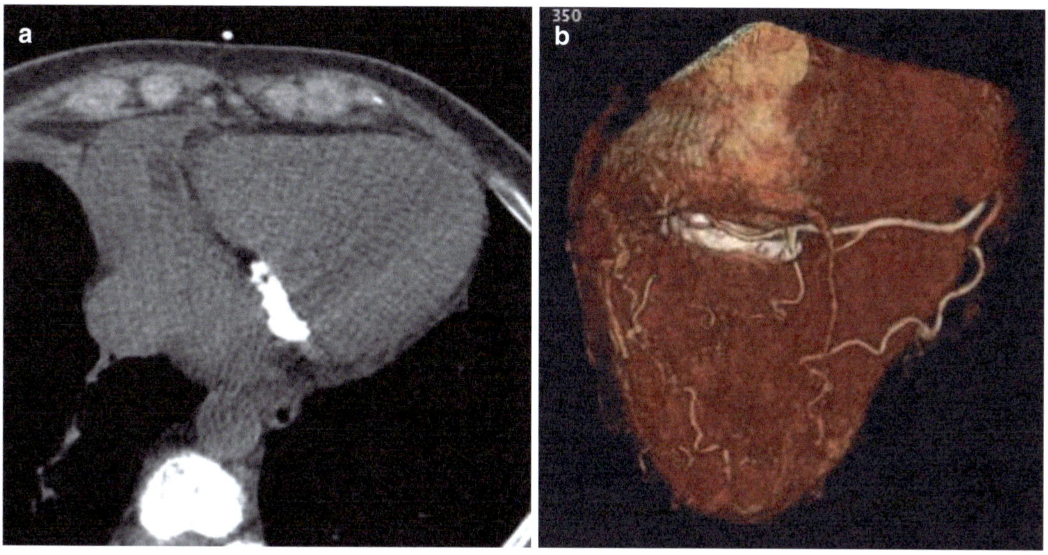

Fig. 13.4 (**a**) Axial and (**b**) 3D reconstruction computed tomography images demonstrating extensive posterior mitral annular calcification

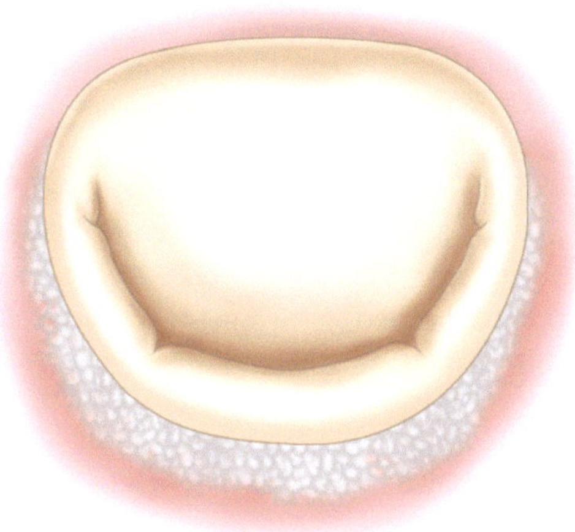

Fig. 13.5 Severe mitral annular calcification, extending greater than 50% of the annular circumference

Surgical Strategy

Mitral valve surgery can be technically very challenging in the presence of extensive calcification of the mitral valve annulus, especially when it extends into the left ventricular myocardium. Serious complications include cardiac rupture at the atrioventricular junction or left ventricular free wall, injury to the circumflex artery and thromboembolic events. In general, the techniques that can be employed to tackle extensive mitral annular calcification are divided into two broad categories, those where the annulus is not debrided and those where the calcification is debrided followed by annular reconstruction.

Mitral Valve Repair Without Annular Decalcification

Mitral valve repair without annular decalcification has the principal advantage that it avoids the risks of atrioventricular disruption and damage to the circumflex artery. These repair techniques include edge-to-edge repair, simple leaflet repair or artificial chordal reconstruction without annuloplasty. Although they can be simple to perform with low operative mortality, their success depends upon the degree of calcification and the amount of flexible leaflet beyond the boundary of the calcium. There is a significant risk of residual or recurrent mitral regurgitation because the isolated mitral repair cannot correct the annular dilatation and leaflet deformation caused by the calcification. In view of this, leaflet augmentation has been suggested as a repair technique to compensate for the leaflet retraction caused by the extensive calcification. Again the success of this will depend upon the amount of useable leaflet that exists beyond the calcified part. Using autologous or bovine pericardium, the leaflet can be extended restoring coaptation. Suturing the pericardium to the atrial wall, thereby excluding the MAC is to be avoided as it can distort posterior leaflet function. Depending on the extent of the calcification, however, these repair techniques without annuloplasty should probably be reserved for high risk, elderly patients; otherwise valve repair with annular decalcification or valve replacement should be performed.

Annular Decalcification and Reconstruction

The posterior leaflet is incised at the edge of the calcified portion of the annulus for the full length of the calcification. This detached region of the posterior leaflet can then be retracted towards the septum with 5/0 polypropylene stay sutures. The atrial endothelium is then incised at the border with the calcified bar. Using a sharp blade, the atrioventricular tissue is separated with controlled dissection by keeping the blade directly on the calcific bar to minimise disruption to the atrioventricular junction (Fig. 13.6).

Generally, there will be a 'tide' of fibrous tissue at the junction with the ventricular muscle that can be kept. This is very valuable for securely holding the sutures in the placement of a pericardial patch. The calcified bar is excised en bloc, which allows resection without calcium fragmentation. En bloc dissection is feasible because the calcific bar is usually encapsulated within a fibrous sheath. Any residual calcification is debrided using a rongeur. It is important to appreciate that extensive debridement of the calcified mitral annulus is a technically complex procedure and can be associated with significant risks, including atrioventricular disruption, circumflex coronary artery injury and ventricular rupture.

Following decalcification, the resultant anatomic separation between the left atrium, left ventricle and mitral annulus exposes the atrioventricular groove and necessitates mitral annular reconstruction. At this stage, the fibrous edges of the atrial and ventricular tissue can usually clearly be identified and used for annular reconstruction. This can be performed using a variety of different techniques, including direct annular suturing, which is not usually recommended, or patch repair. This preserves the integrity of the atrioventricular junction and reduce the risk of atrioventricular disruption.

Occasionally, if partial decalcification has been performed or a small area of the atrioventricular groove has been exposed, direct annular suturing can be performed using either interrupted pledged sutures or figure-of-eight non-pledgeted sutures, placed into the atrial and ventricular fibrous edges (Fig. 13.7). Again, it should be emphasised that this should only be used for very

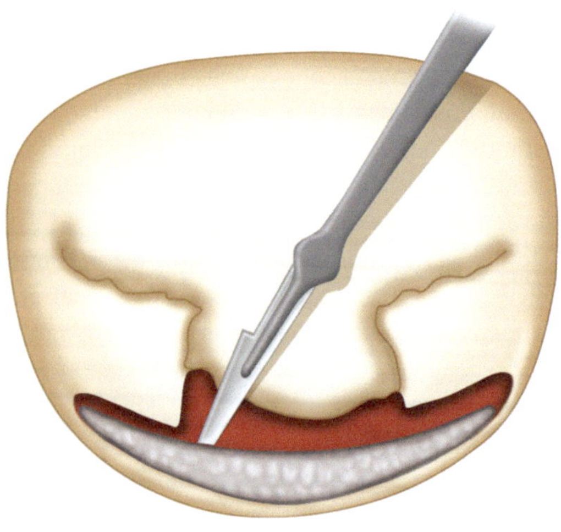

Fig. 13.6 En bloc resection of the mitral annular calcification, using a sharp blade to separate the calcific bar from the atrioventricular tissue

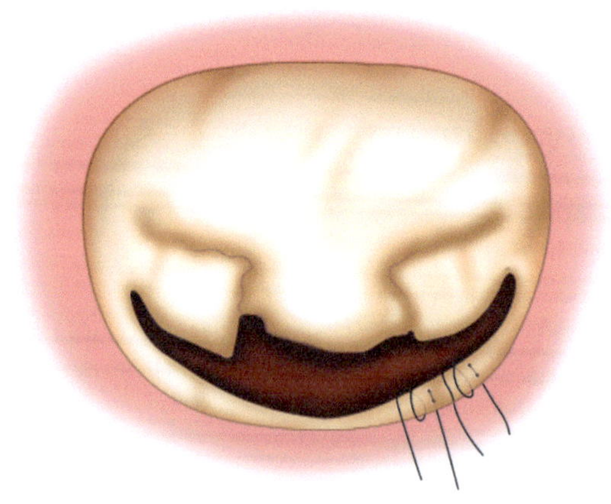

Fig. 13.7 Reconstruction of the atrioventricular junction using figure-of-eight sutures

limited lesions. Any tension at this junctional point of the heart cannot be expected to withstand the significant contractional and torsional forces that exist in the working heart.

In view of this, following decalcification when a significant portion of the atrioventricular groove has been exposed, annular reconstruction is best performed using a large pericardial patch. The patch allows the creation of a new annulus without tension on potentially fragile tissues and excludes the debrided atrioventricular junction, thereby reducing the risk of subsequent atrioventricular disruption. The placement of a generous patch also avoids distortion of the vessels in the atrioventricular groove (circumflex coronary artery and coronary sinus).

Complete decalcification reduces the risk of subsequent patch dehiscence, which may result if the sutures are passed through any remaining brittle calcium. The choice of material used for the patch repair includes fresh or glutaraldehyde-fixed autologous pericardium and bovine pericardium. The rigidity of Dacron makes it a poor material at this site. It will not conform to the atrial and ventricular surfaces, making a leak more likely when the heart is reperfused. It is imperative to use a generous 'over-sized' patch, as a small patch will cause tension at the atrioventricular junction and risk tearing during cardiac contraction. The patch is attached to the ventricular fibrous edge of the incision, as described earlier, or into firm endo/myocardium beyond the area of debridement, using a continuous 4/0 Prolene suture. The superior edge of the patch is then sutured to the atrial margin, taking care not to pick up the contents of the atrioventricular groove.

Depending on the extent of the calcification, mitral valve repair is feasible if the spared leaflet tissue is adequate in length and strength. Following annular decalcification and annular reconstruction, mitral repair may be preferable for the usual reasons. If this is the case, the posterior leaflet may either be reattached to the atrial/patch junction or a pericardial patch extension at the level of the original annulus. If this is anticipated, then a much larger patch can be used and the atrial patch suture line constructed along the pericardium not at its edge but within the body of the patch. The extraneous patch can then be folded over and sutured to the leaflet edge. When completed, any additional repair techniques can be performed. The entire repair should then be stabilised with an annuloplasty ring (Fig. 13.8).

If repair is not feasible following en-bloc resection and pericardial patch repair, then mitral valve replacement is performed by implanting a prosthesis into the reconstructed mitral annulus (Fig. 13.9). The pericardial patch is strong enough to hold the sutures without concern.

Mitral Valve Replacement Without Annular Decalcification

If en-bloc resection and annular reconstruction are deemed too risky, then mitral valve replacement without annular decalcification represents an alternative approach that may reduce the risk of atrioventricular disruption or damage to the circumflex artery. The mitral prosthesis can be implanted using different techniques in an intra-annular or intra-atrial position. The intra-annular technique involves passing the sutures through or around the calcification, with or without fragmentation of the annular calcification but leaving the calcification in situ (Fig. 13.10). The disadvantages of this technique, however, include paravalvar leak, valve dehiscence and embolism from the fragmented calcification, as well as the difficulty in passing valve sutures through the calcified annulus. An alternative intra-annular technique is to pass the sutures through plicated leaflet tissue. Not removing the annular calcification using these intra-annular techniques, however, necessitates implanting a smaller mitral prosthesis, which may result in prosthesis–patient mismatch. There is also a risk that these sutures may tear out as a result of the flexion at that point.

The intra-atrial technique involves implanting the mitral prosthesis about 1 cm lateral to the annulus into the supra-annular left atrial wall. This can be reinforced with plicated leaflet tissue, or using a Dacron or pericardial collar. These intra-atrial techniques, however, transfer ventricular pressures into the atrium and are associated with significant complications, including severe

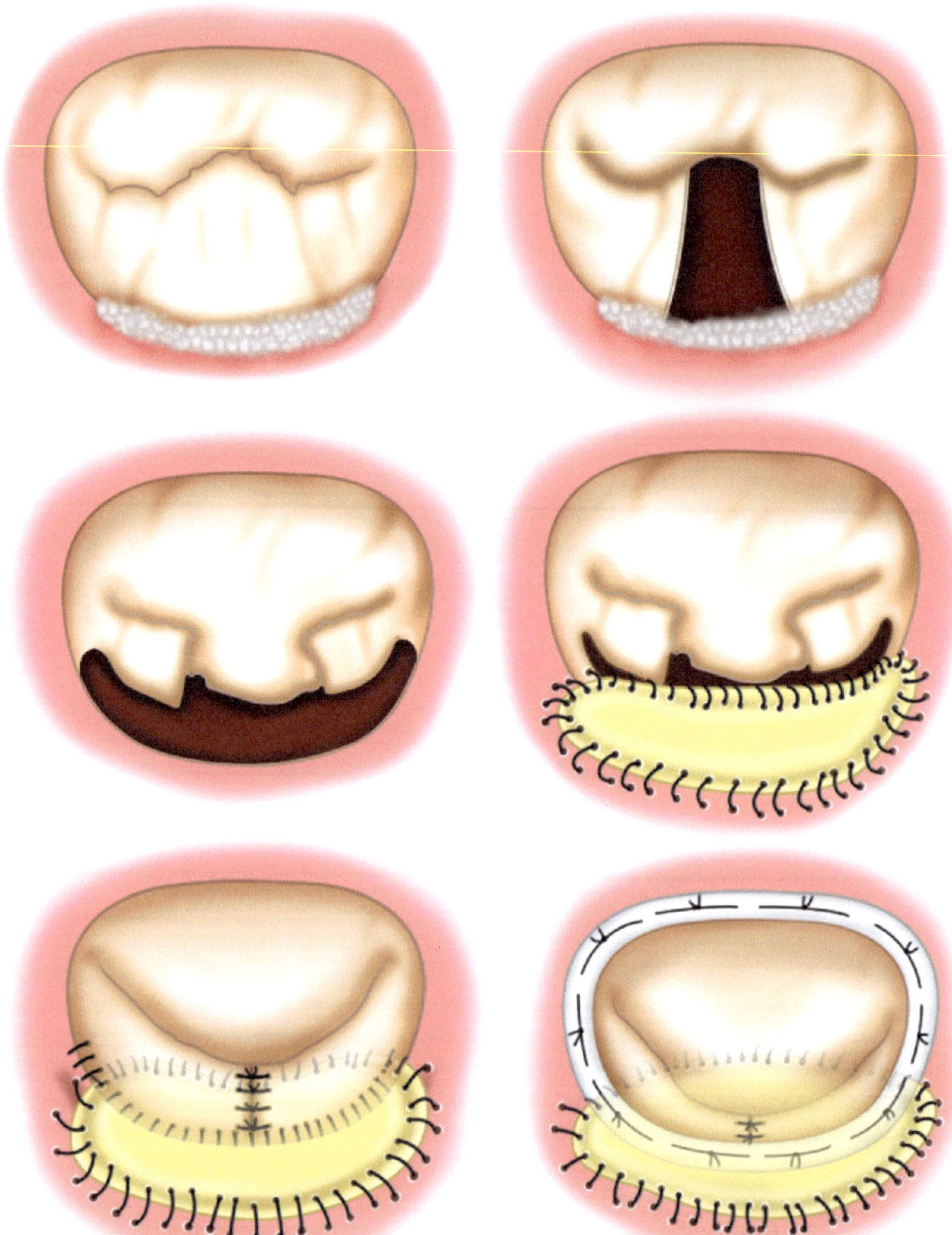

Fig. 13.8 Debridement of mitral annular calcification, annular reconstruction using pericardial patch repair, followed by leaflet repair and implantation of an annuloplasty ring

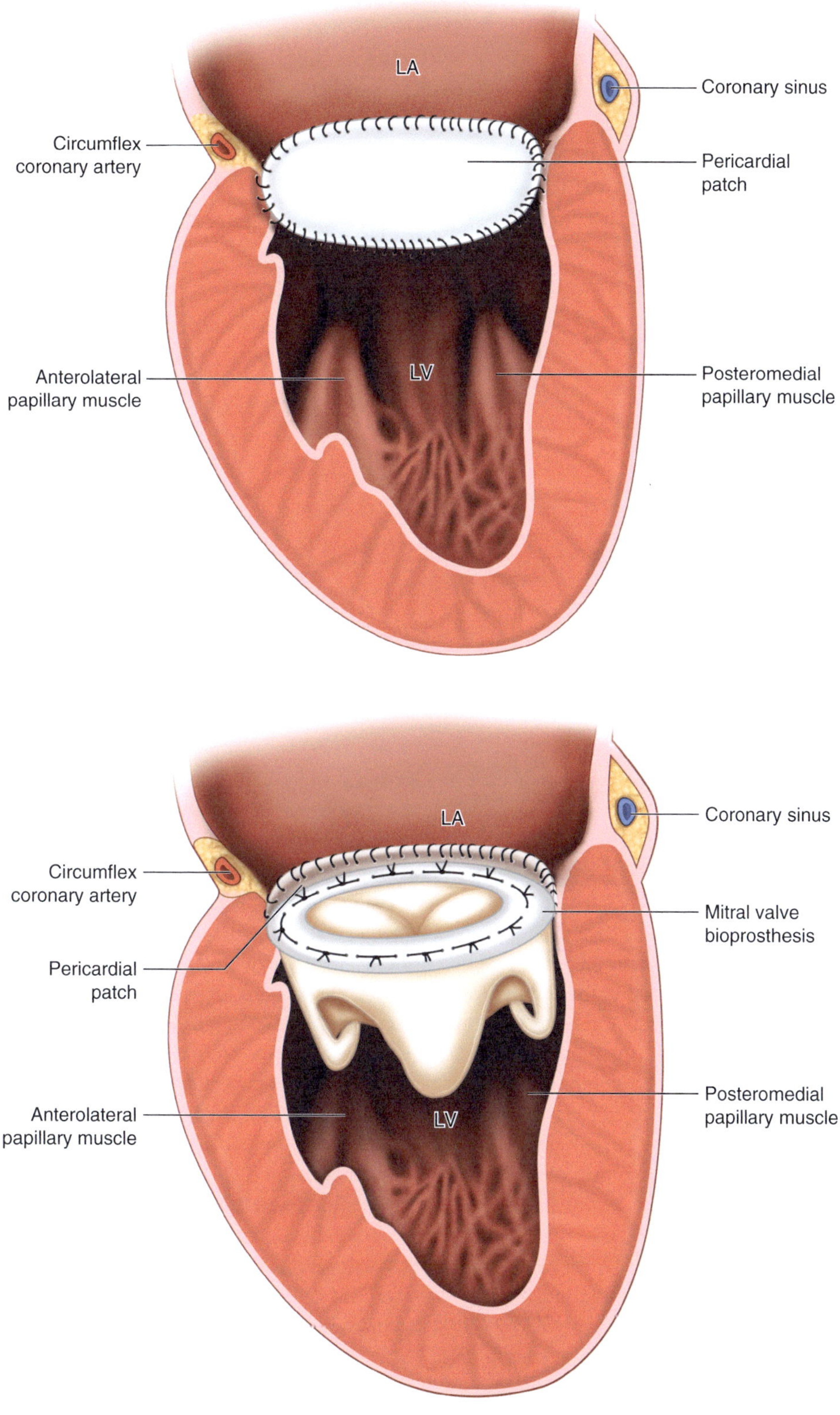

Fig. 13.9 Mitral annular reconstruction using a bovine pericardial patch followed by prosthetic valve implantation. LA left atrium, LV left ventricle

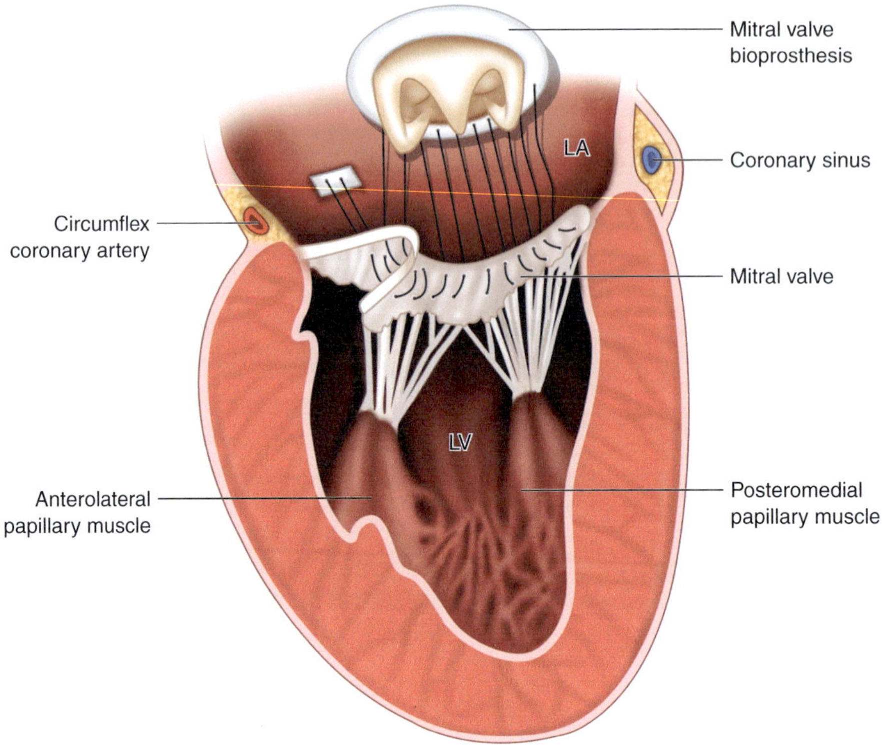

Fig. 13.10 Mitral valve replacement in the presence of extensive mitral annular calcification, implanted using an intra-annular technique by passing the sutures through plicated leaflet tissue. LA left atrium, LV left ventricle

haemorrhage, valve dehiscence, late aneurysm formation and rupture.

Surgical Technique

Following a standard left atriotomy, the junction between the calcified mass and the left ventricular muscle was carefully inspected. It is generally possible to see a whitish area of fibrous tissue, usually extending from the calcium into the ventricular muscle. This fibrous 'tide' is the area that needs to be preserved as far as possible because of its strength in holding sutures. Initially, the remaining pliable posterior leaflet is incised at the junction with the calcium and detached throughout its length. Fine polypropylene sutures are then placed through this incised margin to retract it, whilst the calcium is removed.

The calcium is the approached by cutting onto its edge on the left atrial surface with a No 15 blade scalpel. The blade is often exchanged to maintain sharp dissection. As the endothelium is incised, it is possible to coax the calcium out of the atrial tissue by stroking the atrial tissue away and continuing to gently incise the insinuated tissue (Fig. 13.11a). This is not a forceful movement but a gentle persuasion of the tissues away from the calcium. The incision and plane of dissection must continue along the full extent of the calcific region. As the dissection proceeds, it is common for the atrioventricular fat to become exposed but this should not be a cause for concern, as it is expected (Fig. 13.11b). In addition, it is important to appreciate that the circumflex coronary artery will have been displaced away from this plane by the gradual process of calcification. As the calcified bar is freed from the enveloping tissues, it is possible to grasp it with a pair of heavy forceps. At this stage, it is important not to lever it out of the tissues but to continue with the careful dissection. When it has been freed for approximately two thirds of its depth, it is time to turn attention to the ventricular margin, which is always irregular. An incision is made on the fibrous 'tide' at the margin of the calcification. With a combination of cutting and sweeping, the ventricu-

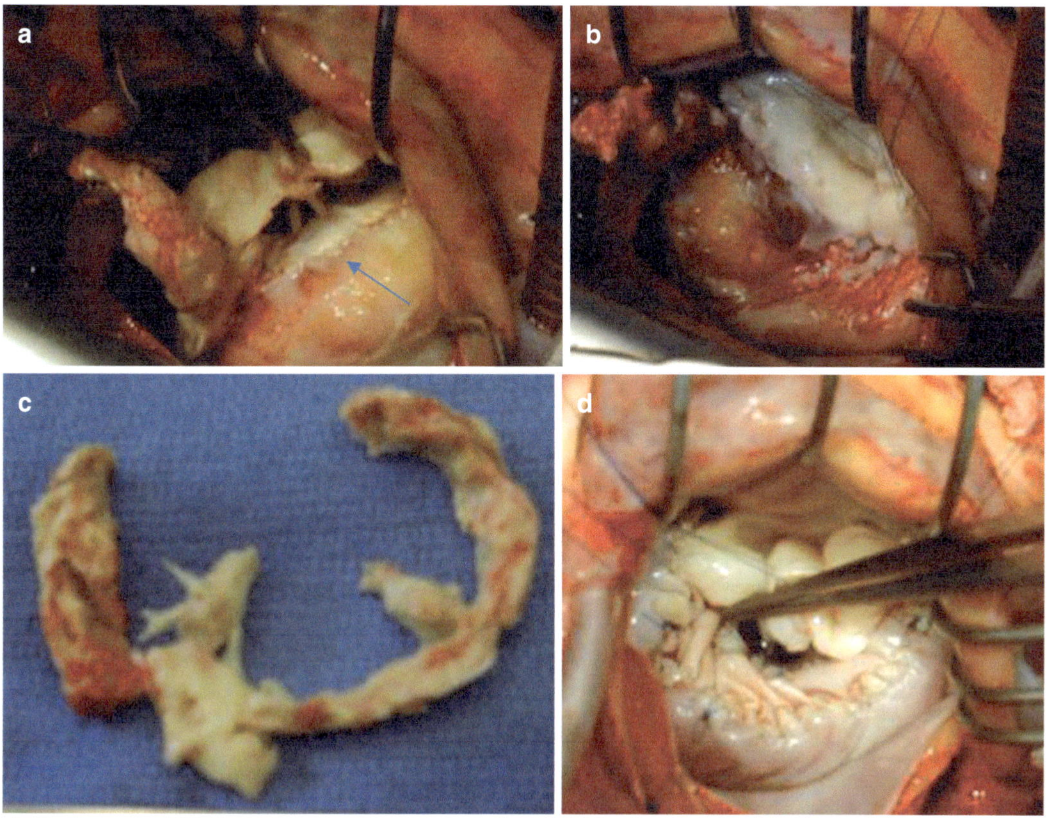

Fig. 13.11 Operative images demonstrating (**a**) and (**b**) excision of the posterior mitral annular calcification en-bloc, using sharp dissection, with the fibrous 'tide' (arrow) and fat within the atrioventricular groove visible, (**c**) excised calcium bar and (**d**) bovine pericardial patch reconstruction of the posterior annulus and atrioventricular groove

lar tissues are swept away from the calcified bar. With care, the calcified mass can be teased out of the surrounding tissues as a single piece. Any residual calcification can be debrided by rongeurs.

Once the calcium bar has been removed (Fig. 13.11c), pliable tissues remain on either side of the atrioventricular groove. Although it is feasible to approximate the atrial tissue to the ventricular muscle with direct sutures, it is quite likely that ventricular and atrial motion will cause these sutures at the atrioventricular junction to tear apart. The ideal solution is to close the defect using a generous pericardial patch, significantly larger than the defect and absolutely not smaller than the defect. The idea is to give a flexible haemostatic platform for the atria and ventricles to move through the phases of the cardiac cycle. The patch is not cut precisely but initially with the appropriate shape for the corner between ventricle and atrium at the inferomedial point. The part of the fibrous tide in the ventricle that has been preserved is used as a secure base for the ventricular sutures. The suture line was then continued along the ventricular margin cephalad to the superior margin. A separate 4/0 Prolene suture was then used along the atrial margin, which provides a secure base to either reattach the posterior mitral leaflet for valve reconstruction or to place sutures for implantation of a prosthesis (Fig. 13.11d). Also if valve insertion is the procedure of choice, the leaflet origins of the chordae to the posterior leaflet can be re-attached to the pericardial neo-annulus preserving valvular-ventricular continuity.

It is important to be aware of the left ventricular outflow tract just beneath the left fibrous trigone, as this is a very vulnerable area and these tissues lead out under the aortic valve towards the left atrial appendage. Intra-mural dissection of the ventricular muscle can lead to disruption and haemorrhage that appears beneath the left atrial appendage, which is very difficult to repair. If the calcification extends deeply into the ventricular muscle, removal of calcific excrescences with a rongeur may be the preferred method. If this is done, it is most important to remove all calcific particles by suction and washing out the ventricle to prevent arterial embolisation to the coronary arteries or to the cerebral circulation.

The posterior leaflet was reattached to the annulus and pericardial patch using 4/0 Prolene. Horizontal mattress annuloplasty sutures (2/0 Ethibond) were then placed around the circumference of the mitral valve, with a 5 mm width and approximately 1 mm apart. To treat the P2 prolapse, both limbs of a CV-4 Gore-Tex neochordae suture (W.L. Gore & Associates, Flagstaff, AZ, USA) were passed through the fibrous part of the papillary muscle head, using a simple U-suture. One of the limbs of the Gore-Tex suture was then passed through the prolapsing P2 segment of the posterior leaflet about 5 mm away from the leaflet edge and 2–3 mm away from the boundary of normal leaflet, from the ventricular side to the atrial side and then through a second time. This was then repeated for the second limb of the Gore-Tex neo-chord.

The provisional height of the Gore-Tex neochordae was then determined by using the level of the annulus as a reference to guide the correct length and tension of the implanted neo-chord. Competency of the mitral valve was then assessed with static testing, by injecting cold saline into the left ventricle, using a bulb syringe. With the left ventricle distended with saline, the depth of coaptation was assessed by colouring the atrial surface of the mitral valve leaflets with a sterile marking pen. The depth of coaptation can be increased to achieve an optimal depth of at least 8 mm by adjusting the length of Gore-Tex beneath the leaflet. An appropriate sized annuloplasty band or ring was then chosen, according to the surface area of the whole mitral valve orifice (i.e. the surface area of the anterior and posterior leaflets together). The annuloplasty ring was then implanted using the 2/0 Ethibond sutures inserted earlier. A final saline test was performed to confirm valve competency and positioning of the coaptation line.

Post-operative Echocardiogram

The post-repair trans-oesophageal echocardiogram (Fig. 13.12) confirmed:

1. Normal physiological functioning of the mitral valve complex, including unrestricted

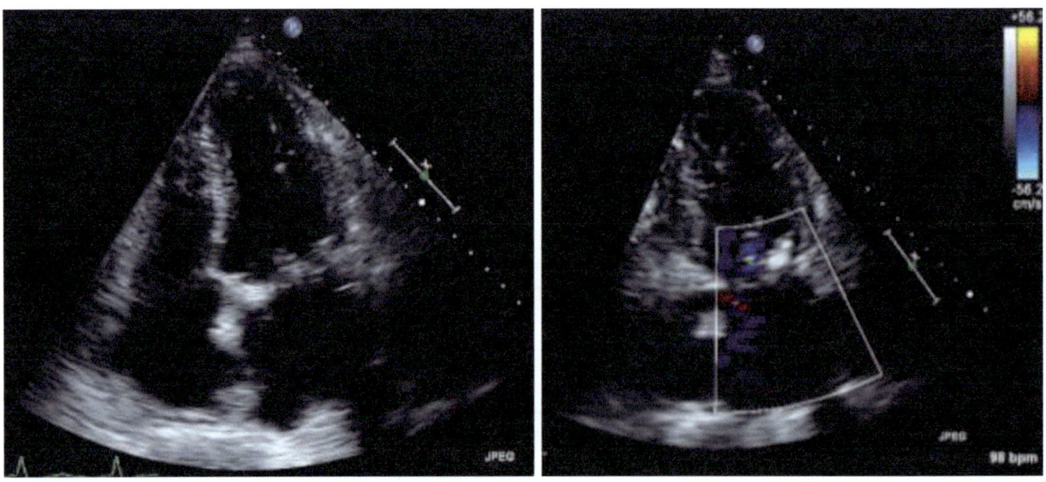

Fig. 13.12 Post-operative trans-thoracic echocardiographical images demonstrating a competent mitral valve, with no residual mitral regurgitation, minimal annular calcification, no SAM and a 9 mm depth of coaptation between the anterior and posterior leaflets

movement of the posterior leaflet, with no residual mitral regurgitation.
2. Minimal residual annular calcification
3. No systolic anterior motion of the anterior mitral valve leaflet (SAM) or left ventricular outflow obstruction (LVOTO).
4. The depth of leaflet coaptation was >8 mm.

Surgical Tips

1. Detaching the posterior leaflet from the annulus gives excellent access to posterior mitral annular calcification
2. The calcium bar should be removed with sharp dissection en-bloc to reduce the risk of fragmentation and embolisation
3. Closure of the defect in the atrioventricular groove should be done with a pericardial patch to restore strength and integrity, thereby reducing the risk of atrioventricular disruption

Comment

The presence of mitral annular calcification in patients undergoing mitral valve surgery is associated with increased operative morbidity and mortality due to the complex nature of surgery required to deal with the calcification. Depending on the extent of the procedure, repair or replacement and extent of the calcification, operative mortality varies between 3% and 9%. The survival has been reported as 93% at 7 years, with an 87% freedom from reoperation at 9 years.

Recommended Reading

Atoui R, Lash V, Mohammadi S, Cecere R. Intra-atrial implantation of a mitral valve prosthesis in a heavily calcified mitral annulus. Eur J Cardiothorac Surg. 2009;36:776–8.

Carpentier AF, Pellerin M, Fuzellier JF, Relland JY. Extensive calcification of the mitral valve: pathology and surgical management. J Thorac Cardiovasc Surg. 1996;111:718–30.

d'Alessandro C, Vistarini N, Aubert S, Jault F, Acar C, Pavie A, Gandjbakhch I. Mitral annulus calcification: determinants of repair feasibility, early and late surgical outcome. Eur J Cardio Thorac Surg. 2007;32:596–603.

David TE, Feindel CM, Armstrong S, Sun Z. Reconstruction of the mitral annulus: a ten years experience. J Thorac Cardiovasc Surg. 1995;110:1323–32.

Feindel CM, Tufail Z, David TE, Ivanov J, Armstrong S. Mitral valve surgery in patients with extensive calcification of the mitral annulus. J Thorac Cardiovasc Surg. 2003;126:777–81.

Stefano SD, Lopez J, Florez S, Rey J, Arevalo A, San Román A. Building a new annulus: a technique for mitral valve replacement in heavily calcified annulus. Ann Thorac Surg. 2009;87:1625–7.

Rheumatic Mitral Valve Disease

14

Keywords
Rheumatic mitral valve disease · Rheumatic fever · Lancefield group A β-haemolytic streptococcal infection · Restricted leaflet motion · Calcified thickened sub-valvular apparatus · Commissural fusion · Commissurotomy · Leaflet augmentation · Mitral valve replacement · Papillary muscle splitting

Case History

A 45 year-old lady presented with a long-standing history of increasing dyspnoea on exertion, associated with fatigue and lethargy. She had a previous history of rheumatic fever as a child and had been followed up with serial echocardiography. Clinical examination revealed a pan-systolic and mid-diastolic murmur, both loudest at the apex.

Echocardiographical Findings

Trans-thoracic echocardiographic images revealed a markedly thickened mitral valve, with retraction and restricted movement of the posterior leaflet on parasternal long-axis (Fig. 14.1a, b) and apical 4-chamber (Fig. 14.1c–e) views. In association, markedly thickened, shortened and fibrotic sub-valvular apparatus was observed, with matted and fused chordae tendineae. Severe mitral regurgitation was also demonstrated on the corresponding colour flow Doppler images across the mitral valve (Fig. 14.1a, b, f). Quantification of the regurgitation, using the PISA method, revealed a regurgitant volume of 65 mL and regurgitant fraction of 56%, associated with a vena contracta of 0.73 cm. Planimetry of the valve demonstrated moderate mitral stenosis (MS), with a mitral valve area of 1.25 cm^2. This was confirmed by Doppler flow, with a pressure half time of 175 ms and a mean pressure gradient across the mitral valve of 8 mmHg. Associated with this, the pulmonary artery pressures were raised at 55/35 mmHg, the left atrium was dilated at 5.36 cm but the left ventricular size and function were preserved, with the left ventricular end-systolic diameter 3.6 cm, left ventricular end-diastolic diameter 5.0 cm and ejection fraction 62%. Trans-oesophageal and three-dimensional (3D) echocardiographical images clearly demonstrate the severely regurgitant and moderately stenotic mitral valve (Fig. 14.2).

N. Moorjani et al., *Operative Mitral and Tricuspid Valve Surgery*,
https://doi.org/10.1007/978-1-4471-4204-1_14

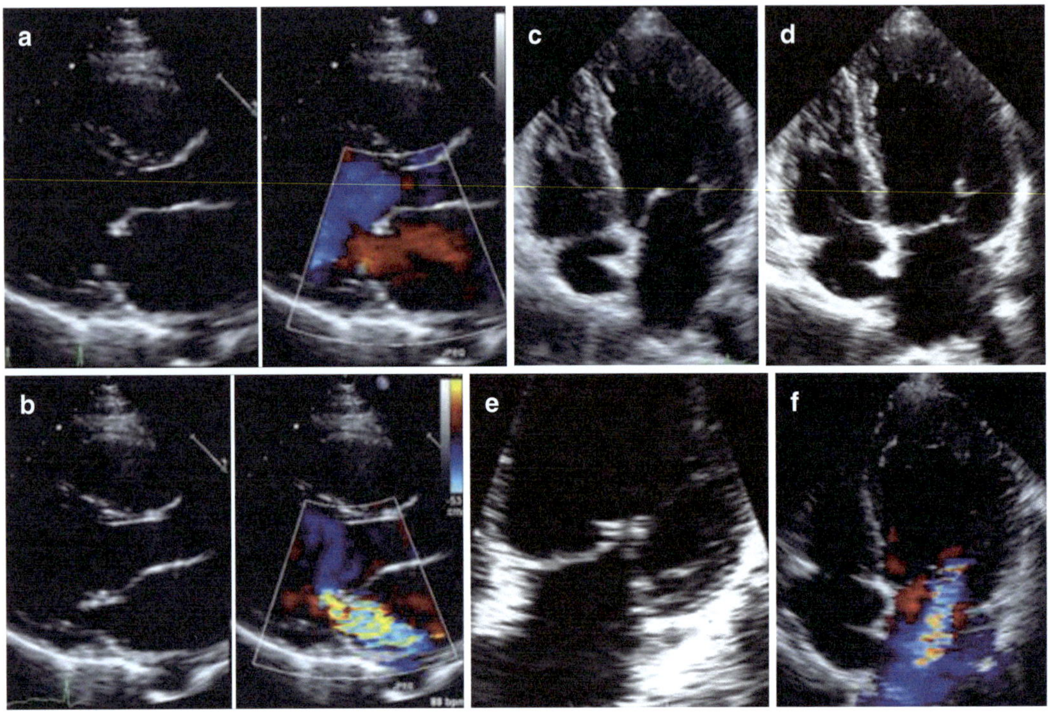

Fig. 14.1 Trans-thoracic echocardiographical images illustrating a markedly thickened and fibrotic mitral valve, with extensive retraction of the posterior leaflet and subvalvular apparatus, associated with restricted opening (hockey-stick appearance) on the parasternal long-axis view and corresponding colour flow Doppler in (**a**) diastole and (**b**) systole. Apical 4-chamber views demonstrating the restricted movement of the posterior leaflet in (**c**) diastole and (**d**) systole, and confirmed on the (**e**) zoomed image with thickened fibrotic leaflet anatomy and a fixed posterior leaflet. (**f**) Apical 4-chamber view with colour flow Doppler demonstrating significant mitral regurgitation

Pathophysiology

Rheumatic fever occurs in 3–4% of patients with untreated Lancefield group A β-haemolytic streptococcal infection, with up to 50% developing some degree of rheumatic heart disease. It is triggered by an autoimmune response against streptococcal antigens with cross-recognition to cardiac tissue, resulting in destruction of valvular and endocardial tissue. Rheumatic heart disease can affect the mitral valve in up to 50% of these patients, and may occur at the level of the leaflets and the subvalvular apparatus. The disease process also invokes a myocarditis, which can cause myocardial fibrosis, a lesion that can have implications in the acute and late phases of the disease with impaired LV function. This rheumatic autoimmune inflammatory process produces a different set of lesions to those in degenerative mitral valve disease and may result in regurgitation, stenosis or both. In the acute phase, mitral regurgitation is predominant, whereas mitral stenosis develops progressively with scarring and eventual calcification of the valve and subvalvular tissues. This tends to worsen with age.

In the acute phase, the rheumatic process produces markedly oedematous leaflets and subvalvular tissues, with characteristic rheumatic nodules (Aschoff bodies) at the free edge of the leaflets, chordal elongation (especially of the anterior leaflet), annular dilatation but minimal calcification and non-fused commissures. Commonly, this is associated with regurgitation of the mitral valve but may also involve the other cardiac valves. Subsequent progressive fibrosis of the leaflets and subvalvular apparatus leads to

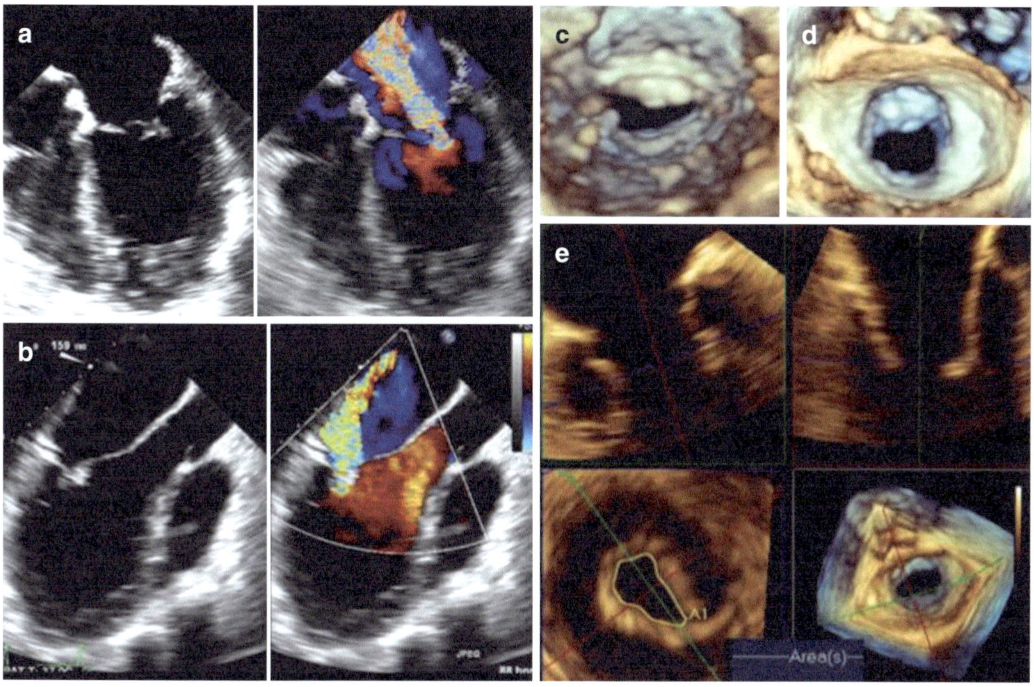

Fig. 14.2 Trans-oesophageal echocardiographical images demonstrating the markedly thickened mitral valve with extensive retraction of the posterior leaflet and subvalvular apparatus on (**a**) mid-oesophageal 4-chamber and (**b**) long-axis views with corresponding colour flow Doppler images. Three-dimensional images confirm the restricted mitral valve orifice with thickened rolled free edges of both leaflets and commissural fusion on (**c**) left ventricular and (**d**) left atrial (surgical) views. (**e**) Three-dimensional data-set analysis of the mitral valve orifice using planimetry confirms a mitral valve area of 1.2 cm^2

restriction of leaflet movement and increasing valvular dysfunction, with a spectrum of severity from those with the disease process limited to fusion of the free edge of the leaflets, with pliable tissue and normal sub-valvular apparatus to those with extensive tissue scarring, fibrosis and retraction resulting in thickened, fused, and calcified leaflets, which are non-pliable and restricted, associated with annular calcification, commissural fusion and calcified sub-valvular apparatus, including shortened and fused chordae tendineae.

Surgical Strategy

Although the prevalence of rheumatic mitral valve disease has been progressively decreasing, it is still one of commonest causes of mitral regurgitation worldwide, especially in the younger population. Reconstruction of the mitral valve in these patients, however, remains controversial because traditionally it has been associated with inferior durability and is technically more challenging due to the complexity of the lesions produced by the rheumatic process. Furthermore, disease progression in younger patients may result in repair failure and the need for reoperation. More recently, however, improved long-term outcomes following repair of rheumatic mitral valve disease have been achieved in the hands of surgeons with greater experience in mitral valve reconstruction. In view of this, experienced surgeons will attempt valve reconstruction in young patients in whom prosthetic valve failure is likely to be high and those where the use of life-long anticoagulants carries significant risk or in young women who wish to become or are already pregnant.

The durability of repair for rheumatic mitral valve disease has improved with appropriate case selection, evolution of repair techniques to optimise the depth of leaflet coaptation, and detailed valvular analysis, which ensures that all components of the mitral apparatus, including leaflets, chordae tendineae, papillary muscles and annulus, involved in the rheumatic disease process are addressed. It is especially important to distinguish retraction of the posterior leaflet from pseudo-prolapse of the anterior leaflet. In terms of case selection, it has been suggested that approximately 75% of regurgitant rheumatic mitral valves may be repairable. This may be true in populations of younger patients particularly in the earlier phase of the disease but patients with severely fibrotic and calcified leaflets with a fused and matted sub-valvular apparatus are less likely to be repairable.

Systematic valve analysis by trans-oesophageal echocardiography and direct inspection, will allow a decision to be made whether valve repair is feasible. The degree of commissural thickening and fusion, leaflet retraction and residual pliability, annular and papillary muscle calcification, and sub-valvular apparatus tethering and shortening will dictate the possibilities for reconstruction.

Increasing Leaflet Mobility

In some patients with pliable leaflets, normal chordae tendineae, with the disease process limited to fusion of the free edge of the leaflets, a commissurotomy taken up to 2–3 mm from the annulus, in combination with splitting of the attached commissural fan chords and papillary muscles, may be sufficient to restore a satisfactory orifice area (Fig. 14.3). Other manoeuvres include releasing the adjacent fused subvalvular apparatus, including papillary muscle splitting and excision of thickened or shortened chordae tendineae, followed by decalcification and peeling off the inflammatory fibrotic layer of the thickened leaflets (leaflet thinning) to improve mobility and pliability. Progression through these steps allow a better assessment of the residual

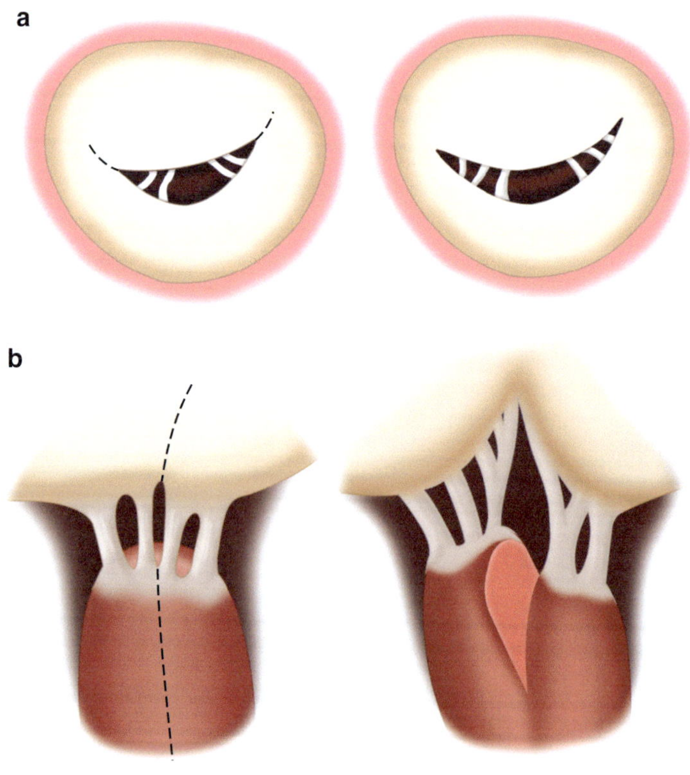

Fig. 14.3 Mobilisation of the fused commissures and sub-valvular apparatus by (**a**) open mitral commissurotomy and (**b**) splitting of the papillary muscle heads

lesions to be dealt with. The key principles are to restore normal leaflet movement as much as possible and restore the depth of coaptation.

Leaflet Augmentation

In patients with more extensive rheumatic mitral disease, fibrosis and calcification of the posterior leaflet results in leaflet retraction and restricted movement. In some patients, leaflet augmentation can be used, thereby providing enhanced mobility and enough tissue to achieve a good depth of coaptation. Posterior leaflet extension may be used if there is adequate pliable tissue at the leading edge of the leaflet for the material to be sutured to and is performed in patients where severe retraction of the leaflet has caused the vertical height of the leaflet to be less than 10 mm. Anterior leaflet extension is performed if the vertical height or the surface area of the leaflet is significantly retracted and stiffened. Either glutaraldehyde-treated autologous pericardium or bovine pericardium can be used for leaflet augmentation. Although both may be subject to late calcification, the onset of this is delayed as compared to that when using untreated autologous pericardium. Newer materials are available but are still subject to study of late results.

The shape of the patch is often recommended as being ovoid in shape. Whereas this may work in some localised areas of P2 contracture, more often the patch needs to extend to the commissures and be more trapezoid in shape to advance the lateral parts of the posterior leaflet (Fig. 14.4). In some cases, if this is not done, it can result in residual regurgitation through either commissure. The exact size and shape of the patch will naturally be determined by the anatomy of the

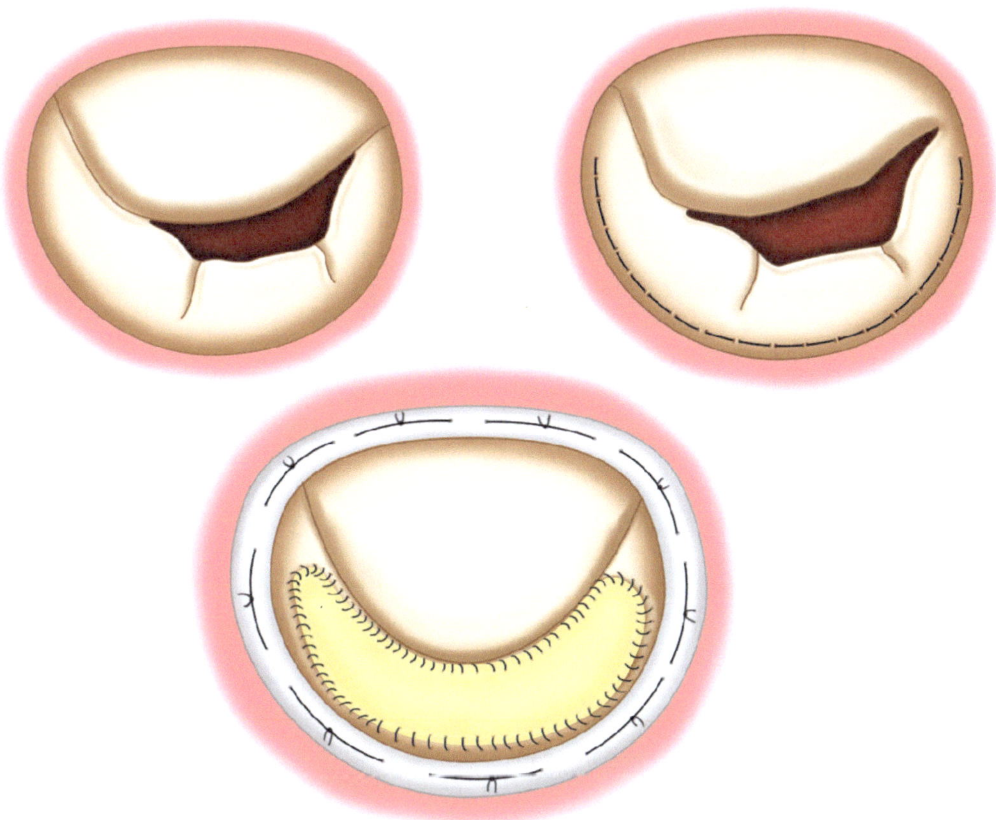

Fig. 14.4 Augmentation of the posterior mitral valve leaflet with a pericardial patch in a patient with rheumatic mitral regurgitation followed by ring annuloplasty

leaflet. The patch advances the line of coaptation towards the anterior leaflet. Any areas of residual prolapse of the anterior or posterior leaflets can be identified at this stage and supported with chordal insertion.

Chordal Replacement

In the younger patient and in the early stages of the disease, mitral regurgitation may be the predominant lesion, with anterior leaflet prolapse being more common. Posterior leaflet prolapse is less frequent because the natural height of the leaflet is less and the disease process causes early contracture of the leaflet. The prolapse is usually more prominent in the medial half of the anterior leaflet (A2, A3), caused by elongation of the chordae tendineae originating from the posteromedial papillary muscle, with stretching of the paramedial chords originating from the anterolateral papillary muscle also present in some patients. This may be managed with Gore-Tex neo-chordae, which are either implanted in parallel with the elongated chords to the originating papillary muscle, or with excision of the diseased native chords. In some patients, the non-elongated native tendinous chords of the posterior leaflet can be used for comparison to determine the height of the Gore-Tex neo-chordae. Although isolated cases of neo-chordal rupture have been described in the literature, there is excellent 20-year data demonstrating the long-term pliability and durability of Gore-Tex chords, including in a younger population. Whilst other techniques such as triangular resection, chordal transfer or chordal shortening can be used in these circumstances, the restricted leaflet tissue most often leaves little tissue available in valves involved in the rheumatic process. Disease progression of pathological chordae will often result in recurrent regurgitation.

In the early phase of the disease, annular dilatation is commonly present and insertion of an annuloplasty ring is indicated. It is important to use the appropriately sized ring, as a ring that is too small may cause an obstruction to left ventricular inflow and potentially a degree of mitral stenosis because of the relative thickness of the leaflets and sub-valvar apparatus. Systolic anterior motion (SAM) of the mitral valve is rare in such cases because the tissue is usually fibrotic and stiff, with reduced height in the posterior leaflet.

Surgical Technique

The mitral valve leaflets and subvalvular apparatus were inspected and correlated with trans-oesophageal echocardiographical findings. Specifically, all the components of the mitral valve apparatus were systematically assessed including the leaflets (for mobility, pliability, calcification, retraction, prolapse and commissural fusion), chordae tendineae and papillary muscles (for fusion, thickening, calcification and shortening) and annulus (for dilatation and calcification). At this stage, it was important to make a judgement to determine whether repair was possible. In this patient, bilateral commissural fusion, associated with thickened, fibrotic and shortened fan chords were identified. In addition, the posterior leaflet was thickened and retracted with a rolled up free edge, associated with thickened, shortened and fused sub-valvar apparatus causing significantly restricted leaflet motion. There was some degree of calcification present in the body of the posterior leaflet and annulus (Fig. 14.5a).

As repair was deemed feasible, horizontal mattress annuloplasty sutures (2/0 Ethibond) were placed around the circumference of the mitral valve, with a 5mm width and approximately 1mm apart to provide much improved access and visualisation of the mitral valve leaflets and subvalvular apparatus. The first step was then to release the fused commissures by incising the leaflet tissue at the commissures. The incision is extended to within 2–3 mm of the annulus to ensure optimal mobilisation of the commissures. Extension of the incision to the annulus will most likely cause regurgitation. In conjunction with this, the sub-valvar apparatus supporting the commissures were also freed by splitting the attached fan-chords and papillary muscles to again increase mobility and pliability at the commissures. The next step was to increase mobility and pliability of the leaflet body and this was achieved by excising

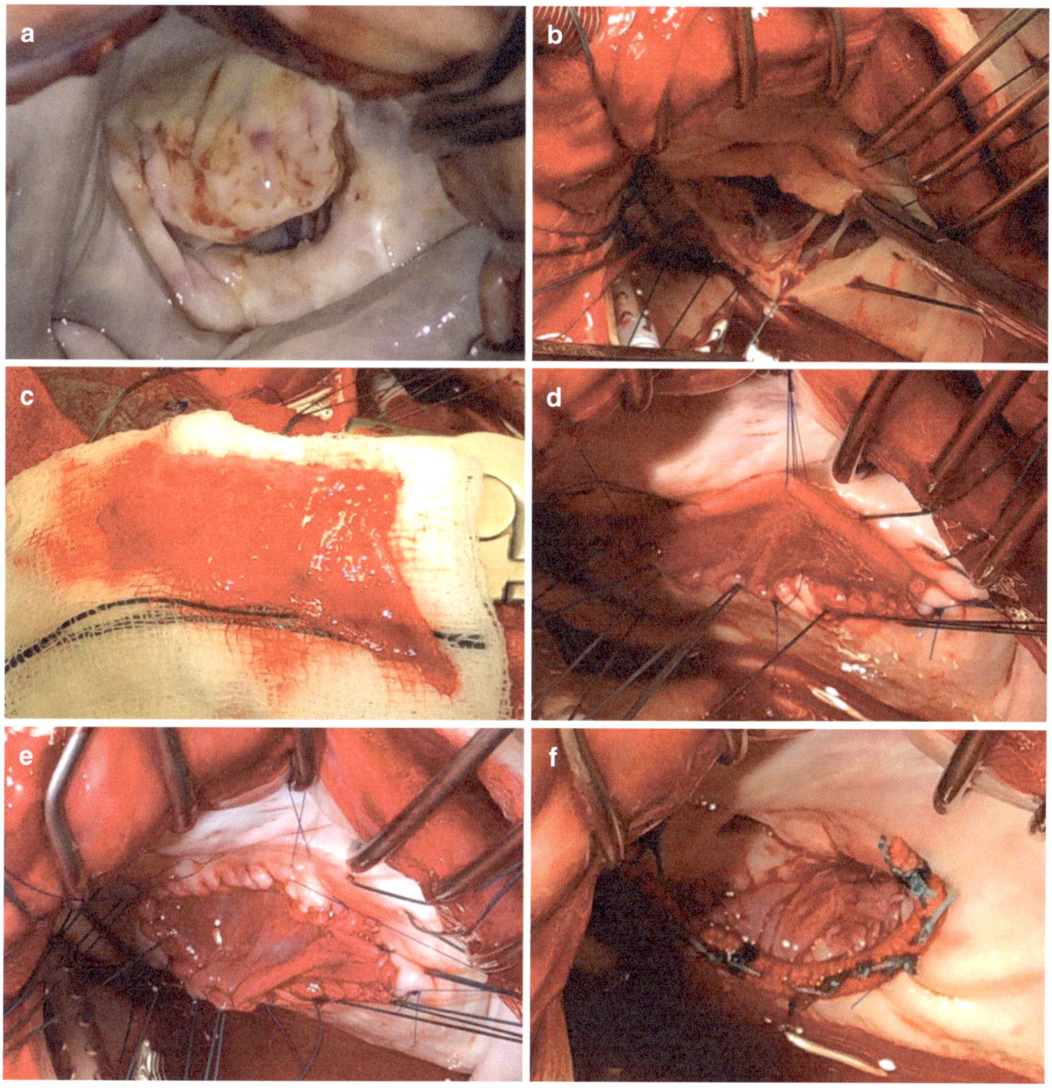

Fig. 14.5 Operative images demonstrating (**a**) a rheumatic mitral valve with commissural fusion, thickened leaflets with rolled up free edges and some degree of calcification, (**b**) detachment of the posterior leaflet from the annulus, (**c**) creation of a trapezoid-shaped autologous pericardial patch, (**d**) attachment of the pericardial patch to the posterior annulus, (**e**) attachment of the pericardial patch to the posterior leaflet, and (**f**) implantation of an annuloplasty band

the attached thickened and shortened secondary chords, as well as some of the primary chords that were causing restricted leaflet movement. The resected primary chords were replaced with CV-4 Gore-Tex sutures implanted from the site of the originating papillary muscle to the site of the resected native chords. In addition, the leaflet body was decalcified and the thickened inflammatory fibrotic layer was peeled (leaflet thinning).

The valve was then reassessed at this stage to determine the degree of residual leaflet restriction and prolapse. It was evident that there was not enough leaflet tissue to achieve an acceptable depth of coaptation because of significant retraction of the posterior leaflet. In view of this, leaflet augmentation was performed using autologous pericardium that had been harvested during the initial stages of the operation. The patch was trimmed, cleared of pericardial fat, soaked in 0.6% glutaraldehyde-buffered solution for 5–10 min at room temperature and then rinsed in 3 baths of normal saline for 5 minutes each. The glutaraldehyde treatment causes cross-linkage of the collagen fibres, thereby making it easier to handle and reducing the likelihood of subsequent calcification. Prolonged treatment with glutaraldehyde leaves the pericardium at an increased risk of fibrosis. The posterior leaflet is then detached from the annulus by making an incision 2 mm away and extending it from commissure to commissure parallel to the annulus, preserving the free edge of the leaflet with the chordae attached (Fig. 14.5b). This allows great access to the left ventricular cavity and the sub-valvar apparatus, through which any additional chordal or papillary muscle releasing manoeuvres can be performed to further improve leaflet mobility and hence depth of coaptation. A slightly oversized patch (25–30mm height) is then fashioned in a roughly trapezoid shape (Fig. 14.5c) and sized so that the height of the new posterior leaflet was 15–20mm (5mm is lost on either side due to the suturing effect) and that it would create a good depth of coaptation with the anterior leaflet. The pericardial patch was attached to the posterior annulus (Fig. 14.5d) and posterior leaflet (Fig. 14.5e), using a continuous 4/0 Prolene suture. The sutures are locked with every bite to reduce the risk of purse-stringing the patch. The smooth side of the patch was placed on the atrial side to reduce the risk of thrombogenesis. As well as increasing the depth of coaptation, leaflet augmentation allows for the insertion of a larger annuloplasty ring or band, thereby reducing the risk of mitral stenosis. The mitral valve orifice was then sized according to the commissural and anteroposterior measurements of the anterior leaflet. An appropriate annuloplasty band was then implanted using the annuloplasty sutures placed earlier (Fig. 14.5f). The band was able to restore the shape of the deformed annulus and support the repair by reducing the tension on the leaflets and chords. Competency of the mitral valve can then be tested by injecting cold saline into the left ventricle using a bulb syringe and any residual valvular pathology addressed, such as with the use of Gore-Tex neo-chordae.

Post-operative Echocardiogram

Following weaning from cardiopulmonary bypass, trans-oesophageal echocardiography (Fig. 14.6) demonstrated:

1. Normal leaflet movement of the repaired valve, ensuring a good depth of coaptation (>8 mm).
2. No residual mitral regurgitation
3. Absence of turbulent flow or a significant gradient across the mitral valve.

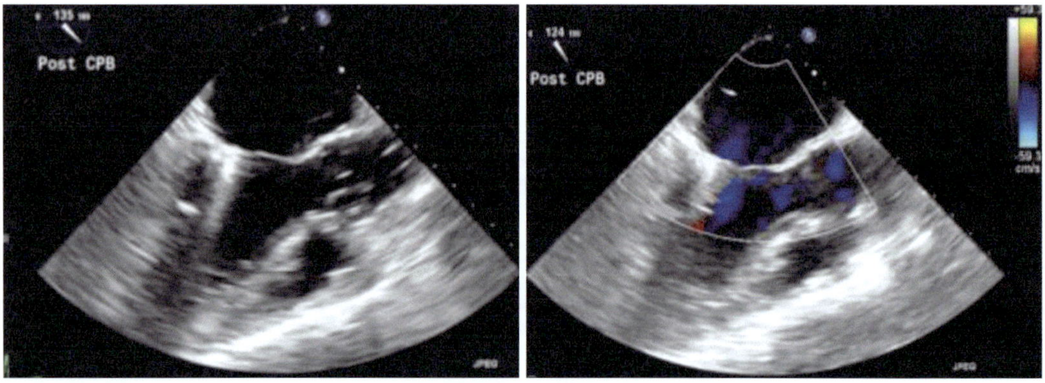

Fig. 14.6 Post-bypass intra-operative trans-oesophageal echocardiographical images demonstrating a competent mitral valve, with a good depth of coaptation and no residual mitral stenosis or regurgitation

Surgical Tips

1. Repair for rheumatic mitral valve disease can produce excellent long term results with appropriate case selection, use of contemporary repair techniques to optimise the depth of leaflet coaptation, and detailed valve analysis, to ensure that all components of the mitral apparatus involved in the rheumatic disease process are addressed.
2. Mobilisation of the fused commissures and supporting sub-valvular apparatus by open mitral commissurotomy and splitting of the papillary muscle heads can significantly increase the mitral valve orifice area
3. Excision of fibrotic and restrictive secondary chords and leaflet thinning (peeling off the thickened fibrotic inflammatory layer from the valve leaflets) can improve leaflet mobility and pliability
4. Leaflet augmentation using a pericardial patch can greatly increase the surface area of the mitral valve orifice and the depth of coaptation
5. Chordal replacement with Gore-Tex neo-chordae may be required following excision of shortened primary chordae or to treat patients with native anterior leaflet prolapse

Comment

Results following repair of rheumatic mitral valve disease have shown a somewhat higher hospital mortality than simple repair for degenerative disease (approximately 2–3%). Studies using contemporary techniques for rheumatic mitral valve repair have demonstrated similar results to those for degenerative mitral valve repair, with mid-term outcome measures reported as freedom from valve failure 92% at 5 years, freedom from reoperation 97% at 5 years and survival 89% at 10 years. In parallel with better surgical techniques, superior anti-failure therapy and rheumatic fever prophylaxis have contributed to improving long-term outcomes.

The mitral valve leaflet and subvalvular apparatus pathology were the most important factors for predicting the success of repair, with the presence of extensive calcification, leaflet retraction and chordal fusion predictors of an increased rate of reoperation. Although it expands the number of patients with potentially reparable valves, performing more complex repair procedures, including leaflet thinning, patch augmentation and chordal replacement, is also a predictor of reduced durability, although it may just be a marker of more advanced disease. The results of rheumatic mitral valve repair vary with the age of the patients, which may also just represent the different stages of the disease.

There are three key factors thought to be responsible for successful mitral valve repair in rheumatic patients, including good patient selection (with suitable mitral valve morphology and the absence of acute rheumatic carditis at the time of surgery), the use of contemporary surgical techniques and prevention of progression of the valve disease (with long-term antibiotic prophylaxis).

Recommended Reading

Antunes MJ. Repair of rheumatic mitral valve regurgitation: how far can we go? Eur J Cardiothorac Surg. 2013;44(4):689–91.

Dillon J, Yakub MA, Nordin MN, Pau KK, Krishna Moorthy PS. Leaflet extension in rheumatic mitral valve reconstruction. Eur J Cardiothorac Surg. 2013;44(4):682–9.

Lee EM, Shapiro LM, Wells FC. Importance of subvalvular preservation and early operation in mitral valve surgery. Circulation. 1996;94(9):2117–23.

Mihos CG, Pineda AM, Capoulade R, Santana O. A systematic review of mitral valve repair with autologous pericardial leaflet augmentation for rheumatic mitral regurgitation. Ann Thorac Surg. 2016;102(4):1400–5.

15 Systolic Anterior Motion of the Mitral Valve

Keywords
Systolic anterior motion (SAM) of the mitral valve · Leaflet height reduction · Gore-Tex neo-chordae · Small annuloplasty ring · Leaflet resection · Left ventricular outflow tract obstruction · Anterior displacement of the coaptation line · Septal hypertrophy · Annuloplasty band

Case History

A 78 year-old female patient presented with a prolonged history of increasing dyspnoea on exertion. She had no history of rheumatic fever or infective endocarditis but was under serial echocardiography follow up with a known murmur.

Echocardiographical Findings

Trans-thoracic apical 4-chamber echocardiographic images revealed the posterior mitral valve leaflet to have an excess of redundant tissue, associated with an increased leaflet height, resulting in displacement of the mitral coaptation line in an anterior direction and subsequent retroflexion of the anterior leaflet during systole (Fig. 15.1a). The presence of some calcification in the posterior annulus can also be seen. Displacement of the anterior leaflet into the outflow tract also caused a failure of mitral valve leaflet coaptation. Subsequent obstruction to flow in the left ventricular outflow tract and mitral regurgitation can be seen on the corresponding colour flow image (Fig. 15.1b). The left ventricular function was preserved, with an ejection fraction 67%, associated with a small left ventricular cavity, with an left ventricular end-diastolic diameter 3.8 cm.

Trans-oesophageal echocardiographical images confirmed the presence of posterior leaflet prolapse, anterior leaflet retroflexion and systolic anterior motion (SAM) of the mitral valve in both the mid-oesophageal long-axis and 5-chamber views (Fig. 15.2a, b). Left ventricular outflow tract obstruction and severe mitral regurgitation can be seen on the corresponding colour flow Doppler images. The left ventricular outflow tract diameter was measured at 1.8 cm and the angle formed by mitral and aortic valves (mitral-aortic angle) was 102°. The distance from the coaptation point of the mitral valve to the point of maximal septal thickness (C-sept) measured at the beginning of systole was 2.2 cm. The length of the anterior mitral valve leaflet was 3.0 cm and posterior leaflet 2.5 cm, measured in systole from the annulus to the coaptation point. Continuous wave Doppler flow across the left ventricular outflow tract in the 5-chamber view confirmed the peak gradient at 62 mmHg. Quantification of the regurgitation, using the PISA method revealed severe MR, with an effective regurgitant orifice area of

N. Moorjani et al., *Operative Mitral and Tricuspid Valve Surgery*,
https://doi.org/10.1007/978-1-4471-4204-1_15

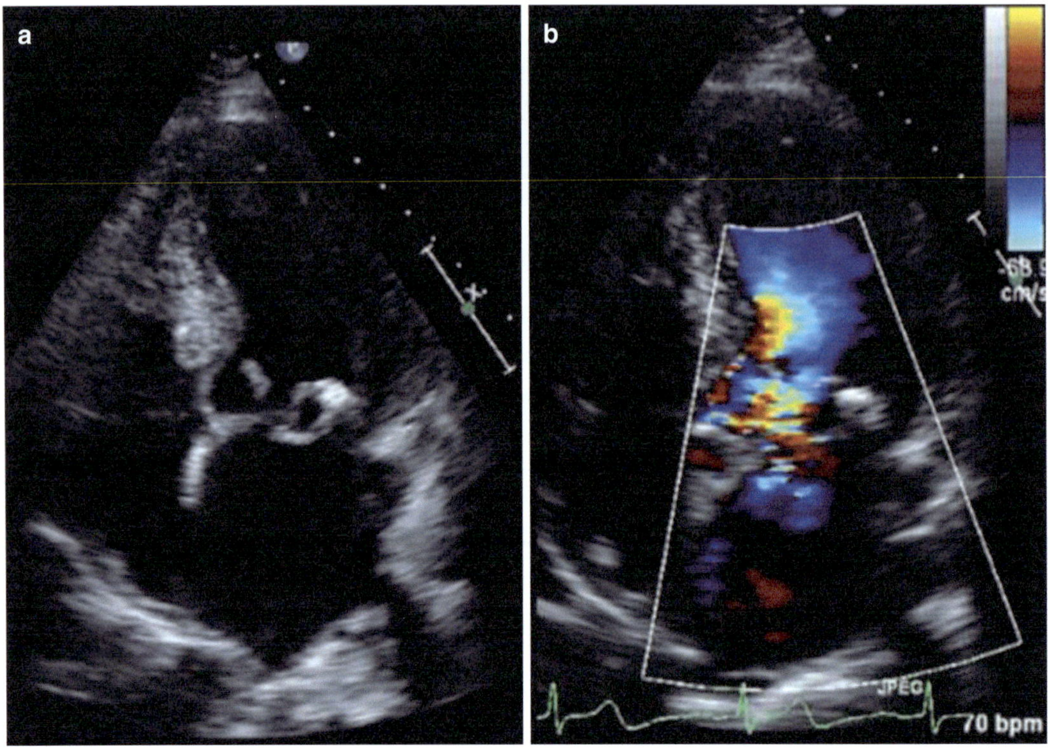

Fig. 15.1 Trans-thoracic echocardiographical images demonstrating (**a**) a tall posterior mitral valve leaflet, anteriorly displaced coaptation line, retroflexion of the anterior leaflet in the left ventricular outflow tract and failure of coaptation of the mitral leaflets on the apical 4-chamber view, resulting in (**b**) severe mitral regurgitation and turbulence in the left ventricular outflow tract on the corresponding colour flow Doppler image

82 mm^2, regurgitant volume of 97 mL and regurgitant fraction of 66%, associated with a vena contracta of 0.91 cm. Three-dimensional images confirm the anteriorly displaced coaptation line caused by redundant tissue in a tall posterior leaflet (Fig. 15.2c).

Pathophysiology

The term systolic anterior motion of the mitral valve is used to define the systolic displacement of the anterior leaflet of the mitral valve into the left ventricular outflow tract. Premature systolic coaptation between the posterior and anterior leaflets, especially if the posterior leaflet is disproportionately tall, will turn the anterior leaflet back onto itself and the blood flow accelerating into the left ventricular outflow tract will then cause the anterior leaflet to hit the septum, thereby obstructing the outflow of blood. At the same time, ventricular displacement of the anterior leaflet will prevent normal closure of the mitral valve orifice leading to mitral regurgitation into the left atrium. Thus, these two lesions always accompany each other in this condition (Fig. 15.3). Anatomical lesions predisposing to SAM are any that lead to this early leaflet coaptation.

It is found occurring naturally in some patients with hypertrophic cardiomyopathy (HCM), which is a genetic disorder characterised by significant left ventricular (LV) hypertrophy and a small, hyperdynamic LV cavity in the absence of a precipitating cause, such as hypertension or aortic stenosis. The hypertrophy is often severe at the level of the basal septum, resulting in significant narrowing of the left ventricular outflow tract (LVOT). During systole, the left ventricular walls, including the basal septum, thicken,

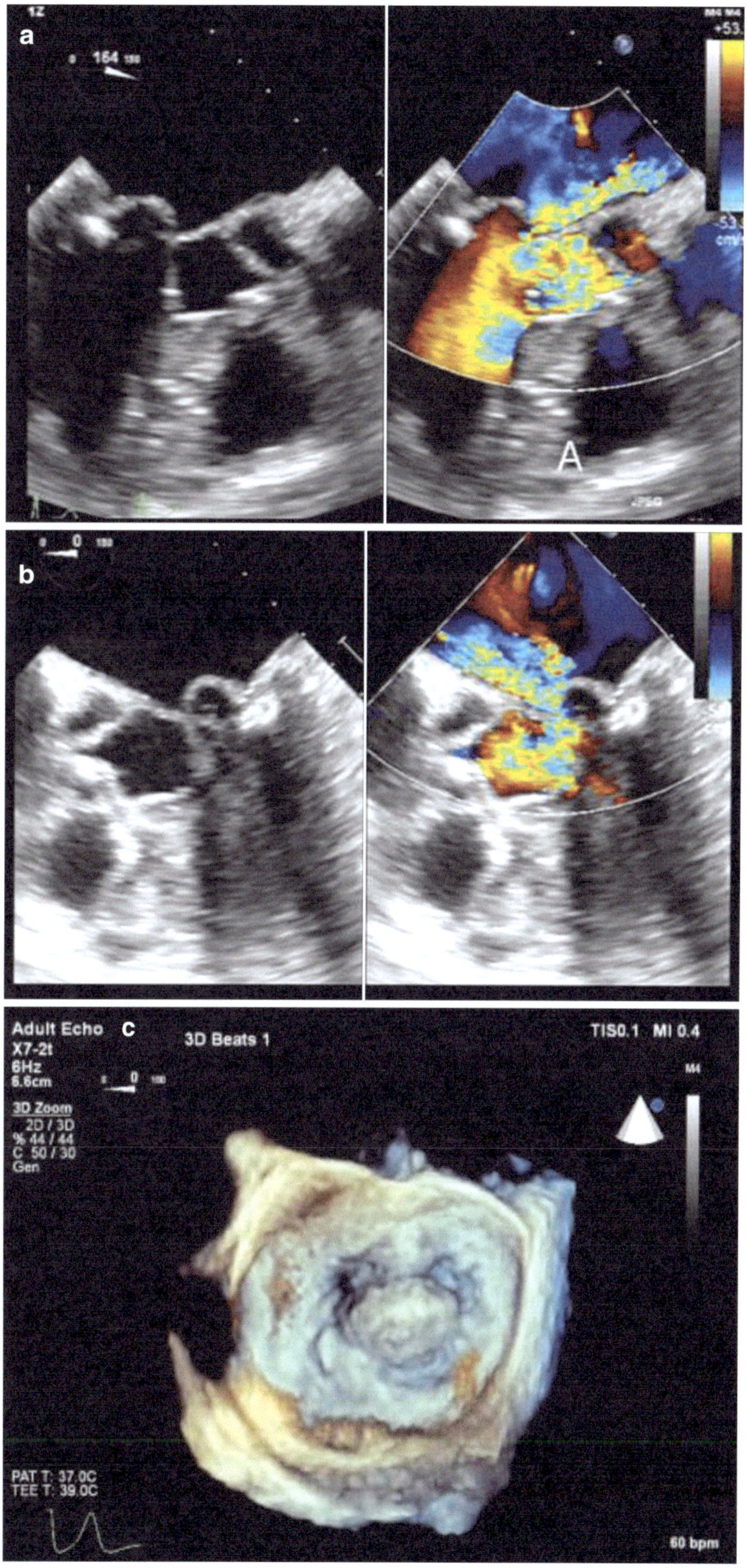

Fig. 15.2 Trans-oesophageal echocardiographical images demonstrating a flail posterior mitral valve leaflet, posterior annular calcification and systolic anterior motion of the anterior leaflet on mid-oesophageal (**a**) long-axis and (**b**) 4-chamber views, with severe mitral regurgitation and turbulence in the left ventricular outflow tract on the corresponding colour flow Doppler views. (**c**) Three-dimensional view demonstrating posterior leaflet prolapse with a large area of redundant tissue and increased leaflet height, displacing the coaptation line towards the left ventricular outflow tract

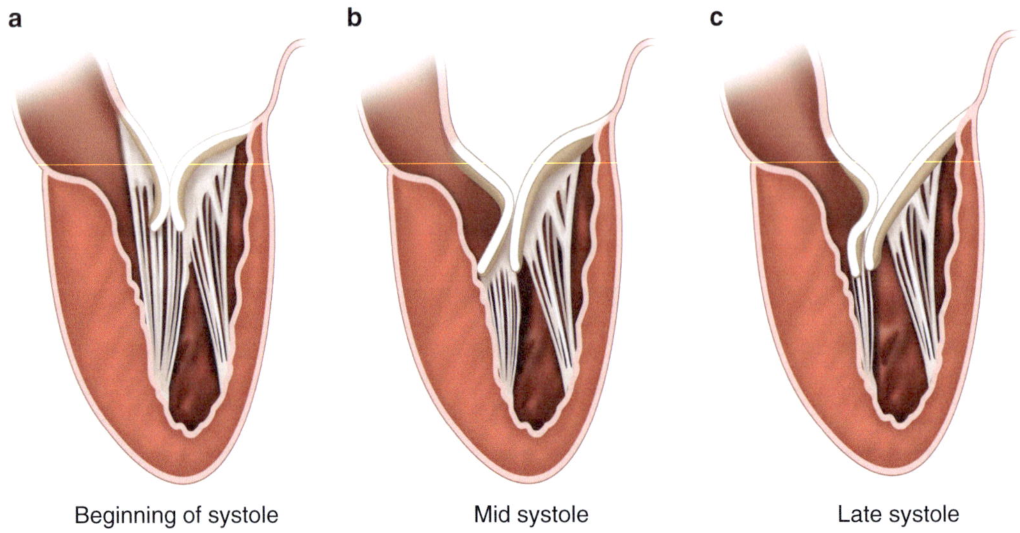

Fig. 15.3 (**a**) Systolic anterior motion (SAM) of the mitral valve resulting in (**b**) left ventricular outflow tract obstruction in mid systole and (**c**) a posterior-directed jet of mitral regurgitation in late systole

thereby further narrowing the LVOT. As well as the basal septum, the other border to the LVOT is formed by the anterior mitral valve leaflet and its subvalvular apparatus. In HCM, the mitral leaflets may be elongated, and the papillary muscles enlarged, closer together and anteromedially displaced. As described above, this produces anterior displacement of the mitral coaptation line. Encroachment of the hypertrophied septal muscle on the outflow tract produces a Venturi effect with flow acceleration, thereby retroverting the anterior leaflet into the outflow tract and causing premature coaptation of the main body of the mitral valve leaflets, rather than their leading edge. In the early stages of HCM, this phenomenon is often transient and volume and pressure dependent, where the presence of SAM is intermittent and can be managed with volume loading and the use of beta-blocker agents. As the outflow tract narrows with increasing septal hypertrophy, this is no longer the case and is an indication for surgery.

Although rare, causes of natural (pre-operative) SAM, other than HCM, include patients where the posterior leaflet and posterior annulus of the mitral valve are calcified (Fig. 15.4). Fixation of the posterior leaflet causes early apposition with the leading edge of the anterior leaflet, causing it to buckle resulting in outflow tract obstruction.

The commonest cause of SAM, however, is iatrogenic during mitral valve reconstruction surgery, with a reported incidence of up to 9% in some studies. It occurs when the orifice of the mitral valve is narrowed and immobilised by the insertion of an annuloplasty ring, fixing the anteroposterior diameter of the valve orifice. This lesion will be inevitable if the posterior leaflet is tall, equal to or greater than the height of the anterior leaflet and by inserting too small an annuloplasty ring. Over-reduction of the orifice area produces crowding of leaflet tissue, which in turn brings about premature leaflet coaptation. This results in folding and retroversion of the anterior leaflet into the outflow tract and subsequent obstruction to blood flow. This situation can easily be created in patients with Barlow's disease, where the posterior leaflet is very tall with excessive leaflet tissue. Perhaps more commonly, however, it is found in non-Barlow's patients with a very tall P2 because the mitral valve orifice in Barlow's disease is usually 20–40% greater than that in posterior leaflet prolapse, allowing a greater distance from the coaptation point to the outflow tract. It can be created when using either a rigid or a flexible annuloplasty ring, indicating that the ring type is not the issue. It is a function of either early coaptation between leaflets because of an abnormally tall

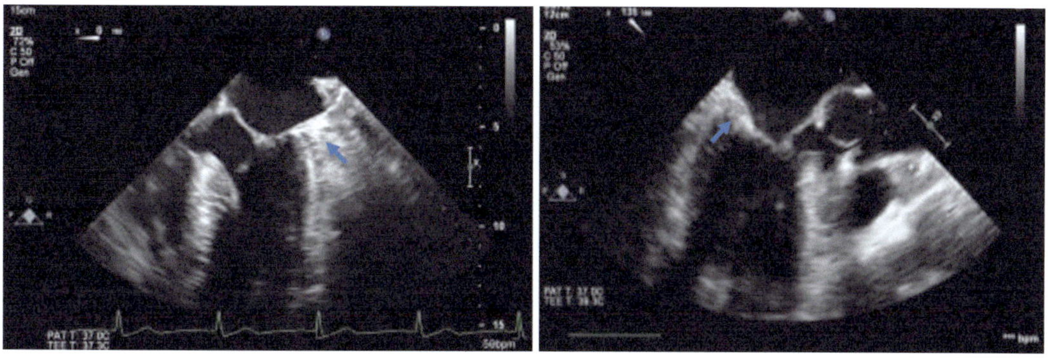

Fig. 15.4 Trans-oesophageal echocardiographical images of a patient with calcification of the posterior mitral valve annulus (arrows) forcing the posterior leaflet into the anterior leaflet with premature closure, resulting in retroversion of the anterior leaflet and subsequent SAM

posterior leaflet or too much leaflet tissue in too small an orifice. The use of an annuloplasty ring that is too small for the orifice will pull the posterior annulus towards the outflow tract, which will have the effect of causing premature contact between the posterior and anterior leaflets of the valve, pushing the anterior leaflet into the outflow tract. The flowing blood then causes it to buckle and to fold into the outflow tract causing obstruction (Fig. 15.5).

There are pre-operative echocardiographic warning signs for producing iatrogenic SAM following mitral valve repair (Fig. 15.6). The first is the relative heights of the anterior and posterior leaflets. If they are equal in height or, of more concern, if the posterior leaflet is taller than the anterior, then after restoring normal leaflet coaptation, any reduction of the mitral orifice area with an annuloplasty ring smaller in diameter than that will create the right conditions for SAM to occur.

The other anatomical condition that will increase the risk of post reconstruction SAM is the relationship of the anterior leaflet with the septum at the end of diastole. If the ventricular surface of the anterior leaflet kisses the septum in diastole, then drawing the posterior annulus towards the outflow tract without addressing posterior leaflet height will cause early contact between the two leaflets and SAM will ensue. Either or both of these anatomical situations must be recognised (Table 15.1, Fig. 15.7).

SAM nearly always occurs at the level A1/A2 and P1/P2. The presence of the mitral leaflets in the LVOT during systole results in obstruction to left ventricular outflow and failure of mitral valve leaflet closure. The subsequent mitral regurgitation jet is posteriorly-directed because of the channel created by the leaflets tips as they are dragged into the LVOT and occurs in mid-late systole after the onset of SAM and LVOTO. The haemodynamic effects of SAM depend on the extent and duration of mitral leaflet-septal contact and range from minimal impact on blood flow to significant left ventricular outflow obstruction and impaired cardiac output. SAM represents a dynamic phenomenon that is affected by preload, contractility and afterload. It can be precipitated or exacerbated by decreased left ventricular end-diastolic volume, increased inotropy, decreased systemic vascular resistance or increased chronotropy.

Surgical Strategy

Surgical management of SAM secondary to HCM requires an appreciation of the contribution of the septal hypertrophy and abnormalities of the mitral valve complex to the systolic displacement of the mitral valve leaflets. The traditional operative management of HCM involves a septal myectomy to increase the distance between septum and anterior mitral valve leaflet. Surgery is performed through the aortic annulus, with the aortic valve leaflets displaced using a leaflet retractor. Access to the septal muscle can be

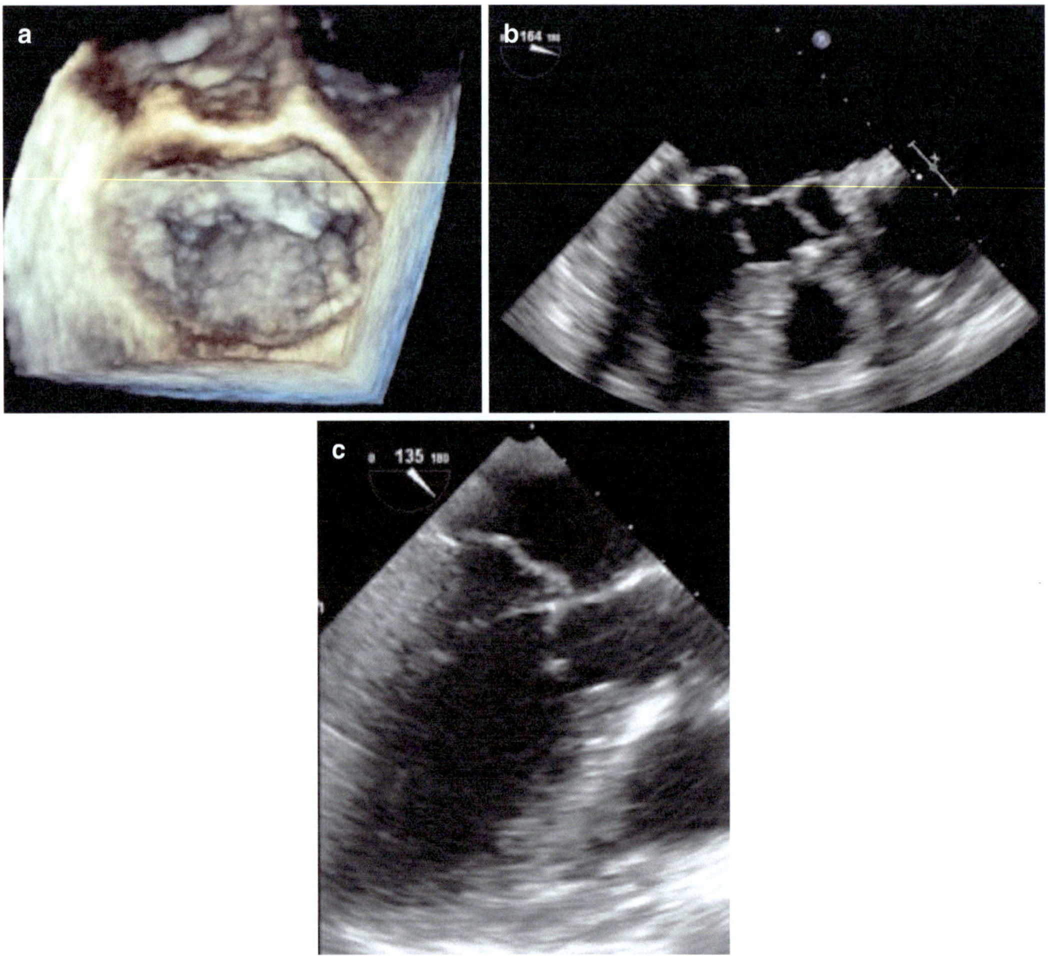

Fig. 15.5 Trans-oesophageal echocardiographical images demonstrating the posterior leaflet height significantly greater than the anterior leaflet, where the posterior leaflet can be seen to be pushing the anterior leaflet into the outflow tract on (**a**) 3D surgical, and (**b**) and (**c**) long-axis views

improved by pulling on a long-handled trefoil sharp hook placed into the ventricular septum. The hook also defines the orientation of the resection and prevents the muscle being pushed away by the blade during incision. Two parallel incision lines are placed using a No 15 blade; one beneath the mid-point of the right coronary sinus and other beneath the commissure between the right and left coronary cusps. The incisions are commenced 3–5 mm beneath the aortic annulus, to maintain the integrity of the conducting tissue and aortic annulus, and extended to the base of the papillary muscle. The muscle mass is then resected by connecting the two incisions. The depth of the resection depends on the thickness of the septum but often 1.0–1.5 cm can be resected in patients with septal thickness of 2.0–2.5 cm. Echocardiographical visualisation before bypass and digital palpation from the ventricular cavity during the procedure can help to guide the depth of resection. The first incision often provides the best resection, as subsequent attempts are made in shredded muscle. Trans-oesophageal echocardiography is used to determine the adequacy of resection, resolution of LVOTO, as well as the presence of any aortic regurgitation or ventricular septal defect.

An alternative approach to treat SAM caused by a tall posterior mitral valve leaflet in the presence of HCM is by simply reducing the height of

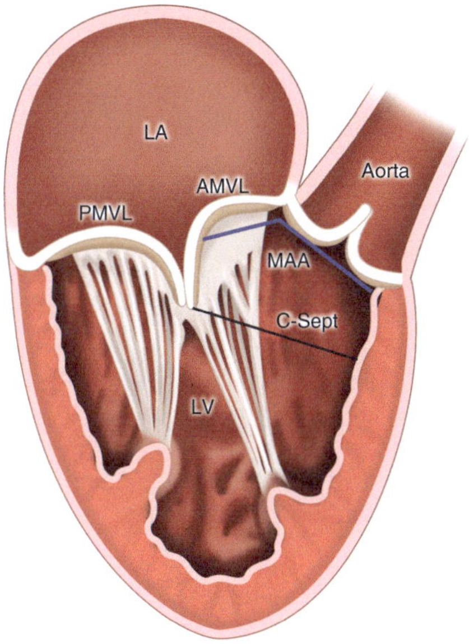

Fig. 15.6 Echocardiographic measurements to help predict the risk of post-mitral repair SAM. LA left atrium, LV left ventricle, PMVL posterior mitral valve leaflet, AMVL anterior mitral valve leaflet, C-Sept coaptation to septal distance, MAA mitral-aortic angle

Table 15.1 Risk factors contributing to the development of SAM

Structural factors	Geometric factors
Small, hyperdynamic left ventricle	Anterior displacement of the coaptation line
Displacement of the papillary muscles	Reduced aorto-mitral angle
Septal hypertrophy	Low anterior: posterior leaflet length ratio
Redundant anterior or posterior MV leaflet tissue	Under-sizing of the mitral annuloplasty ring

the posterior leaflet (leaflet displacement) and not resecting any septal muscle. The posterior leaflet is detached from the annulus and an appropriate amount of basal tissue (closest to the annulus) is resected, before reattaching the posterior leaflet. The asymmetrical heights of the various segments of the posterior leaflet may require an asymmetrical excision of tissue to produce a symmetrical residual posterior leaflet following resection. Simply detaching and reattaching the posterior leaflet reduces the height of the leaflet by 3–6 mm, depending on the depth of suture placement from the leaflet edge during reattachment. This brings the line of coaptation towards the posterior annulus, thereby reducing the risk of anterior displacement of the mitral valve during systole into the left ventricular outflow tract. Leaflet displacement can also be performed by making an incision at the point that the posterior leaflet is tallest, from the free edge to the annulus. Both edges are then detached from the annulus and a triangle of tissue is resected from the inferior leaflet edge (the portion to the right of the valve from the surgeon's perspective) to reduce its height, so that it matches the height of the other side of the incision (Fig. 15.8a). The leaflets are then sutured back to the annulus and to each other (Fig. 15.8b, c). Both of these techniques of leaflet displacement move the coaptation line posteriorly and thereby prevent SAM.

Post-mitral Repair SAM

Ideally, consideration of the risk factors would have been made to prevent the occurrence of post-mitral repair SAM. In patients with a large posterior leaflet height and reduced anterior: posterior leaflet height ratio, consideration should be given to reducing the posterior leaflet height to <1.5 cm and posterior displacement of the coaptation line with neo-chordae, resection or sliding plasty. Similarly, in patients with a large anterior leaflet and small annulus, consideration should be given to implanting a non-rigid annuloplasty ring or band sized to the whole mitral orifice, rather than the anterior leaflet alone.

Despite these considerations, a small number of patients may still present with SAM following mitral repair. In these patients, the management depends on the degree of SAM and its persistence. Initially, conservative measures can be tried, including increasing the ventricular preload with fluid administration, reduction or removal of any inotropic agents, such as adrenaline or dopamine, or increasing the afterload on the ventricle

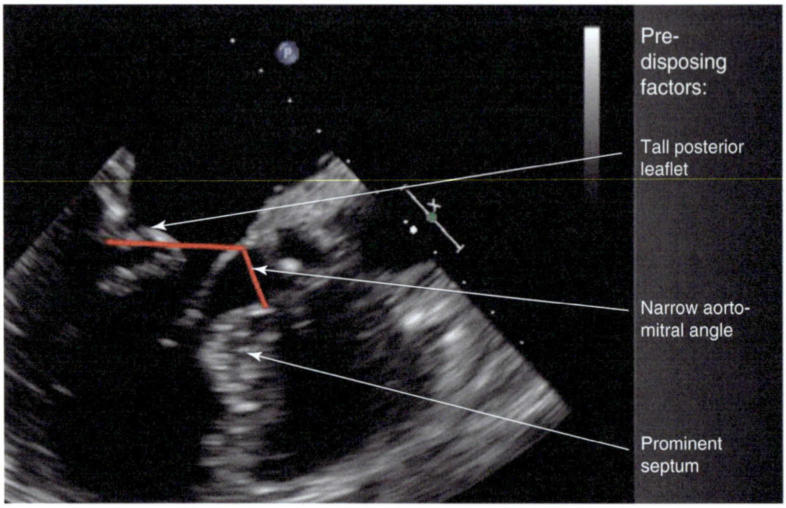

Fig. 15.7 Trans-oesophageal echocardiographical image demonstrating some of the pre-disposing factors for SAM, including a tall posterior leaflet, narrow aorto-mitral angle and prominent septal knuckle

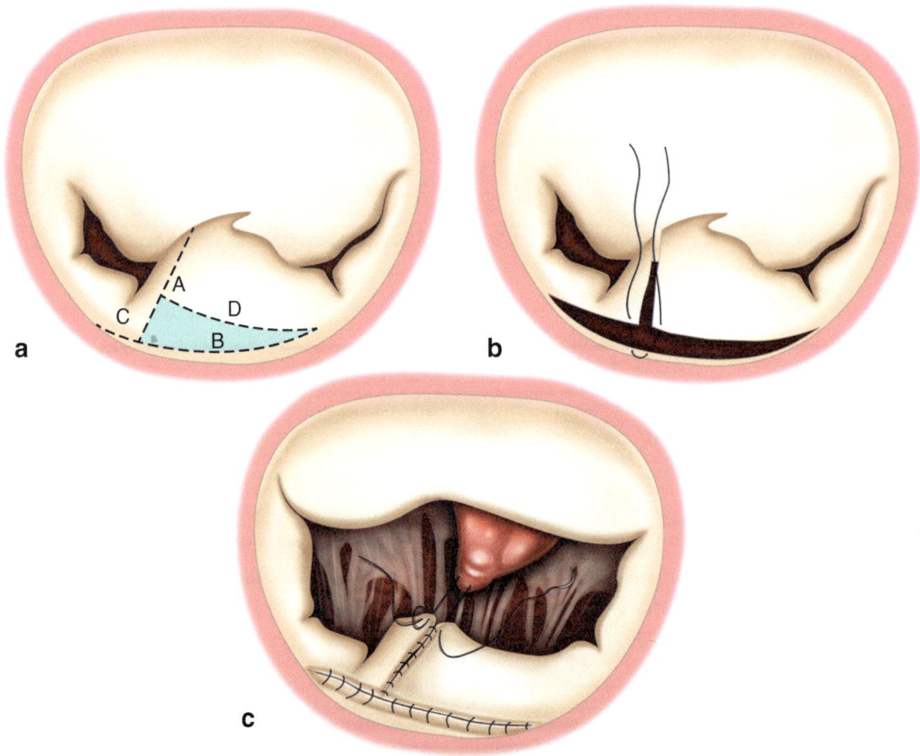

Fig. 15.8 Asymmetric leaflet height reduction, where (**a**) the leaflet is divided asymmetrically from the free edge to the annulus, with a triangle of leaflet then resected at the base of the leaflet, (**b**) the edges are re-approximated and (**c**) sutured back to the annulus, with neo-chords inserted, as required

with the administration of a vasoconstriction agent, such as noradrenaline. In addition, to increase left ventricular filling time, the heart rate is reduced by decreasing any external pacing or administering a negative chronotropic agent, such as a beta-blocker. Cardiac dys-synchrony can also exacerbate SAM and hence atrioventricular pacing should be optimised.

If conservative measures are not able to eliminate SAM, then further surgical intervention should be employed. In this situation, it is important to understand the anatomical factors causing SAM in the individual patient to choose the appropriate corrective technique. In addition, consideration should be made regarding the ease and durability of re-repair, as well as the additional ischaemic and cardiopulmonary bypass time required for re-repair, in the context of clamp and bypass times of the initial repair and underlying biventricular function. Re-repair techniques include removing the annuloplasty ring, reducing or further reducing the height of the posterior leaflet using leaflet resection or neo-chord insertion, and implanting a larger annuloplasty ring. Alternatively, a flexible band can be implanted to release the constraint on the dynamic changes of the anterior annulus. If SAM persists despite medical and surgical attempts at eliminating SAM, or re-repair is not considered feasible, then the insertion of a mitral prosthesis should be considered. In this setting, it is important to resect any components of the anterior mitral valve leaflet and sub-valvular apparatus contributing to the SAM and if necessary, maintain anterior annulo-ventricular continuity with additional Gore-Tex sutures implanted onto the anterior annulus. The key to prevent a disappointing progression from repair to re-repair and then valve insertion is to really understand the anatomy of the valve at the outset and deal with it accordingly.

Surgical Technique

Horizontal mattress band annuloplasty sutures (2/0 Ethibond) were placed around the mitral valve annulus. Stay sutures (5/0 Prolene) were placed on the anterior and posterior leaflets to extend them and to open them out. Using gentle traction on the posterior leaflet stay sutures and posterior annuloplasty sutures, the height of the posterior leaflet was measured (Fig. 15.9a). The posterior leaflet was then incised horizontally, at the mid-point of its insertion to the annulus, using a N°11 blade. The incision was continued parallel to the posterior annulus, just short of both commissures, thereby detaching the posterior leaflet from the annulus (Fig. 15.9b). A strip of tissue, approximately 25% of the height of the leaflet, was then excised from the base of the posterior leaflet, to reduce its height. It is important not to remove too much, as simply by detaching and reattaching the leaflet reduces the height by 3–6 mm in the suture line. The secondary and tertiary chords were preserved and, if necessary, reattached to the annulus. This moved the line of coaptation posteriorly, thereby reducing the risk of SAM and subsequent left ventricular outflow tract obstruction. The extent of resection depends on the degree of excess tissue of the posterior leaflet, ensuring that height of the posterior leaflet is <15 mm throughout its circumference. The posterior leaflet was reattached to the posterior annulus, using 4/0 Prolene (Fig. 15.9c).

The degree of prolapse of the anterior and posterior mitral valve leaflets was then reassessed with a reduced posterior leaflet height. In this patient, it was apparent that Gore-Tex neo-chordae were only required for the posterior leaflet. Using gentle traction on the anterior and posterior leaflet stay sutures, both the anterolateral and posteromedial papillary muscles could be accessed. Pledgeted CV-4 Gore-Tex neo-chordae were passed through the fibrous part of the papillary muscles using a horizontal mattress technique (Fig. 15.9d). Gore-Tex neo-chordae placed to the right of the midline on the posterior leaflet were anchored to the posteromedial papillary muscle, whilst those placed to the left of the midline were anchored to the anterolateral papillary muscle. The native chordae were also used as a guide to determine which head of the papillary muscles to insert the neo-chordae. The free ends of the neo-chordae were then placed through the leaflets approximately 5 mm from the free edge using a single-loop technique. The leaflet was drawn down with forceps whilst pulling up on the neo-chords until it was at the appropriate coaptation height, usually just beneath the annular plane. Competency of the mitral valve was then assessed with static testing, by injecting cold saline into the left ventricle using a bulb syringe. The free ends of the Gore-Tex neo-chordae were

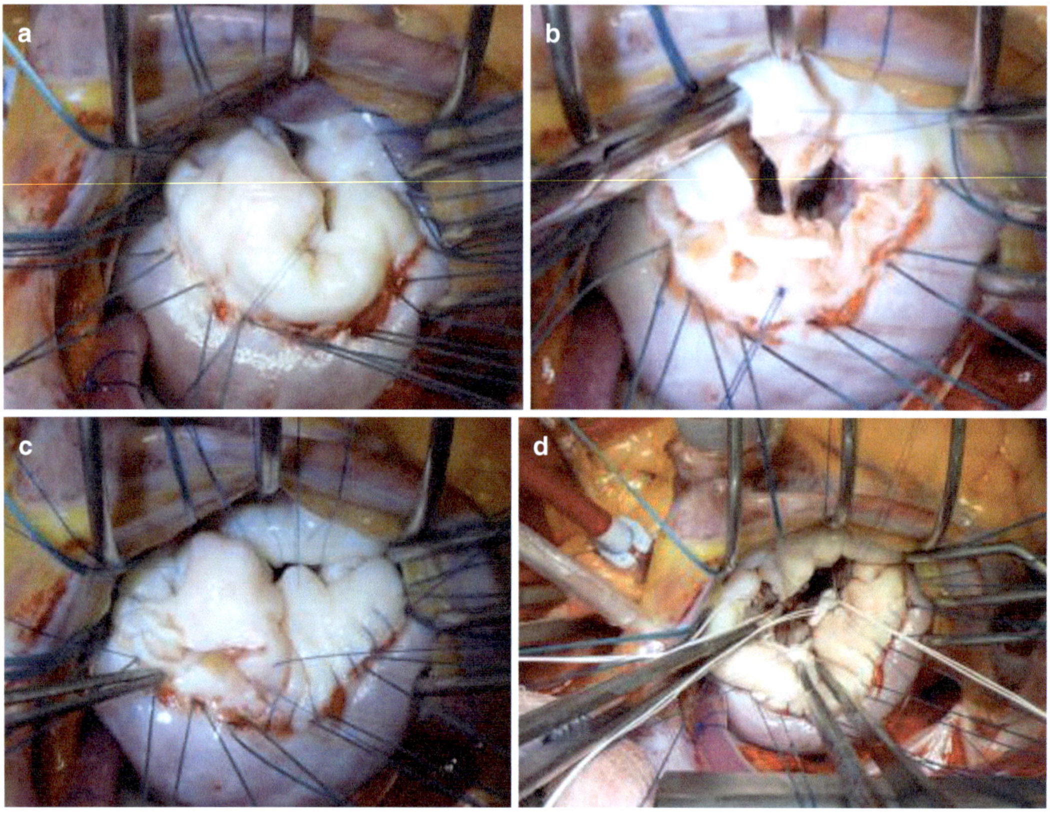

Fig. 15.9 Operative images demonstrating the surgical management of SAM, including (**a**) placement of horizontal mattress annuloplasty sutures, demonstrating a very tall posterior leaflet, (**b**) detachment of the posterior leaflet from the annulus, whilst preserving the tertiary chords, (**c**) reattachment of the leaflet following excision of the basal section of the leaflet, and (**d**) neo-chordal implantation

then tied with the leaflets at the annular plane and when competency of the mitral valve had been achieved. Each neo-chordae was tied with a total of 12 knots (6 in each direction) to ensure that the Gore-Tex knots did not loosen. With a left ventricle distended with saline, the depth of coaptation was assessed by colouring the atrial surface of the mitral valve leaflets with a sterile marking pen. The depth of coaptation can be increased to achieve an optimal depth of at least 8 mm, if necessary, by implanting additional Gore-Tex neo-chordae.

An appropriate sized annuloplasty ring or band was then chosen, according to the surface area of the whole mitral valve orifice (i.e. the surface area of the anterior and posterior mitral valve leaflets together), with the ventricle distended with saline. This is a crucial step, as choosing a ring or band that is based simply on the height of the anterior leaflet alone will crowd the leaflet tissue and make the anterior leaflet susceptible to displacement into the left ventricular outflow tract during systole. In this patient, a fully flexible annuloplasty band was used, extending from trigone to trigone. This minimizes the risk of excessive reduction of the anteroposterior distance of the mitral orifice, which otherwise would increase the risk of SAM. The annuloplasty band was then tied in situ using the horizontal mattress 2/0 Ethibond sutures placed earlier. Injecting cold saline again allowed the mitral valve to be assessed for competency, adequate depth of coaptation (>8 mm), that the coaptation line runs parallel to the posterior annulus and that the height of the posterior leaflet was <15 mm.

Post-operative Echocardiogram

The post-repair trans-oesophageal echocardiogram (Fig. 15.10) confirmed:

1. Normal physiological functioning of the mitral valve complex with no residual mitral regurgitation.
2. Absence of septal-mitral contact during systole or of any left ventricular outflow obstruction.
3. The depth of leaflet coaptation was >8 mm.
4. The height of the posterior leaflet was <15 mm.

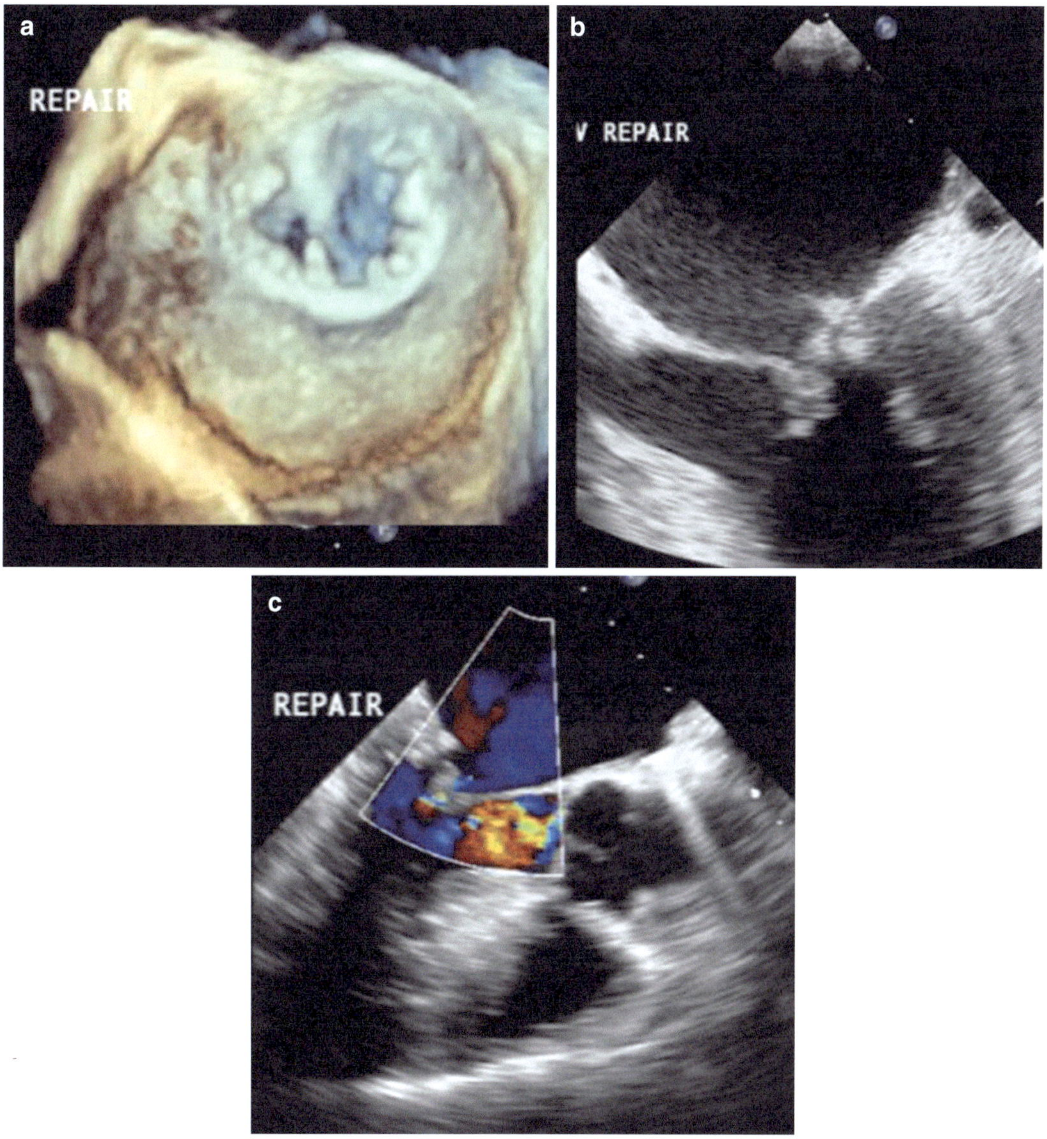

Fig. 15.10 Post-bypass intra-operative trans-oesophageal echocardiographical images demonstrating (**a**) the annuloplasty band in-situ on the 3D surgical view; (**b**) no SAM and 10 mm depth of coaptation between the anterior and posterior leaflets on the mid-oesophageal 5-chamber view; and (**c**) a competent mitral valve with no residual regurgitation on the mid-oesophageal long-axis view, using colour flow Doppler

Surgical Tips

1. Systolic anterior motion of the mitral valve caused by a tall posterior leaflet in the presence of septal hypertrophy can be managed by posterior displacement of the coaptation line to reduce the height of the posterior leaflet and without the need of a septal myectomy
2. Ensure that the height of the posterior leaflet is less than 1.5 cm and no more than 50% of the height of the anterior leaflet
3. An annuloplasty ring or band should be sized to the whole mitral valve orifice to avoid crowding of leaflet tissue and anterior displacement of the mitral leaflets
4. Avoid the use of a complete rigid annuloplasty ring as it increases the risk of excessive reduction of the anteroposterior distance of the mitral orifice and impairs the normal dynamic changes of anterior annulus that occur during the cardiac cycle

Comment

Results of posterior leaflet displacement surgery for patients with systolic anterior motion secondary to enlarged posterior mitral valve leaflets and hypertrophic cardiomyopathy are associated with excellent outcomes, with in-hospital mortality <1% and a low peri-operative complication rate.

Recommended Reading

Bothe W, Kvitting JP, Swanson JC, Goktepe S, Vo KN, Ingels NB, Miller DC. How do annuloplasty rings affect mitral leaflet dynamic motion? Eur J Cardiothorac Surg. 2010;38:340–9.

Crescenzi G, Landoni G, Zangrillo A, Guarracino F, Rosica C, La Canna G, Alfieri O. Management and decision-making strategy for systolic anterior motion after mitral valve repair. J Thorac Cardiovasc Surg. 2009;137:320–5.

Gersh BJ, Maron BJ, Bonow RO, Dearani JA, Fifer MA, Link MS, Naidu SS, Nishimura RA, Ommen SR, Rakowski H, Seidman CE, Towbin JA, Udelson JE, Yancy CW, American College of Cardiology Foundation/American Heart Association Task Force on Practice Guidelines. ACCF/AHA guideline for the diagnosis and treatment of hypertrophic cardiomyopathy: a report of the American College of Cardiology Foundation/American Heart Association Task Force on Practice Guidelines. Developed in collaboration with the American Association for Thoracic Surgery, American Society of Echocardiography, American Society of Nuclear Cardiology, Heart Failure Society of America, Heart Rhythm Society, Society for Cardiovascular Angiography and Interventions, and Society of Thoracic Surgeons. J Am Coll Cardiol. 2011;58:e212–60.

Hwang HJ, Choi EY, Kwan J, Kim SA, Shim CY, Ha JW, Rim SJ, Chung N, Kim SS. Dynamic change of mitral apparatus as potential cause of left ventricular outflow tract obstruction in hypertrophic cardiomyopathy. Eur J Echocardiogr. 2011;12:19–25.

Iacovoni A, Spirito P, Simon C, Iascone M, Di Dedda G, De Filippo P, Pentiricci S, Boni L, Senni M, Gavazzi A, Ferrazzi P. A contemporary European experience with surgical septal myectomy in hypertrophic cardiomyopathy. Eur Heart J. 2012;33:2080–7.

Maslow AD, Regan MM, Haering JM, Johnson RG, Levine RA. Echocardiographic predictors of left ventricular outflow tract obstruction and systolic anterior motion of the mitral valve after mitral valve reconstruction for myxomatous valve disease. J Am Coll Cardiol. 1999;34:2096–104.

Messmer BJ. Extended myectomy for hypertrophic obstructive cardiomyopathy. Ann Thorac Surg. 1994;58:575–7.

Quigley RL. Prevention of systolic anterior motion after repair of the severely myxomatous mitral valve with an anterior leaflet valvuloplasty. Ann Thorac Surg. 2005;80:179–82.

Seeburger J, Passage J, Borger MA, Mohr FW. A new concept for correction of systolic anterior motion and mitral valve regurgitation in patients with hypertrophic obstructive cardiomyopathy. J Thorac Cardiovasc Surg. 2010;140:481–3.

Varghese R, Itagaki S, Anyanwu AC, Trigo P, Fischer G, Adams DH. Predicting systolic anterior motion after mitral valve reconstruction: using intraoperative transesophageal echocardiography to identify those at greatest risk. Eur J Cardiothorac Surg. 2014;45:132–47.

Vriesendorp PA, Schinkel AF, Soliman OI, Kofflard MJ, de Jong PL, van Herwerden LA, Ten Cate FJ, Michels M. Long-term benefit of myectomy and anterior mitral leaflet extension in obstructive hypertrophic cardiomyopathy. Am J Cardiol. 2015;115:670–5.

16 Tricuspid Regurgitation

Keywords
Tricuspid regurgitation · Functional regurgitation · Ring annuloplasty · De Vega suture annuloplasty · Edge-to-edge repair · Leaflet extension · Chordal replacement · Atrioventricular node

Case History

A 74 year-old gentleman presented with a progressive history of increasing exertional dyspnoea, associated with peripheral oedema. He had no previous history of rheumatic fever or infective endocarditis. Clinical examination revealed a pansystolic murmur audible over the apex and at the left sternal edge. Coronary angiography demonstrated no obstructive coronary artery disease.

Echocardiographical Findings

Trans-thoracic echocardiography revealed marked tricuspid annular dilatation (end-systolic diameter of 4.8 cm), with normal movement of the tricuspid valve leaflets and no evidence of prolapse or restriction on the apical 4-chamber view (Fig. 16.1a). In addition, severe mitral regurgitation was identified, secondary to prolapse of the P2 scallop of the posterior mitral valve leaflet. Colour flow Doppler flow across the tricuspid valve in the apical 4-chamber view demonstrated a central jet of severe tricuspid regurgitation (TR), confirming annular dilatation as the dominant lesion and the absence of coaptation as the cause of the regurgitation (Fig. 16.1b). Quantification of the regurgitation, using the PISA method, revealed severe TR, with an effective regurgitant orifice area of 52 mm^2 and regurgitant volume of 74 mL, as well as a vena contracta of 0.82 cm (Fig. 16.1b). The right atrium was markedly enlarged (diameter 5.8 cm), whereas the right ventricle was contracting well and not dilated. Three-dimensional (3D) image of the tricuspid valve from the right ventricle confirmed the central loss of coaptation (Fig. 16.1c).

Trans-oesophageal echocardiographical images confirmed the tricuspid annular dilatation, with the leaflets reaching the annular plane during systole but with a poor depth of coaptation on the 45° and 135° orthogonal views (Fig. 16.2a, b), resulting in severe tricuspid regurgitation on the corresponding colour flow Doppler images (Fig. 16.2c, d). No underlying structural disease of the leaflets or subvalvular apparatus could be identified.

N. Moorjani et al., *Operative Mitral and Tricuspid Valve Surgery*,
https://doi.org/10.1007/978-1-4471-4204-1_16

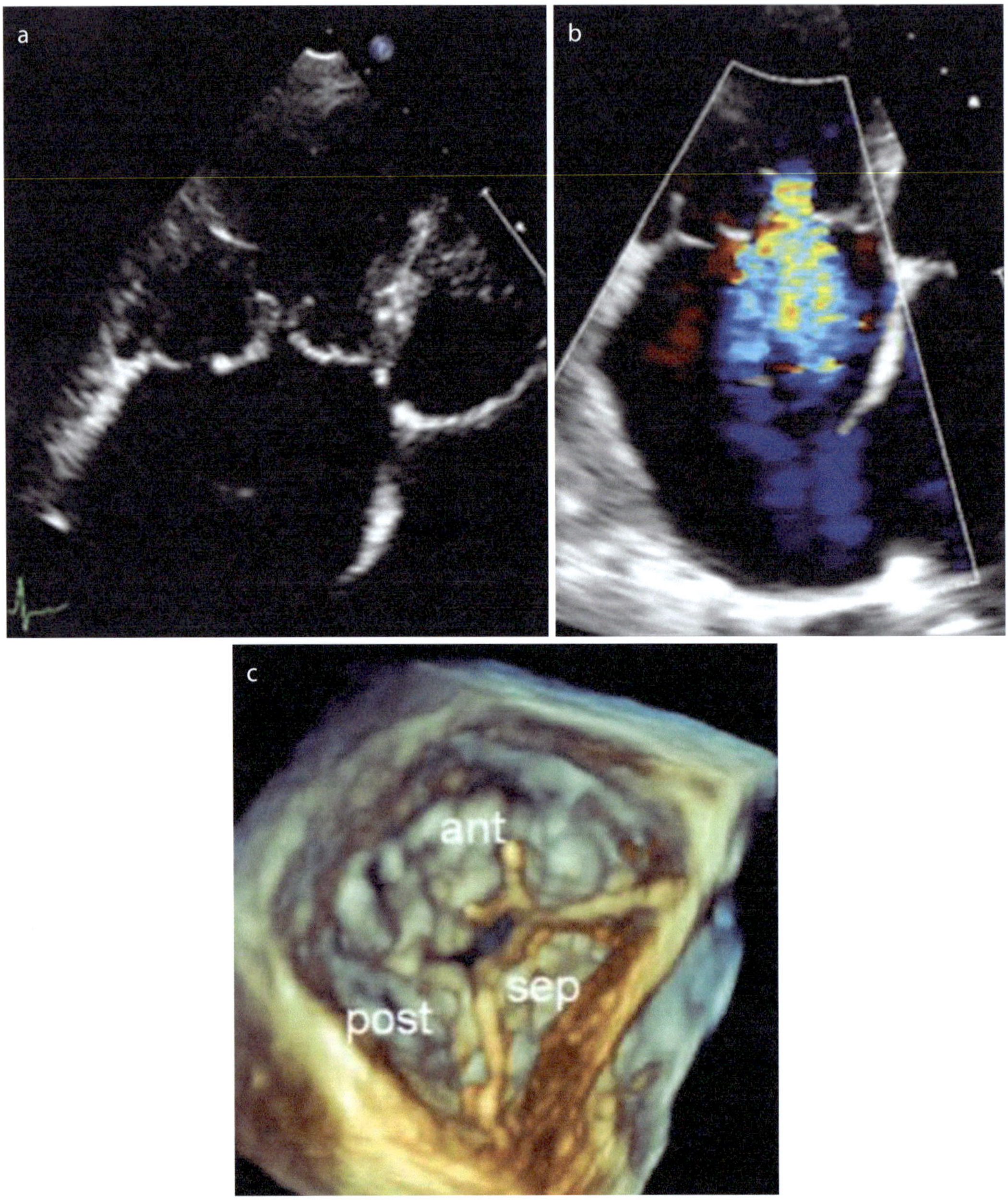

Fig. 16.1 Trans-thoracic echocardiographical images demonstrating (**a**) loss of leaflet coaptation, secondary to tricuspid annular dilatation, on an apical 4-chamber view, resulting in (**b**) severe tricuspid regurgitation on the corresponding colour flow Doppler image. (**c**) 3D image of the tricuspid valve viewed from right ventricular side clearly demonstrating central loss of leaflet coaptation. Ant anterior leaflet, post posterior leaflet, sep septal leaflet

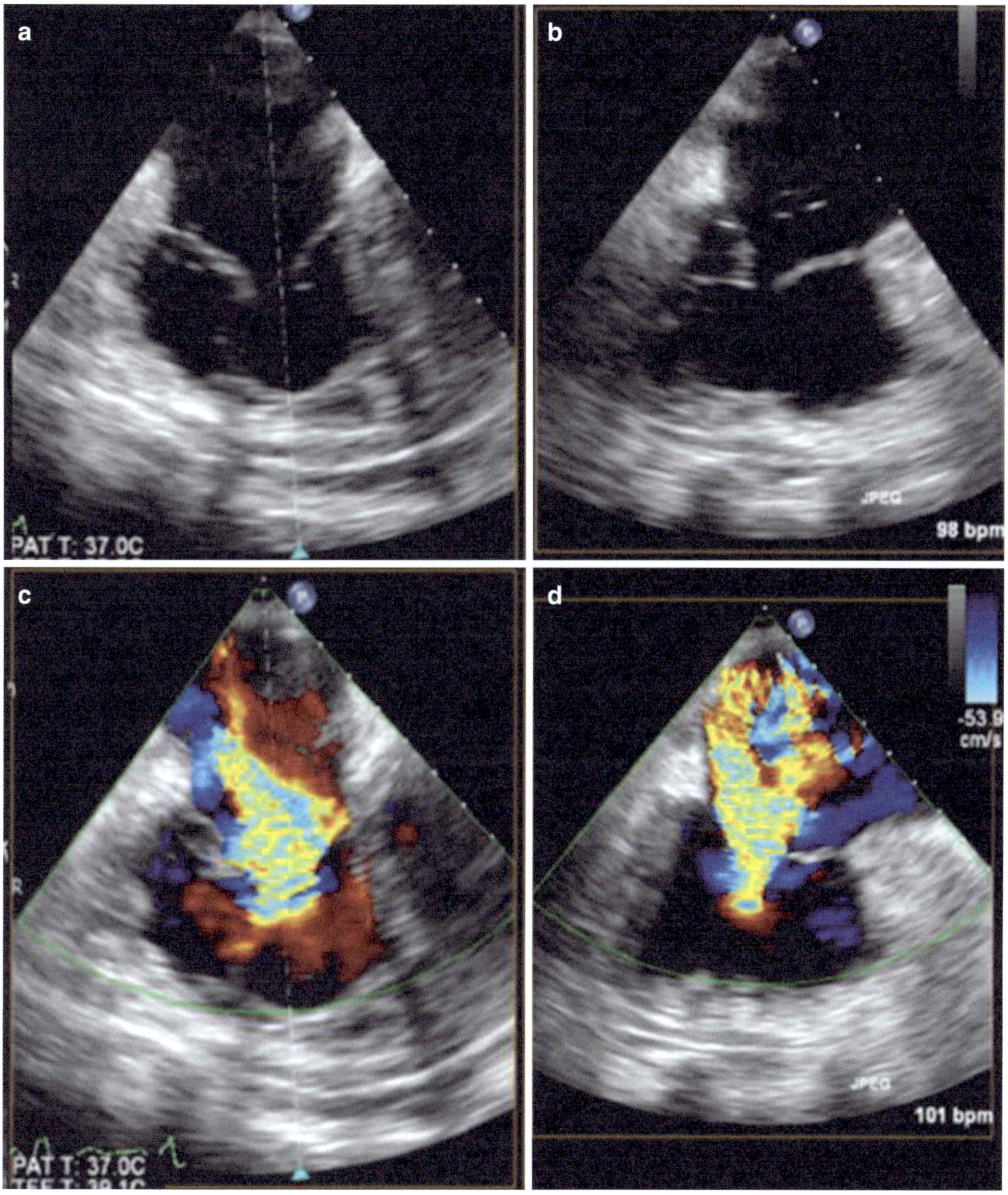

Fig. 16.2 Trans-oesophageal echocardiographical images demonstrating loss of leaflet coaptation, secondary to annular dilatation on orthogonal (**a**) 45° and (**b**) 135° views, resulting in severe tricuspid regurgitation on (**c**, **d**) the corresponding colour flow Doppler images

Pathophysiology

The aetiology of tricuspid regurgitation is categorised using a functional classification that describes leaflet motion, similar to mitral regurgitation. Type I tricuspid regurgitation involves normal leaflet motion and can be caused by annular dilatation, the presence of a pacemaker lead, cleft leaflet or leaflet perforation (with endocarditis). Type II tricuspid regurgitation represents excessive leaflet motion and can be caused by chordal elongation (leaflet prolapse) with degenerative tricuspid valve disease or chordal rupture (flail leaflet) with endocarditis, trauma or degenerative disease. Type III tricuspid regurgitation represents restricted leaflet motion (leaflet tethering) and can be caused by papillary muscle displacement (with right ventricular remodelling), rheumatic valve disease, carcinoid valve disease, radiation or the presence of pacemaker leads.

Functional or secondary tricuspid regurgitation represents the commonest aetiology in clinical practice, accounting for over 80% of cases and is caused by a combination of annular dilatation and leaflet tethering. The development of functional tricuspid regurgitation occurs as a result of right ventricular remodelling. Initially, ventricular enlargement results in tricuspid annular dilatation in a septo-lateral direction (Fig. 16.3). This corresponds to the right ventricular margin of the valve from the aortic root to the ventricular septum. The septal annulus does not dilate because of the fibrous skeleton of the heart.

Further right ventricular enlargement and subsequent tricuspid annular dilatation causes flattening of the otherwise multi-planar tricuspid annulus, which in turn produces impaired leaflet coaptation and tricuspid regurgitation.

As this process progresses, the dilating right ventricle causes papillary muscle displacement, with leaflet tethering and further annular dilatation, resulting in increasing tricuspid regurgitation. Right ventricular remodelling is most commonly due to left heart disease. Mitral valve regurgitation of any aetiology will produce back pressure across the pulmonary circulation and varying degrees of pulmonary hypertension. In addition, functional tricuspid regurgitation can be caused by atrial fibrillation induced atrial and ventricular enlargement, with subsequent annular dilatation. The stage at presentation will determine whether annular dilatation alone or in combination with leaflet tethering are responsible for the regurgitation and therefore the complexity of the valve repair procedure, whether annuloplasty alone or adjunctive repair techniques will be required.

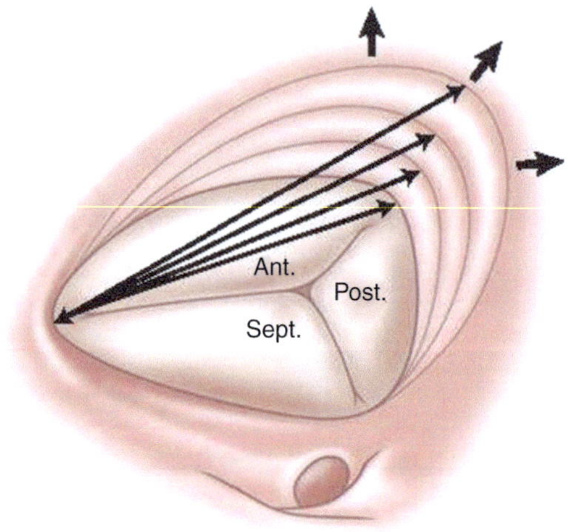

Fig. 16.3 Dilatation of the tricuspid valve annulus, which occurs in a septo-lateral direction, due to the relatively fixed attachment of the septal leaflet to the fibrous skeleton of the heart

It was previously thought that surgical correction of the left-sided valve pathology in patients with severe functional tricuspid valve regurgitation would result in resolution of the tricuspid regurgitation by decreasing pulmonary arterial pressures and subsequent right ventricular reverse remodelling. In the absence of surgical intervention on the tricuspid valve, however, as tricuspid annular dilatation is an on-going process, up to 40% of patients undergoing isolated left-sided valve surgery develop significant tricuspid regurgitation during long-term follow-up. Severe residual functional tricuspid valve regurgitation secondary to left-sided valve disease is associated with reduced functional outcome and long-term survival. Furthermore, patients undergoing reoperation for tricuspid valve surgery who have previously undergone left-sided valve surgery is associated with a high mortality, suggesting an aggressive approach to intervention on the tricuspid valve at the time of left-sided valve surgery.

Surgical Strategy

According to the American Heart Association/American College of Cardiology and the European Society of Cardiology, tricuspid valve surgery is recommended for isolated surgery in patients with symptomatic severe TR or asymptomatic severe TR with evidence of RV dysfunction or dilatation. In patients undergoing cardiac surgery for left-sided valve surgery, concomitant intervention on the tricuspid valve is indicated in the presence of moderate (or greater) TR or a dilated TV annulus. This is defined as >40 mm or 21 mm/m^2 end-systolic diameter from the mid-septal annulus to the mid-anterior annulus on pre-operative echocardiography 4-chamber view or >70 mm from the anteroseptal commissure to the anteroposterior commissure on intra-operative direct measurement. In patients who have previously undergone left-sided valve surgery, subsequent intervention on the TV is indicated in patients with symptomatic severe TR but in the absence of severe pulmonary arterial hypertension or right ventricular dysfunction. In addition to the guidelines, it has been suggested that tricuspid valve surgery should also be performed at the time of left-sided valve surgery in a patient with a tricuspid valve annulus >35 mm in the presence of atrial fibrillation, pulmonary hypertension, right ventricular dysfunction or enlargement and rheumatic valve disease. The presence of right atrial dilatation, significant peripheral oedema, ascites or hepatic congestion can also be used as a marker of tricuspid valve severity.

The principles of tricuspid valve surgery include treating the underlying valvular pathology and correction of any annular dilatation. In patients with type I regurgitation caused by annular dilatation, suture annuloplasty or ring annuloplasty is usually sufficient to restore valvular competency. Endocarditis destruction of the valve causing leaflet perforation usually requires pericardial patch closure of the defect in the leaflet, supported by ring annuloplasty (see Chap. 17). Severe tricuspid regurgitation caused by pacing wires traversing the valve orifice that interfere with leaflet coaptation and produce leaflet tethering can be removed, placed outside the annuloplasty ring or replaced with permanent epicardial pacing leads. In patients with type II tricuspid regurgitation caused by leaflet prolapse or flail leaflet secondary to degenerative valve disease, they can be treated with Gore-Tex neochordae implantation. Finally, patients with type III regurgitation caused by leaflet tethering may be repairable with leaflet augmentation or downsizing annuloplasty but in severe cases caused by carcinoid syndrome, radiation or rheumatic valve disease for example, valve replacement is often required.

In patients with functional tricuspid regurgitation, the main principles of treatment include restoration of annular geometry and size by suture or ring annuloplasty to improve leaflet coaptation. If severe leaflet tethering is present, adjunctive surgical techniques may be required in addition to annuloplasty, including leaflet augmentation or the 'clover' edge-to-edge technique, or in some patients if the valve is not repairable valve replacement will be necessary. In addition, optimisation of right ventricular function is important, which is facilitated by correcting any left-sided valve disease, thereby reducing RV afterload.

The most stable results of tricuspid valve repair have recently been shown to be with the use of an annuloplasty ring, most commonly the Carpentier tricuspid annuloplasty ring, which is bi-planar and rigid. Intuitively, one might think that an annuloplasty ring, which is flexible at its interface with the right ventricular part of the annulus would reduce the risk of dehiscence but as yet there are no data to support this inference. Recent studies have demonstrated the inherently unstable nature of suture annuloplasty repairs of the tricuspid valve of all types. As they, however, continue to be used, they are described here for completeness.

Suture Annuloplasty

Two principle methods of suture annuloplasty are in common usage. The first and perhaps the most commonly used is the de Vega technique (Fig. 16.4). In this procedure, two weaving 4/0 Prolene purse-string sutures are placed from the anteroseptal commissure to the posteroseptal commissure to cinch the anterior and posterior tricuspid valve annulus. This effectively reduces the valve orifice area, thereby increasing leaflet coaptation.

The second is sometimes described as the Kay technique of commissural exclusion but is commonly performed as exclusion of the posterior leaflet by annular plication (Fig. 16.5). This localised annuloplasty technique does not address progressive dilatation of the right ventricular annulus. Although both techniques are relatively simple and quick to perform, they are probably less reproducible than ring annuloplasty in the hands of the occasional tricuspid surgeon.

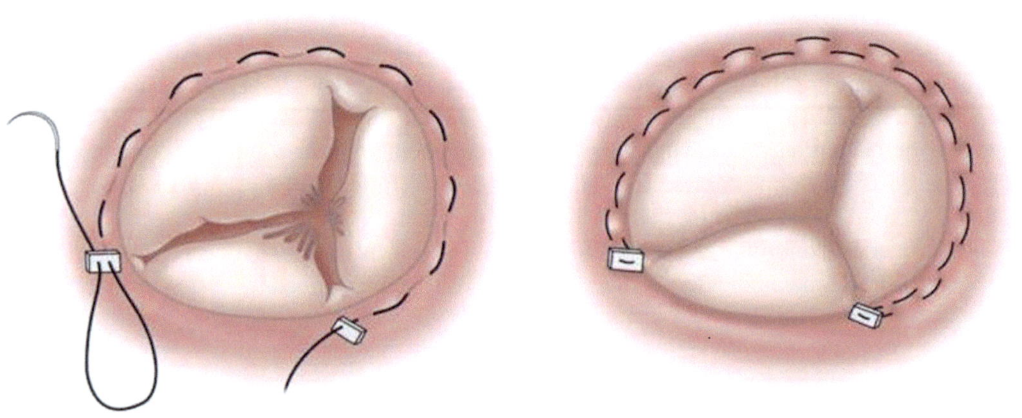

Fig. 16.4 De Vega suture annuloplasty technique, where (**a**) two weaving 4/0 Prolene purse-string sutures are placed from the anteroseptal commissure to the posteroseptal commissure and (**b**) tied in situ to cinch the anterior and posterior tricuspid valve annulus

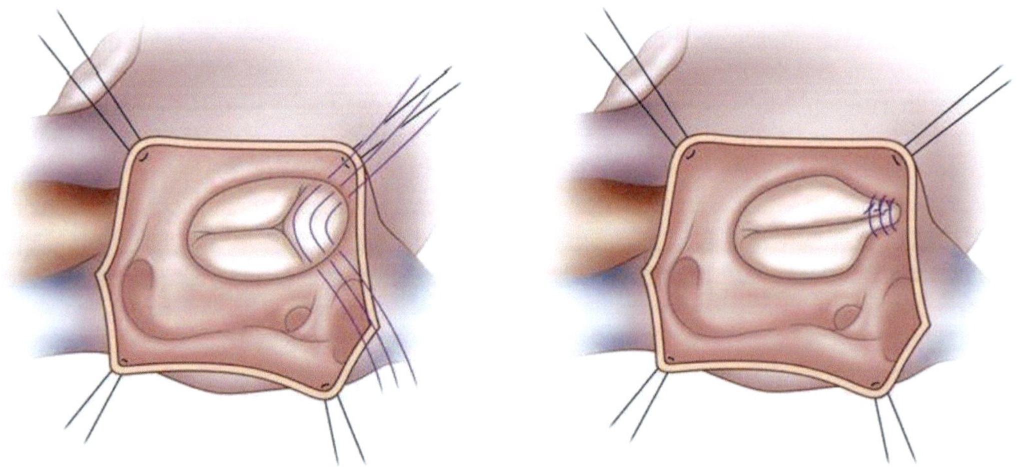

Fig. 16.5 Kay annuloplasty technique, which uses (**a**) annular plication to compress the posterior tricuspid valve annulus, resulting in (**b**) exclusion of the posterior leaflet

Ring Annuloplasty

In view of the problems with suture annuloplasty, ring annuloplasty is recommended as the treatment of choice for annular dilatation, as it is more reproducible at reducing annular size, thereby increasing the surface area of coaptation and achieving valve competency. Tricuspid valve annuloplasty rings are incomplete to avoid damaging the conduction tissue that sits at the apex of the 'triangle of Koch', adjacent to the medial aspect of the septal annulus (Fig. 16.6). As tricuspid annular dilatation takes place in the region of the right ventricular origin, the use of incomplete rings achieves the desired reduction in annular size. Tricuspid annuloplasty rings may be rigid, semi-rigid or flexible. Flexible bands have the advantage of preserving the dynamic changes of the tricuspid annulus that occur during the cardiac cycle. It has been argued by some that flexible rings are less able to protect the annulus against future dilatation, predisposing the patient to recurrent regurgitation. The contrary argument against rigid rings, however, is that the constant movement that they are subjected to at the right ventricular interface is more likely to give rise to ring dehiscence. Distortion of the annular plane in chronic regurgitation may be better addressed by the multi-planar nature of the rigid rings restoring natural coaptation. If the right ventricle is not irreversibly dilated, however, then the flexible ring will allow more natural reverse remodelling. There are as yet no convincing answers to these important questions and so, as with much of surgery, the choice of the type of ring will remain in the preference of the surgeon.

Although tricuspid valve annuloplasty alone is sufficient at restoring valve competency in the majority of patients, there are several risk factors for recurrent regurgitation, including leaflet tethering with a coaptation height >1 cm, atrial fibrillation, large annular size, raised pulmonary artery pressure and the presence of pacemaker leads traversing the valve orifice. In view of this, adjunctive techniques are sometimes required in addition to ring annuloplasty, especially in patients with leaflet tethering secondary to right ventricular dilatation, to produce a competent valve, including edge-to-edge repair and leaflet augmentation.

Edge-to-Edge Repair

The edge-to-edge repair ('clover' technique) uses the same principles of the equivalent mitral repair technique by approximating the free edges of the three leaflets, producing a clover-shaped triple-orifice valve (Fig. 16.7). The

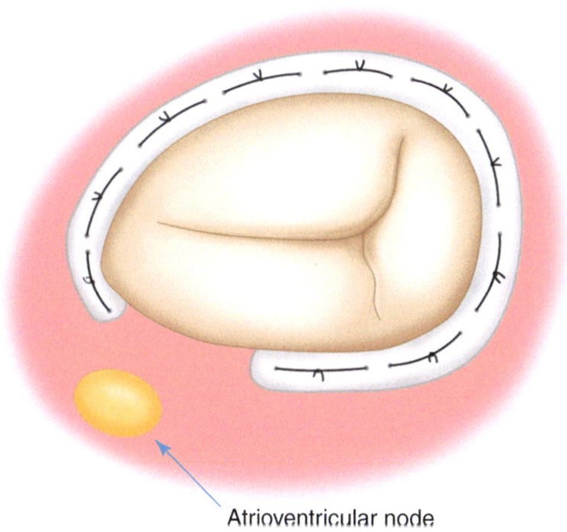

Fig. 16.6 Tricuspid valve ring annuloplasty with an incomplete ring to avoid damage to the conducting system and especially atrioventricular node (AVN), which sit in close proximity to the medial part of the septal annulus

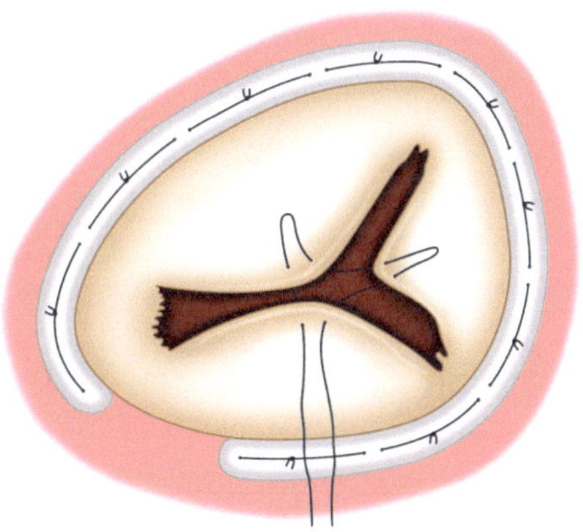

Fig. 16.7 Edge-to-edge repair ('clover' technique), where the free edges of the three leaflets are approximated using a 5/0 Prolene suture, producing a clover-shaped triple-orifice valve

durability and long-term outcome of this technique has not yet been firmly established.

Leaflet Extension

Depending on the presence and location of leaflet tethering (coaptation distance >8 mm, tenting area >1.6 cm^2), augmentation of the affected leaflet has been suggested as an adjunct to increase the depth of coaptation. It is important all the leaflets are pliable, and that there is no leaflet or annular calcification. The affected leaflet is detached at its attachment to the annulus, from commissure to commissure. Annuloplasty sutures are then placed to enhance exposure, allowing a long oval-shaped autologous or bovine pericardial patch to be implanted, using a continuous locking 5/0 Prolene suture (Fig. 16.8). It is important to oversize the patch to ensure that there is no tension on the leaflet causing restricted leaflet motion. Long-term follow-up is required to establish whether the pericardial patch remains pliable to maintain adequate leaflet motion.

Chordal Replacement

Chordal replacement is used in patients with a prolapsed or flail tricuspid valve leaflet due to chordal elongation or rupture, respectively. The diseased chordae are replaced with Gore-Tex polytetrafluoroethylene (PTFE) sutures (W.L. Gore & Associates, Flagstaff, AZ, USA).

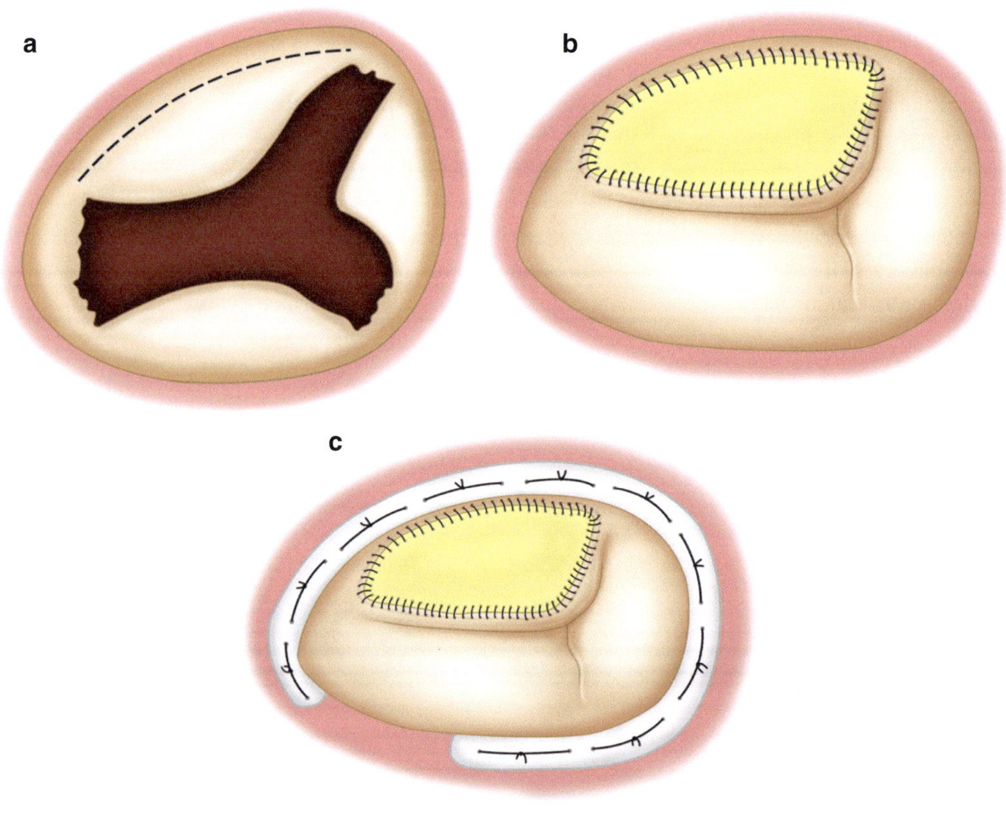

Fig. 16.8 Patch augmentation of the anterior tricuspid valve leaflet. (**a**) Detachment of the anterior leaflet at the annulus from commissure to commissure, (**b**) implantation of a bovine pericardial patch using a continuous 5/0 polyprolpylene suture and (**c**) implantation of an annuloplasty ring

As it does not require the excision of valve tissue, it preserves leaflet anatomy and mobility, as well as maintaining the maximal orifice area of the tricuspid valve. Chordal replacement is performed by passing both limbs of a pledgeted CV-4 Gore-Tex neo-chordae through the fibrous part of the papillary muscle head that was providing chordal support to the prolapsing leaflet. Both limbs of the Gore-Tex sutures are then passed through the prolapsing segment 5 mm from the free edge. The height of the Gore-Tex neo-chordae is determined by functional assessment, using saline inflation of the right ventricle to adjust the height of the neo-chord.

Tricuspid Valve Replacement

In patients with extensive disease of the valve where repair is not feasible, such as marked leaflet tethering, extensive calcification, carcinoid or rheumatic valve disease, replacement of the tricuspid valve is indicated. The choice between a mechanical or biological stented valve remains controversial. Although both have similar outcomes for survival, it has always been assumed that mechanical valves are prone to thromboembolic complications in the low-pressure right-sided circulation. Although mechanical valves have a greater theoretical durability over bioprostheses, recent reported results suggest little difference between the two in longevity in the tricuspid position.

There is a reported increase in the rate of heart block in patients undergoing tricuspid replacement due to the proximity of the sutures to the conducting system at the apex of the triangle of Koch. In view of this, sutures positioned at the medial aspect of the septal annulus are placed very carefully close to the annulus, including leaflet tissue, to avoid the conducting tissue (Fig. 16.9). In addition, subsequent placement of a transvenous endocardial pacing system can damage the leaflets of a tissue valve and result in early structural valve deterioration due to the lead causing leaflet fibrosis and distortion. A transvenous pacing system cannot be used if a mechanical tricuspid valve prosthesis is implanted. In view of this, permanent epicardial pacing wires should be placed at the time of tricuspid valve replacement surgery. If a transvenous system is already in situ, the pacing wire can be excluded from the orifice of the valve by imbricating the annulus over it and then placing the valve sutures as usual. As with the mitral valve, tricuspid valve replacement should be performed with retention of all of the subvalvular apparatus in place, thereby maintaining annular-ventricular continuity and preserving ventricular function.

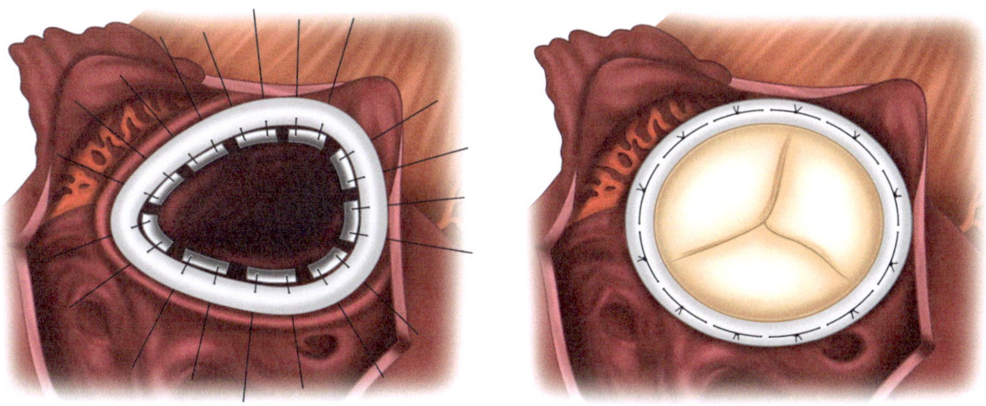

Fig. 16.9 Tricuspid valve replacement using interrupted pledgeted horizontal mattress sutures

Surgical Technique

The leaflets and the subvalvular apparatus of the tricuspid valve were assessed and correlated with the trans-oesophageal echocardiographical findings. Marked annular dilatation was observed with normal leaflet motion and no evidence of leaflet prolapse or restriction (Fig. 16.10a). Horizontal mattress annuloplasty sutures (2/0 Ethibond) were placed around the circumference of the tricuspid valve, with a 5 mm width and approximately 1 mm apart. These sutures were placed from the mid-point of the septal leaflet on the lateral half of the septal annulus, as well as the entire anterior and posterior annulus. No sutures were placed on the medial part of the septal annulus to avoid the Bundle of His and the atrioventricular node, which sit at the apex of the triangle of Koch. A 32 mm MC3 tricuspid annuloplasty ring (Edwards Lifesciences, Irvine, CA) was then chosen according to the surface area of the anterior leaflet and the distance between the anteroseptal and the posteroseptal commissures. The sutures were passed through the ring (Fig. 16.10b) and tied down in situ. Competency of the tricuspid valve was then assessed with static testing, by injecting cold saline into the right ventricle, using a bulb syringe, whilst occluding the main pulmonary artery (Fig. 16.10c).

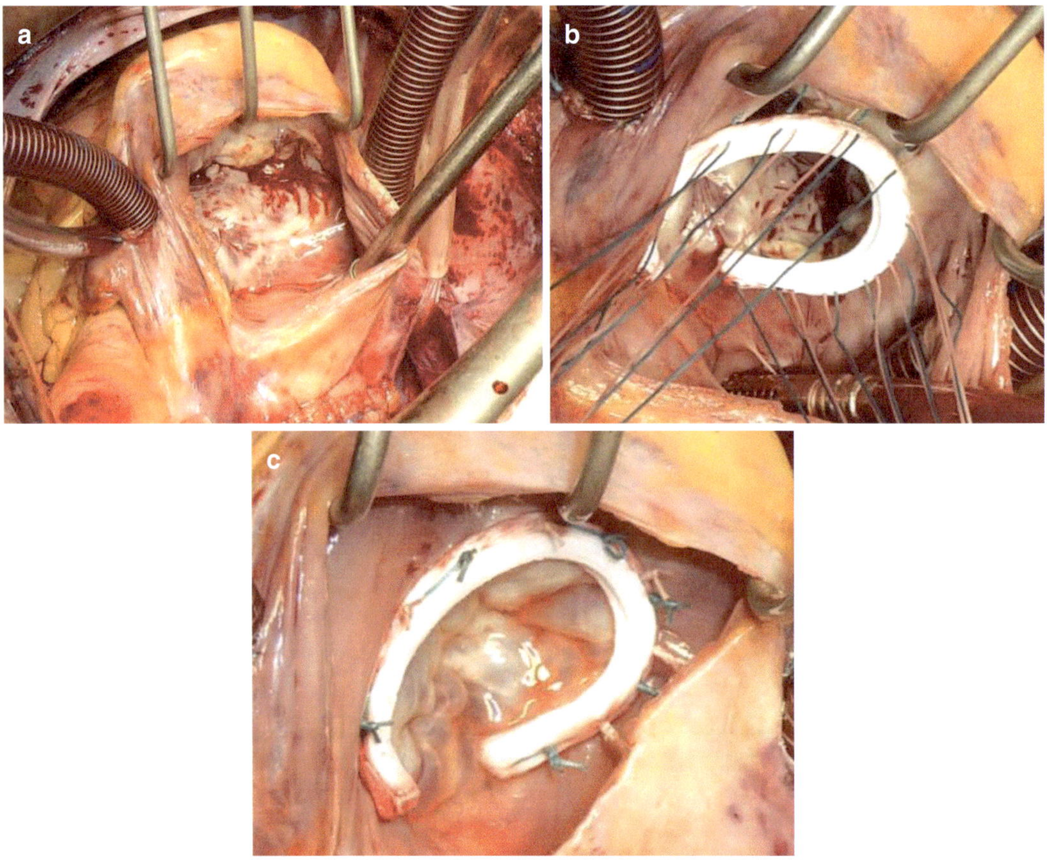

Fig. 16.10 Operative images illustrating (**a**) analysis of the tricuspid valve, demonstrating isolated annular dilatation, with no evidence of leaflet prolapse or restriction, (**b**) implantation of a 32 mm MC3 tricuspid annuloplasty ring (Edwards Lifesciences, Irvine, CA) and (**c**) a competent tricuspid valve following static testing

Post-operative Echocardiogram

The post-repair trans-oesophageal echocardiographical images (Fig. 16.11) confirmed:

1. Normal physiological functioning of the tricuspid valve complex with no residual tricuspid regurgitation.

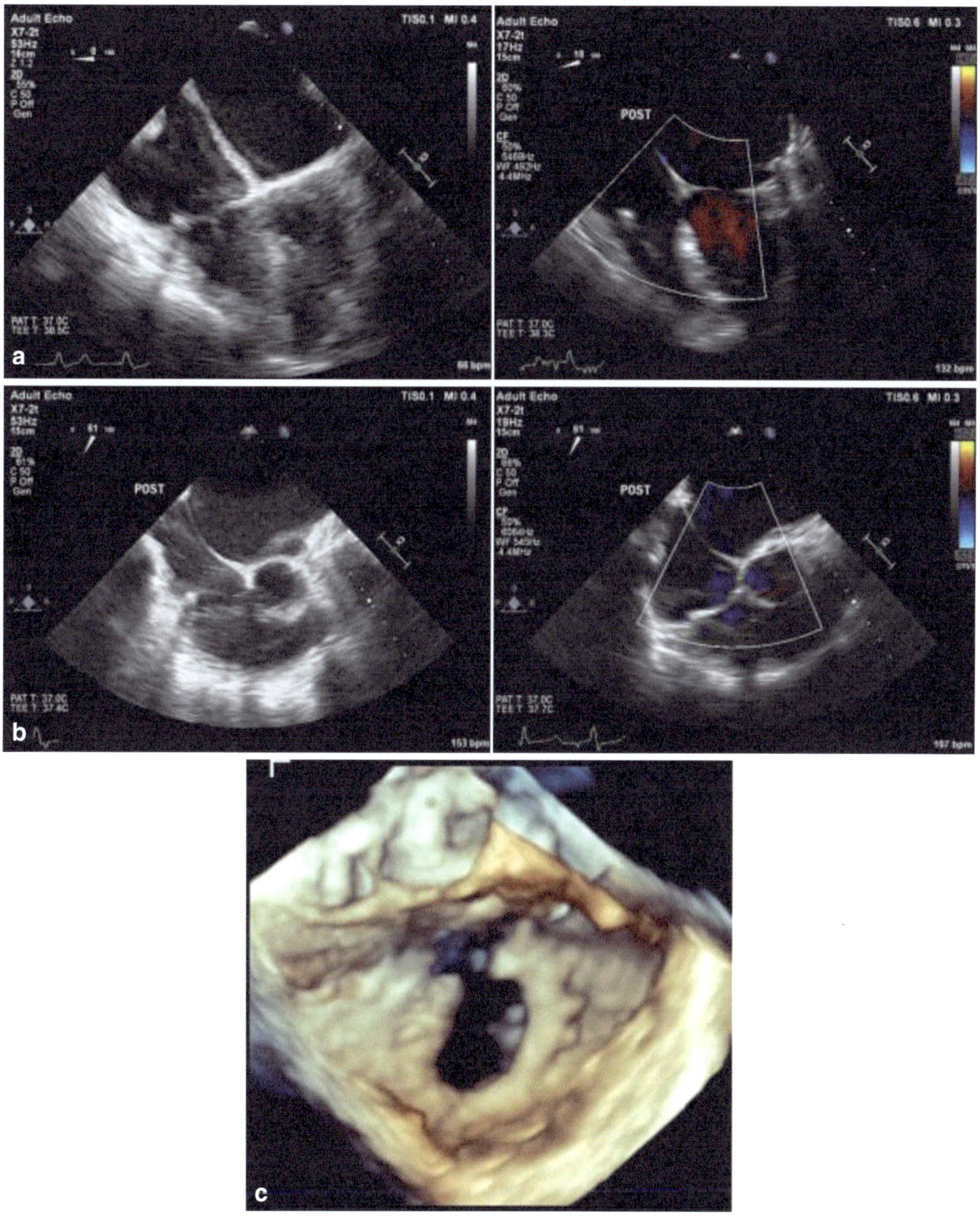

Fig. 16.11 Post-bypass intra-operative trans-oesophageal echocardiographical images demonstrating excellent depth of coaptation between the leaflets on the mid-oesophageal (**a**) 4-chamber and (**b**) right ventricular inflow/outflow views, and a competent tricuspid valve, with no residual tricuspid regurgitation on the corresponding colour flow Doppler views. (**c**) Three-dimensional right atrial view demonstrating the annuloplasty ring in situ

2. The diameter of the tricuspid valve annulus reduced to 32 mm.
3. No evidence of tricuspid stenosis
4. The depth of leaflet coaptation was 8 mm.

Surgical Tips

1. Identify the underlying pathophysiological mechanism to determine whether annuloplasty ring implantation alone will be sufficient
2. Accurate sizing of the tricuspid valve using the surface area of the anterior leaflet and the distance between the anteroseptal and posteroseptal commissures
3. Obtaining an adequate depth of coaptation (>8 mm) is important for the long-term durability of the procedure.

Comment

Although concomitant mitral and tricuspid valve surgery is documented to be associated with a greater operative mortality than mitral valve surgery alone, it is mainly a reflection of a more advanced disease process, including worsening ventricular function, higher pulmonary artery pressures and the presence of hepatic or renal congestion. The addition of tricuspid valve repair at the time of left-sided valve surgery, however, can be performed following removal of the aortic cross-clamp during the reperfusion time and is actually associated with a minimal incremental risk of morbidity or mortality. Although there are some risks specific to tricuspid valve surgery, including damage to the right coronary artery, aortic valve and conducting system, these are relatively rare. Concomitant tricuspid valve surgery at the time of left-sided valve surgery is associated with an 85% freedom from moderate or severe TR at 10 years, compared to 50% for those where the tricuspid valve is not operated on. The risk factors for recurrence include the presence of severe tethering of the tricuspid leaflets (coaptation distance >0.76 cm and tenting area >1.63 cm^2), severe preoperative tricuspid regurgitation, pulmonary hypertension, pacemaker leads, left ventricular dysfunction, and the use of suture rather than ring annuloplasty.

Ring annuloplasty has been shown to be associated with a greater freedom from recurrent significant tricuspid regurgitation than suture annuloplasty, using the De Vega or Kay annuloplasty techniques (17% vs. 33% at 8 years), especially in patients with severe tricuspid annular dilatation or pulmonary hypertension. As well as being more durable, ring annuloplasty is associated with better long-term and event-free survival at 15 years. As regards ring prosthesis type, rigid and semi-rigid rings are associated with greater freedom from recurrent significant tricuspid regurgitation than flexible bands.

The operative mortality for isolated tricuspid valve surgery traditionally has been reported as 5–10% and maybe higher in patients undergoing reoperation or with evidence of right ventricular dysfunction or severe pulmonary hypertension. Following surgery, the predominant causes of death in these patients include low cardiac output syndrome, right ventricular dysfunction, and secondary renal and hepatic impairment. Late referral of these patients also contributes to the operative mortality risk.

Recommended Reading

Hwang HY, Kim KH, Kim K, Ahn H. Propensity score matching analysis of mechanical versus bioprosthetic tricuspid valve replacements. Ann Thorac Surg. 2014;97(4):294–1299.

Parolari A, Barili F, Pilozzi A, Pacini D. Ring or suture annuloplasty for tricuspid regurgitation? A meta-analysis review. Ann Thorac Surg. 2014;98(6):2255–63.

Rodés-Cabau J, Taramasso M, O'Gara PT. Diagnosis and treatment of tricuspid valve disease: current and future perspectives. Lancet. 2016;388(10058):2431–42.

Rogers JH, Bolling SF. Valve repair for functional tricuspid valve regurgitation: anatomical and surgical considerations. Semin Thorac Cardiovasc Surg. 2010;22(1):84–9.

Shinn SH, Schaff HV. Evidence-based surgical management of acquired tricuspid valve disease. Nat Rev Cardiol. 2013;10(4):190–203.

Taylor JT, Chidsey G, Disalvo TG, Byrne JG, Maltais S. Contemporary management of tricuspid regurgitation: an updated clinical review. Cardiol Rev. 2013;21(4):174–83.

Zhu TY, Wang JG, Meng X. Is a rigid tricuspid annuloplasty ring superior to a flexible band when correcting secondary tricuspid regurgitation? Interact Cardiovasc Thorac Surg. 2013;17(6):1009–14.

17 Tricuspid Valve Infective Endocarditis

Keywords
Infective endocarditis · Vegetation · Leaflet reconstruction · Autologous pericardium · Bovine pericardium · Tricuspid regurgitation · Tricuspid valve replacement · Bacteraemia · Embolisation · Leaflet resection · Intravenous drug abuser (IVDA)

Case History

A 28 year-old gentleman presented with a 6-week history of fever, night sweats and some dyspnoea on exertion. He had no previous history of rheumatic fever but was an intravenous drug abuser. Clinical examination revealed a pyrexia of 38.7 °C and a pan-systolic murmur. Blood cultures isolated *Staphylococcus aureus*, associated with a raised white blood cell count (19,200/μL) and C-reactive protein (245 mg/dL).

Echocardiographical Findings

The trans-thoracic echocardiographic right ventricular inflow view revealed the presence of a large vegetation on the anterior tricuspid valve leaflet associated with normal movement of tricuspid valve leaflets (Fig. 17.1a). Doppler flow across the tricuspid valve in this view demonstrated significant tricuspid regurgitation (TR), through a perforation in the anterior leaflet (Fig. 17.1b). This was also observed on the parasternal short-axis view at the level of the aortic valve (Fig. 17.1c), where the vegetation can be seen as a mobile mass attached to the atrial surface of the anterior leaflet and measures 2.5 cm in length (Fig. 17.1d).

Quantification of the regurgitation, using the PISA method, revealed severe TR, with a regurgitant volume of 74 mL and regurgitant fraction of 59%, associated with a vena contracta of 0.82 cm. The right atrium was not enlarged, whereas the right ventricle was dilated with impaired function.

Trans-oesophageal echocardiographical images confirm the presence of the vegetation on the atrial side of the anterior leaflet and the severe tricuspid regurgitation (Fig. 17.2).

Pathophysiology

Isolated tricuspid valve infective endocarditis (IE) is uncommon and accounts for approximately 5–10% of all cases of infective endocarditis. The principle risk factor for the development of infective endocarditis of this valve is intravenous drug abuse (IVDA). Other risk factors include the presence of prosthetic material on the right side of the heart, such as an indwelling central venous catheter, prosthetic tricuspid valve or annuloplasty ring, pacemaker or defibrillator, and right-sided cardiac lesions,

N. Moorjani et al., *Operative Mitral and Tricuspid Valve Surgery*,
https://doi.org/10.1007/978-1-4471-4204-1_17

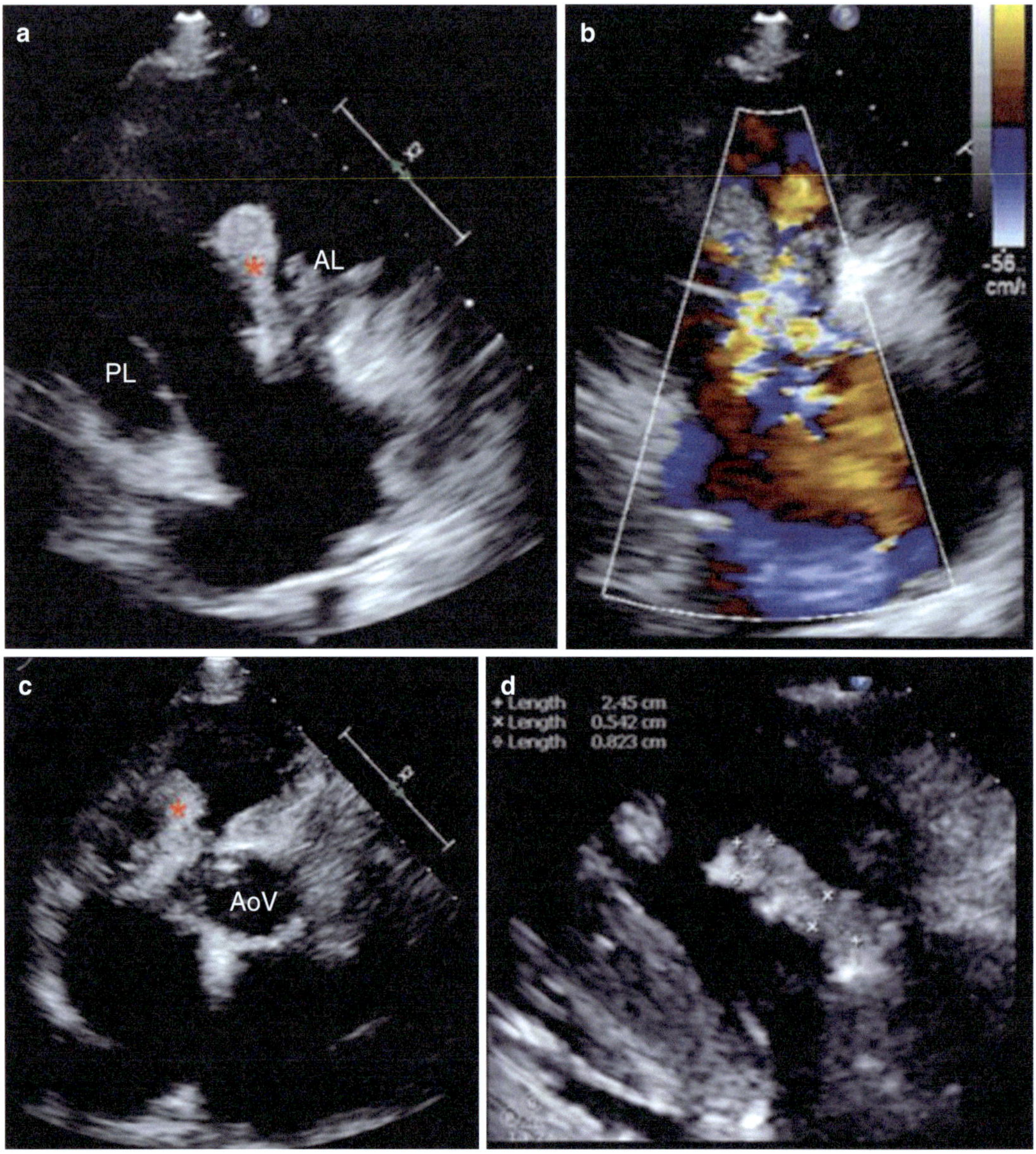

Fig. 17.1 Trans-thoracic echocardiographical images demonstrating a large vegetation (red star) lying on the atrial side of the anterior tricuspid valve leaflet on (**a**) the right ventricular inflow view, resulting in severe tricuspid regurgitation through the leaflet on (**b**) the corresponding colour flow Doppler view. The vegetation can also be seen on (**c**) the parasternal short-axis view at the level of the aortic valve and (**d**) measures 2.45 cm in length. AL anterior tricuspid valve leaflet, PL posterior tricuspid valve leaflet, AoV aortic valve

such as tricuspid valve regurgitation. These predispose the patient to the development of platelet-fibrin thrombus formation, with subsequent bacteraemia allowing colonisation of the pre-existing thrombus, resulting in vegetation formation. The organisms are able to multiply within the platelet-fibrin thrombus, as they are 'protected' from the body's immune system.

The commonest causative organism is *Staphylococcus aureus*, which accounts for 70–80% of cases of tricuspid valve endocarditis and is associated with a higher morbidity and mortality than other pathogens. Other organisms responsible for tricuspid valve IE include coagulase-negative *Staphylococcus, Streptococcus*, HACEK organisms (*Haemophilus aphrophilus, Actinobacillus*

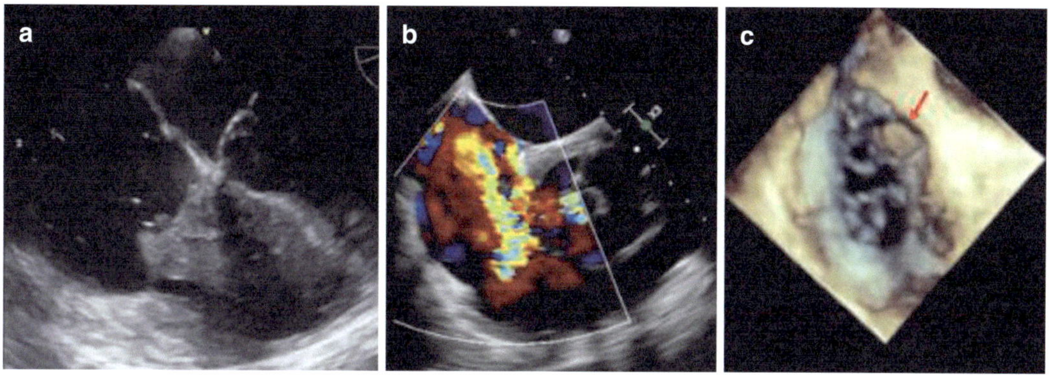

Fig. 17.2 Trans-oesophageal echocardiographical images demonstrating (**a**) a large vegetation lying on the atrial side of the anterior tricuspid valve leaflet on the 4-chamber view, (**b**) resulting in severe tricuspid regurgitation through the leaflet on the right ventricular inflow-outflow view with colour flow Doppler. (**c**) The vegetation (red arrow) can also be seen on the 3D right atrial view (with ventricular septum to the left of the image)

actinomycetemcomitans, Cardiobacterium hominis, Eikenella corrodens and *Kingella kingae*), *Enterococci* spp. and fungi. The pathological effects of tricuspid valve infective endocarditis are secondary to the spread of infection causing local valve destruction, such as leaflet perforation. Peri-annular abscess formation is uncommon in the tricuspid position. Embolisation of the vegetation can result in septic pulmonary emboli, with subsequent respiratory impairment and, if large, right ventricular dysfunction. In comparison to left-sided lesions, the low-pressure circulation of the right heart can better tolerate acute valve regurgitation, especially as the patient population is younger.

In view of this, as tricuspid valve infective endocarditis is thought to be more indolent, the majority of patients can be managed conservatively. Medical management includes a 6-week course of organism-directed antibiotic therapy, diuretics and supportive ventilation, as required. This is usually very effective, with an in-hospital mortality of less than 5%. Surgery, however, is required in up to 20% of patients with:

- Uncontrolled sepsis or fever that persists for more than 3 weeks despite appropriate antibiotic therapy
- Right-sided heart failure despite appropriate medical therapy
- Recurrent pulmonary emboli
- Peri-annular abscess formation
- Fungal infective endocarditis of the tricuspid valve
- Concomitant left-sided infective endocarditis
- Vegetation greater than 20 mm diameter

The urgency of surgery depends on a number of factors, including the cause of the disease (presence of a prosthetic valve or unsuccessful percutaneous removal of trans-venous pacing leads), infecting organism (*Staphylococcus aureus* or fungi), response to antibiotic therapy and extension of the infective process (increasing size of vegetation or peri-annular abscess). Although patients with healed endocarditis have better outcomes than those with active endocarditis, with lower complication rates, hospital length of stay and operative mortality, this needs to be balanced with the risks of delaying surgery to complete the course of antibiotic therapy. In particular, the risks of deteriorating ventricular function, extension of the disease into the annulus and embolisation needs to be considered.

Surgical Strategy

As with all patients requiring operative intervention for infective endocarditis, the main principles of surgery include eradication of the infection with excision of the vegetation and radical debridement of the affected tissue to prevent further access of the infection into the circulation; removal of any prosthetic material that may have been responsible for the infective process, such as pacing leads; closure or correction of any defects, such as an abscess or fistula; minimise the implantation of prosthetic material, especially in intravenous drug abusers; and haemodynamic correction with restoration of valve function. In addition, high-dose intravenous organism-specific antibiotic therapy is administered post-operatively, usually for 6 weeks.

The surgical options in the treatment of tricuspid valve endocarditis include valve excision alone, valve repair (using autologous or bovine pericardium) or replacement with a prosthetic valve (mechanical or biological). Whilst simply excising leaflet tissue has the benefit that it can be performed quickly without myocardial ischaemia, it will leave the patient with significant residual tricuspid regurgitation. Although it was used in the past as a prosthetic-free solution to reduce the risk of reinfection in patients associated with recurrent intravenous drug abuse, it is rarely used in contemporary practice due to the significant haemodynamic consequences of right ventricular volume overload and failure, especially in patients with raised pulmonary artery pressures.

In view of this, excision and debridement of all infected tissue followed by tricuspid valve reconstruction, with minimal use of prosthetic material, is the preferred surgical option, especially if less than 50% of the valve tissue has been destroyed by the infective process. The valve repair techniques employed to restore the functional competence of the valve are similar to those used following endocarditis destruction of the mitral valve, including leaflet reconstruction, implantation of artificial neo-chordae and annuloplasty, or a combination of the techniques.

Leaflet Reconstruction

In patients where the regurgitation is caused by leaflet destruction, it is important to assess whether it is possible to resect the infected tissue with a clear margin, whilst leaving enough native tissue to form a competent valve (Fig. 17.3a).

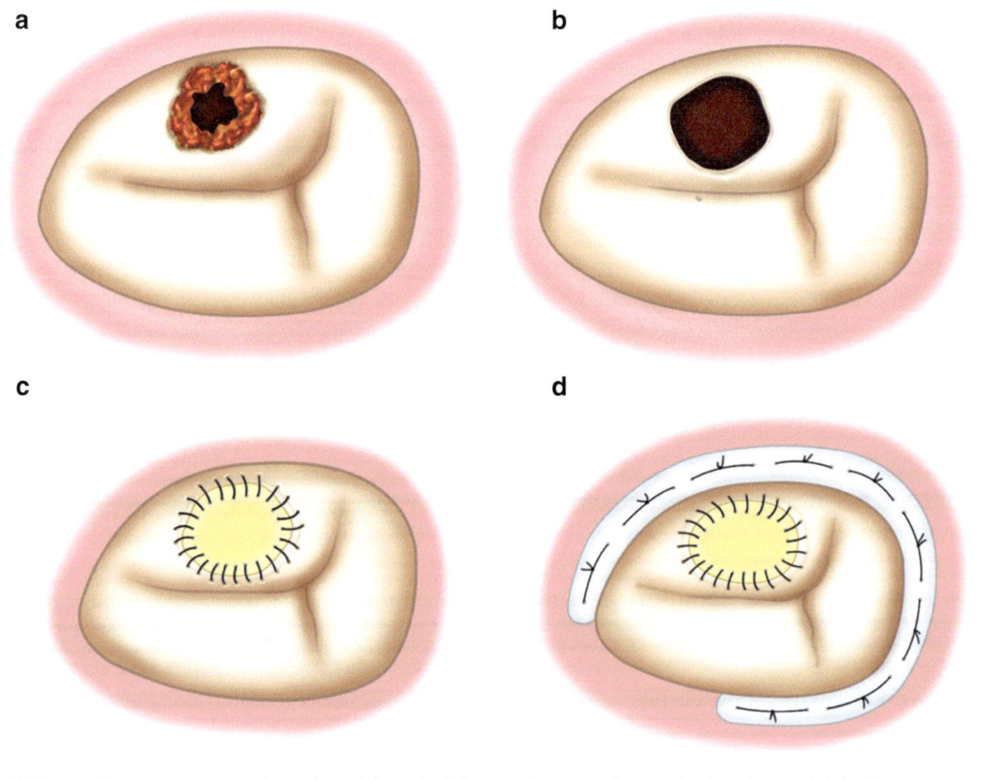

Fig. 17.3 Leaflet reconstruction by pericardial patch. (**a**) Infective endocarditis destruction of the anterior tricuspid valve leaflet, (**b**) radical debridement of the vegetation and surrounding infective tissue, (**c**) leaflet reconstruction using a bovine pericardial patch, and (**d**) ring annuloplasty

If the valve is deemed repairable, all macroscopically infected and inflamed tissue is excised with a 2 mm margin (Fig. 17.3b), to ensure that the residual native tissue is free from infection and that the residual tissue will be strong enough to hold suture material. All resected tissue should be sent for microbiological analysis.

Repair of a defect in the leaflets is usually possible, even if up to 50% of the leaflet body is involved, so long as the leading edge of the leaflet, along the coaptation line, is intact. The defect in the leaflet body can be repaired with autologous or bovine pericardium. The pericardium is implanted using a continuous locking 5/0 Prolene suture, to avoid purse-stringing the patch (Fig. 17.3c). It is important to oversize the patch to ensure that there is no tension on the leaflet causing restricted leaflet motion. In some patients, Gore-Tex neo-chordae are required to support the free edge of the leaflet. Once the repair procedure has been completed, the annulus is stabilised with an annuloplasty (Fig. 17.3d). This may be a situation where the de Vega technique is used because of the desire to leave as little prosthetic material as possible in the heart.

If the free edge of the leaflet is involved (Fig. 17.4a), an option is debridement of the infected tissue by quadrangular resection (Fig. 17.4b). Following annular plication, leaflet reconstruction is performed using 5/0 polypropylene suture (Fig. 17.4c), and supported by ring annuloplasty (Fig. 17.4d).

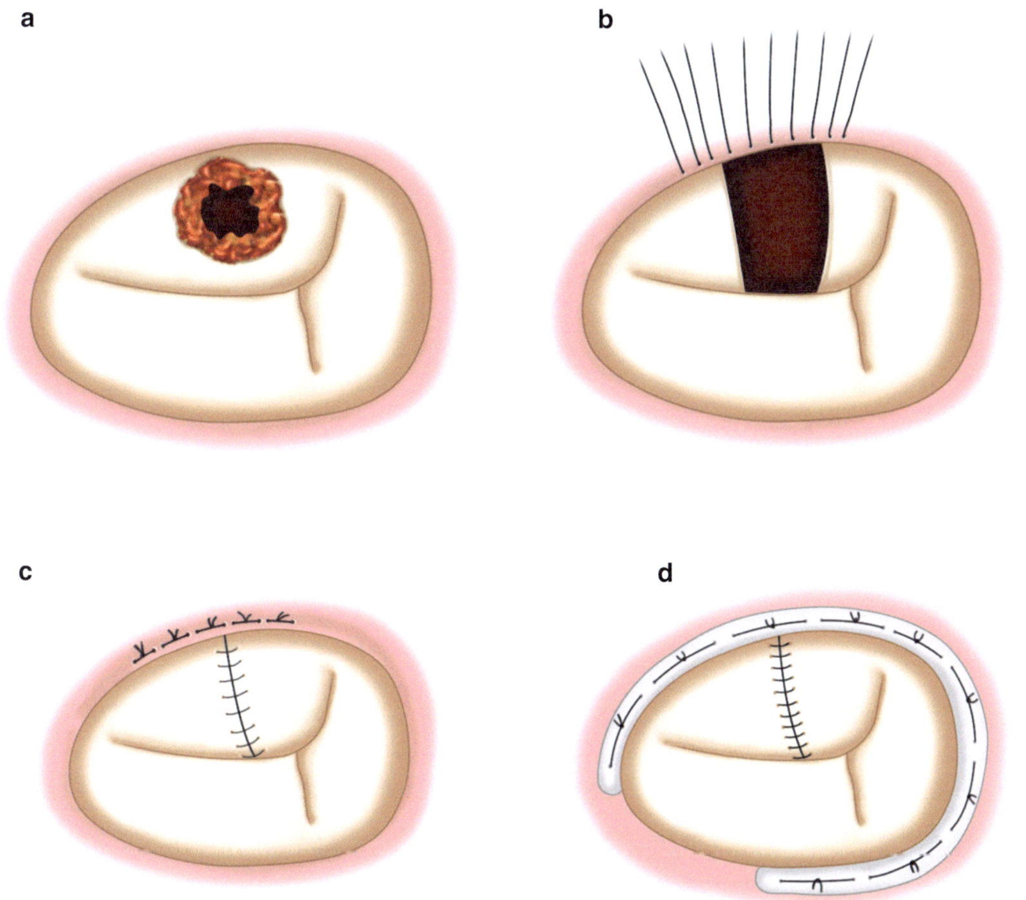

Fig. 17.4 Leaflet reconstruction by quadrangular resection. (**a**) Infective endocarditis destruction of the anterior tricuspid valve leaflet, (**b**) radical debridement of the infective tissue by quadrangular resection and placement of annular compression sutures, (**c**) reconstruction of the anterior leaflet using 5/0 polypropylene suture, and (**d**) ring annuloplasty

Bicuspidisation Annuloplasty (Posterior Leaflet Exclusion)

This technique, also known as the Kay annuloplasty, represents a non-prosthetic option for repair of the tricuspid valve following infective endocarditis destruction of the posterior leaflet (Fig. 17.5a). After complete resection of the leaflet (Fig. 17.5b), pledgeted horizontal mattress compression annuloplasty sutures are used to plicate the posterior annulus (Fig. 17.5c), thereby effectively excluding it from the functioning valve orifice and creating a 'bileaflet' tricuspid valve (Fig. 17.5d). This technique cannot, however, be used for repair following resection of the anterior or septal leaflets.

Down-Sizing Annuloplasty

This can be achieved using sutures alone (De Vega annuloplasty), thereby avoiding the implantation of prosthetic material, or by ring annuloplasty. In the De Vega annuloplasty, the anterior and posterior annulus is compressed by placing two weaving 4/0 Prolene purse-string sutures, from the anteroseptal commissure to the posteroseptal commissure. This decreases the tricuspid valve orifice thereby increasing leaflet coaptation. This technique, however, has been shown to be associated with progressive dilatation of the tricuspid annulus and recurrent regurgitation in a significant number of cases. There are, however, strong advocates of this

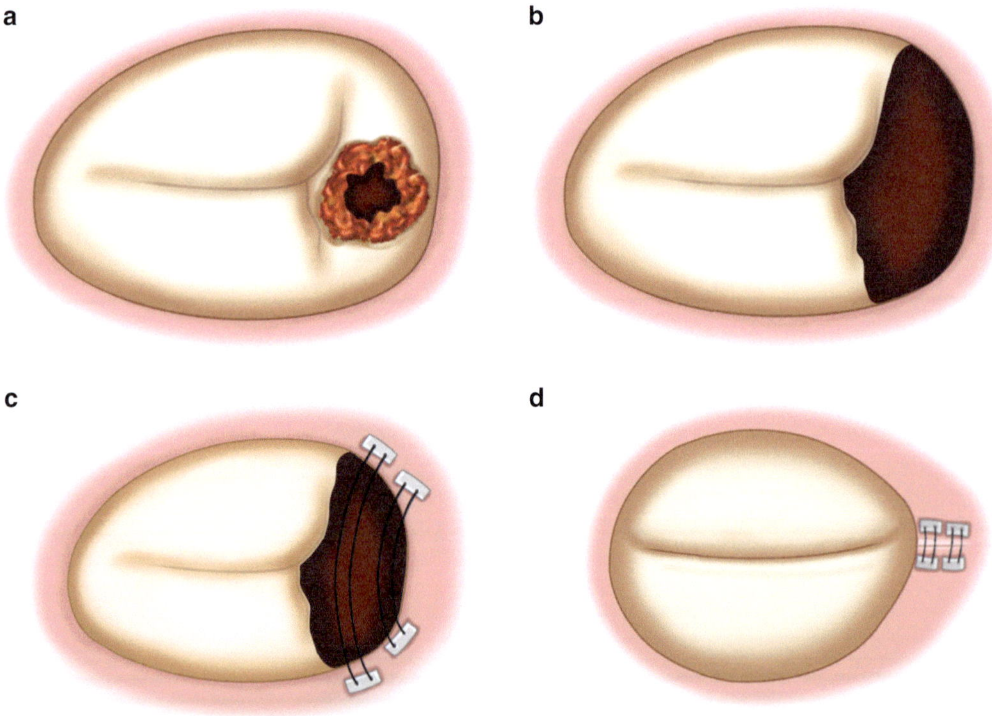

Fig. 17.5 (**a**) Infective endocarditis destruction of the posterior tricuspid valve leaflet, (**b**) radical debridement of the vegetation and surrounding infective tissue, (**c**) placement of pledgeted annular plication sutures at the posterior annulus, and (**d**) exclusion of the posterior annulus to create a 'bileaflet' tricuspid valve

procedure and undoubtedly in experienced hands it can be made to work satisfactorily. Much of its appeal in the setting of endocarditis is the minimal amount of exposed prosthetic tissue in the atrium at the end of the procedure.

Perhaps the majority of surgeons advocate the use of a prosthetic annuloplasty ring to achieve the most reliable and persistent desired reduction in annular orifice area. An appropriately selected prosthetic ring will restore an approximation of the normal shape of the tricuspid annulus, thereby preserving leaflet motion, increasing the surface area of coaptation and achieving valve competency. Although the avoidance of prosthetic material in these patients is perceived to be beneficial, there is no evidence that using an annuloplasty ring increases the risk of recurrent endocarditis but it probably increases the longevity of the repair. The prosthetic ring size is determined by measuring distance between the anteroseptal and the posteroseptal commissures, as well as the surface area of the anterior leaflet.

Tricuspid Valve Replacement

If repair is not possible due to extensive destruction of the valve from the endocarditic process involving more than 50% of the valve area, the choice between a mechanical or biological stented valve remains controversial. Although both have similar outcomes for survival and valve-related complications, mechanical valves are believed to have greater durability. There is, however, evidence of excellent long-term durability of a tricuspid valve bioprosthesis in the low-pressure right-sided circulation. The disadvantage of using a mechanical prosthesis in the tricuspid position in these patients, especially with a high proportion of intravenous drug users, is the need for and complications of lifelong anticoagulation, where compliance may be an issue. In addition, there is the presence of foreign material and the risk of thrombosis in the low-pressure right-sided circulation. Other options that have been described for tricuspid valve replacement in these patients include using a cryopreserved mitral homograft or an inverted stentless aortic valve.

It is important to note that there is a significantly increased rate of heart block in patients undergoing tricuspid valve replacement, as compared to tricuspid valve repair. Subsequent placement of a transvenous endocardial pacing system is not only a risk of recurrent infection to the bioprosthetic valve but also a risk factor for valve dysfunction secondary to damage of the leaflets at the time of pacemaker insertion and early structural valve deterioration, due to the lead causing leaflet fibrosis and distortion. The use of a transvenous pacing system also is not feasible if a mechanical tricuspid valve prosthesis is implanted. In view of this, permanent epicardial pacing wires are usually placed at the time of surgery following tricuspid valve replacement for infective endocarditis.

Intravenous Drug Abuse

Management of tricuspid valve infective endocarditis in intravenous drug abusers can be somewhat challenging due to a number of factors, including delayed presentation resulting in more extensive valve destruction and multivalve involvement, polymicrobial infection involving resistant organisms, poor compliance with medical therapy and the risk of recurrent endocarditis. Despite this, the management strategy and indications for surgery remain the same. Although valve repair would confer many benefits, the extensive destruction associated with delayed presentation may prevent valve reconstruction from being feasible. If replacement is required, a bioprosthesis is recommended due to the poor compliance with anticoagulation therapy. Due to the young age of these patients, this strategy, however, will often require re-operation due to the risk of structural valve degeneration. Although valvectomy (valve excision without replacement) can be used in these patients, it results in long-term severe tricuspid regurgitation and a poor prognosis related to right-heart failure. This patient group should be discussed in a multi-disciplinary team environment with social services involvement to discuss the support mechanisms available, the risk of returning to intravenous drug abuse and the likely compliance with antibiotic or anticoagulation therapy.

Surgical Technique

Following median sternotomy, a large piece of autologous pericardium was harvested and soaked in 0.5% glutaraldehyde solution for 5–10 min. The patient was placed on cardiopulmonary bypass with bicaval venous cannulation, with caval snares, and ascending aortic arterial return, ensuring minimal cardiac manipulation to avoid fragmentation and embolisation of the vegetation.

Following a standard right atriotomy, the tricuspid valve was inspected to identify the vegetation and assess the leaflets and the subvalvular apparatus for endocarditic destruction, as well as the presence of any peri-annular abscesses. This was correlated with the trans-oesophageal echocardiographical findings. A 2.5 × 2 cm vegetation was identified on the atrial surface of the anterior leaflet, associated with perforation of the body of the leaflet (Fig. 17.6a). The infective process had spread into adjacent areas of the anterior leaflet but was not involving the chordae tendineae or the other leaflets.

Horizontal mattress annuloplasty sutures (2/0 Ethibond) were placed around the circumference of the tricuspid valve, with a 5 mm width and approximately 1 mm apart. These sutures were placed from the mid-point of the septal leaflet counter-clockwise around the tricuspid annulus to the anteroseptal commissure. No sutures were placed on the medial part of the septal tricuspid valve annulus to avoid the Bundle of His and the atrioventricular node, which sit at the apex of the triangle of Koch.

Stay sutures (5/0 Prolene) were placed around the chordae tendineae attached on either side of the perforated area of the anterior leaflet. Gentle traction on these stay sutures gave better access and visualisation of the anterior leaflet. The vegetation and any residual infected leaflet

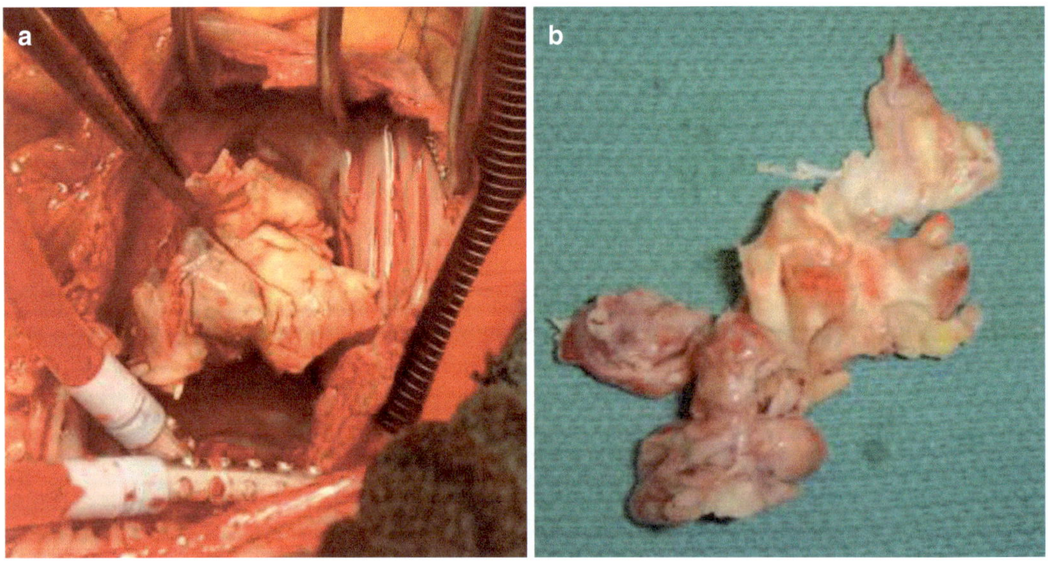

Fig. 17.6 Operative images illustrating (**a**) large vegetation lying on the atrial surface of the anterior tricuspid valve leaflet and (**b**) resected vegetation and surrounding infected tissue

surrounding the perforation were debrided and sent for microbiological analysis (Fig. 17.6b). All viable leaflet tissue that was not involved in the infective process was preserved. At this stage, it was important to assess the degree of destruction to the surrounding tissues and whether enough of the valve and sub-valvular structures remained intact and free from the infective process to produce a competent valve by repair.

A slightly over-sized glutaraldehyde-preserved autologous pericardial patch was then fashioned and used to close the defect in the anterior leaflet using a continuous locking 5/0 Prolene suture with a tension-free anastomosis. Competence of the tricuspid valve was then assessed with static testing, by injecting cold saline into the right ventricle, using a bulb syringe. The appropriate sized annuloplasty ring was then chosen, according to the surface area of the anterior leaflet and the distance between the anteroseptal and the posteroseptal commissures, and tied down in situ.

Following implantation of the annuloplasty ring, injecting cold saline again allowed the tricuspid valve to be assessed for competency. The right atrium was then closed with a two-layer continuous 4/0 Prolene suture, followed by placement of temporary epicardial right atrial and right ventricular pacing wires.

Post-operative Echocardiogram

The post-repair echocardiographical images (Fig. 17.7) confirmed:

1. No residual vegetation
2. Competency of the tricuspid valve with trace tricuspid regurgitation.

Surgical Tips

1. It is crucial to remove all the infected tissue before assessing whether valve reconstruction is feasible
2. Valve excision without repair or replacement should be avoided due to the long term effects of long-standing severe tricuspid regurgitation and subsequent right ventricular dysfunction
3. Ideally, valve repair should be performed minimising implantation of any prosthetic material by using native tissue, such as autologous pericardium
4. Valve repair should probably be supported by an annuloplasty ring, as simple annuloplasty suture (De Vega annuloplasty) leads to progressive annular dilatation and tricuspid regurgitation

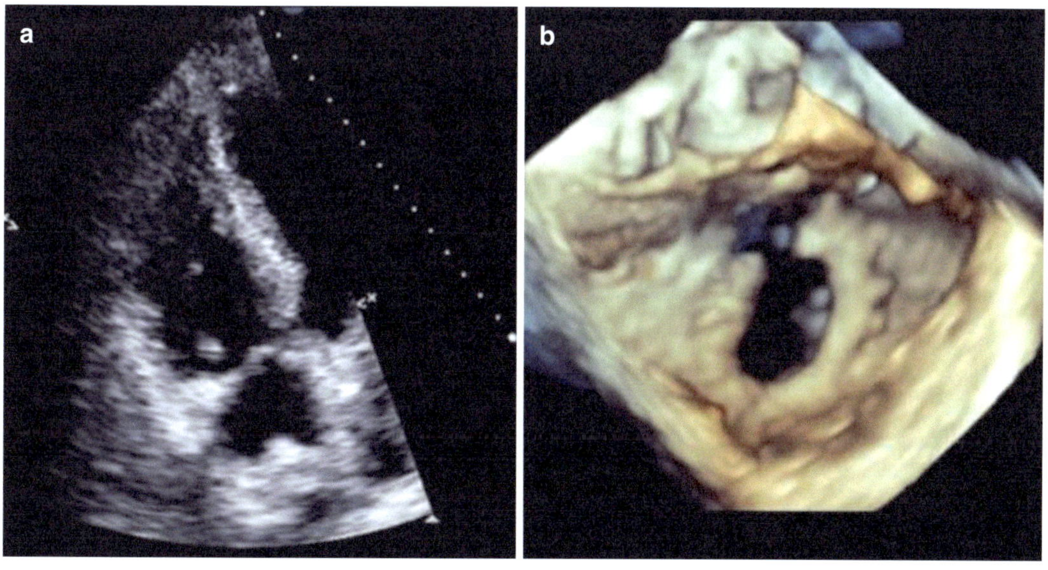

Fig. 17.7 Post-repair echocardiographical images demonstrating (**a**) good coaptation of the leaflets and no residual vegetation on the trans-thoracic apical 4-chamber view, and (**b**) the annuloplasty ring in situ on the 3D right atrial view

Comment

Operative surgery for tricuspid valve infective endocarditis can be performed with reasonable short and long-term results. Operative mortality in contemporary series varies between 5–10%. Long-term survival for patients who have undergone surgery for tricuspid valve endocarditis has been reported as 58% at 20 years, with risk factors for poor prognosis including intravenous drug abusers, *Staphylococcus aureus* or fungal infecting organisms, vegetation greater than 20 mm and the presence of concomitant left-sided endocarditis. The long-term outcome of patients undergoing valve reconstruction is thought be improved as compared to those undergoing replacement because of the risk of prosthetic valve endocarditis (especially in intravenous drug abusers), structural valve deterioration in patients undergoing bioprosthesis implantation and anticoagulation-related complications in patients undergoing mechanical prosthesis implantation. Although it is laudable to attempt to minimise the implantation of prosthetic material, repair is not feasible in all patients, depending on the extent of destruction caused by the infective process, and replacement should be performed if repair is likely to leave residual regurgitation.

Recommended Reading

Akinosoglou K, Apostolakis E, Koutsogiannis N, Leivaditis V, Gogos CA. Right-sided infective endocarditis: surgical management. Eur J Cardiothorac Surg. 2012;42(3):470–9.

Arbulu A, Holmes RJ, Asfaw I. Tricuspid valvulectomy without replacement. Twenty years' experience. J Thorac Cardiovasc Surg. 1991;102(6):917–22.

Athan E, Chu VH, Tattevin P, Selton-Suty C, Jones P, Naber C, Miró JM, Ninot S, Fernández-Hidalgo N, Durante-Mangoni E, Spelman D, Hoen B, Lejko-Zupanc T, Cecchi E, Thuny F, Hannan MM, Pappas P, Henry M, Fowler VG Jr, Crowley AL, Wang A, ICE-PCS Investigators. Clinical characteristics and outcome of infective endocarditis involving implantable cardiac devices. JAMA. 2012;307(16):1727–35.

Gaca JG, Sheng S, Daneshmand M, Rankin JS, Williams ML, O'Brien SM, Gammie JS. Current outcomes for tricuspid valve infective endocarditis surgery in North America. Ann Thorac Surg. 2013;96(4):1374–81.

Gottardi R, Bialy J, Devyatko E, Tschernich H, Czerny M, Wolner E, Seitelberger R. Midterm follow-up of tricuspid valve reconstruction due to active infective endocarditis. Ann Thorac Surg. 2007;84:1943–8.

Habib G, Hoen B, Tornos P, Thuny F, Prendergast B, Vilacosta I, Moreillon P, de Jesus Antunes M, Thilen U, Lekakis J, Lengyel M, Müller L, Naber CK, Nihoyannopoulos P, Moritz A, Zamorano JL, ESC Committee for Practice Guidelines. Guidelines on the prevention, diagnosis, and treatment of infective endocarditis (new version 2009): the Task Force on the Prevention, Diagnosis, and Treatment of Infective Endocarditis of the European Society of Cardiology (ESC). Endorsed by the European Society of Clinical Microbiology and Infectious Diseases (ESCMID) and the International Society of Chemotherapy (ISC) for Infection and Cancer. Eur Heart J. 2009;30(19):2369–413.

Heydari AA, Safari H, Sarvghad MR. Isolated tricuspid valve endocarditis. Int J Infect Dis. 2009;13(3):e109–11.

Kang DH, Kim YJ, Kim SH, Sun BJ, Kim DH, Yun SC, Song JM, Choo SJ, Chung CH, Song JK, Lee JW, Sohn DW. Early surgery versus conventional treatment for infective endocarditis. N Engl J Med. 2012;366(26):2466–73.

Nishimura RA, Otto CM, Bonow RO, Carabello BA, Erwin JP 3rd, Guyton RA, O'Gara PT, Ruiz CE, Skubas NJ, Sorajja P, Sundt TM 3rd, Thomas JD, Anderson JL, Halperin JL, Albert NM, Bozkurt B, Brindis RG, Creager MA, Curtis LH, DeMets D, Guyton RA, Hochman JS, Kovacs RJ, Ohman EM, Pressler SJ, Sellke FW, Shen WK, Stevenson WG, Yancy CW, American College of Cardiology; American College of Cardiology/American Heart Association; American Heart Association. 2014 AHA/ACC guideline for the management of patients with valvular heart disease: a report of the American College of Cardiology/American Heart Association Task Force on Practice Guidelines. J Thorac Cardiovasc Surg. 2014;148(1):e1–e132.

Wang TK, Oh T, Voss J, Pemberton J. Characteristics and outcomes for right heart endocarditis: six-year cohort study. Heart Lung Circ. 2014;23(7):625–7.

Weymann A, Borst T, Popov AF, Sabashnikov A, Bowles C, Schmack B, Veres G, Chaimow N, Simon AR, Karck M, Szabo G. Surgical treatment of infective endocarditis in active intravenous drug users: a justified procedure? J Cardiothorac Surg. 2014;9:58.

18 Atrial Fibrillation Surgery

Keywords
Atrial fibrillation · Ablation · Pulmonary vein isolation · Posterior left atrial box lesion set · Cox-maze IV procedure · Focal areas of automaticity · Thromboembolism · Macro re-entry circuits · Bipolar radiofrequency ablation · Cryoablation · Left atrial appendage excision

Case History

A 65 year-old gentleman presented with a progressive history of increasing exertional dyspnoea, associated with frequent palpitations. He had no previous history of rheumatic fever or infective endocarditis but had been diagnosed with atrial fibrillation 6 months previously. Medical management included amiodarone therapy and an electrical cardioversion, which had failed to provide sustained freedom from the atrial arrhythmia. In view of this, he was also being managed with warfarin anti-coagulation therapy. His electrocardiogram had shown absence of P waves and an irregular ventricular response, consistent with his atrial fibrillation (Fig. 18.1). Cardiac catheterisation had demonstrated no obstructive coronary artery disease. Trans-thoracic and trans-oesophageal echocardiography had revealed an anterior directed jet of severe mitral regurgitation caused by prolapse of the posterior mitral valve leaflet, dilated left atrium (diameter 5.64 cm), enlarged left ventricle (left ventricular end-diastolic diameter 6.1 cm) and impairment of left ventricular function (ejection fraction 48%).

Pathophysiology

Atrial fibrillation (AF) is defined as a supraventricular arrhythmia where asynchronous atrial activation occurs, resulting in impaired atrial mechanical function. It can be categorised as first diagnosis, paroxysmal, persistent, long-standing persistent and permanent AF. First diagnosis AF represents the first episode of AF irrespective of duration or severity. Paroxysmal AF usually self-terminates within 48 h, whereas persistent AF is defined as an episode of AF that lasts longer than 7 days or requires pharmacological or electrical cardioversion after 48 h from onset. Long-standing persistent AF represents AF that has been present for more than 1 year but where a rhythm control strategy is still considered, whereas permanent AF is where a rhythm control strategy (including chemical and electrical cardioversion) has failed and is no longer pursued. AF can also be classified as primary or secondary, where primary AF occurs in patients with no underlying cardiac disease, whilst secondary AF is associated with pre-existing cardiac disease.

N. Moorjani et al., *Operative Mitral and Tricuspid Valve Surgery*,
https://doi.org/10.1007/978-1-4471-4204-1_18

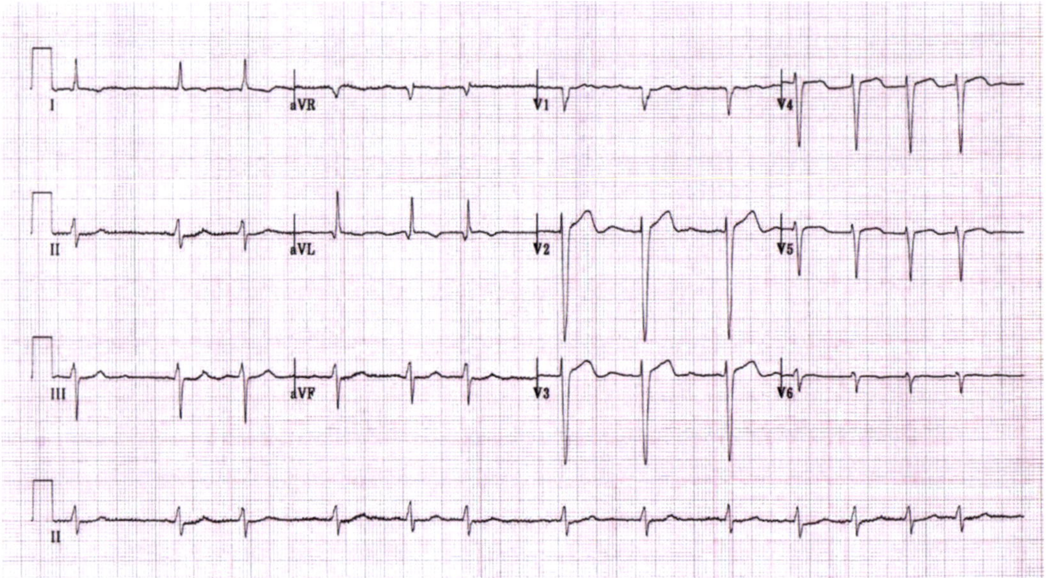

Fig. 18.1 Electrocardiogram demonstrating the absence of P waves with an irregular ventricular response, consistent with atrial fibrillation

Although the exact underlying mechanisms for the development of AF are not completely understood, AF is thought to be initiated by focal areas of automaticity of ectopic atrial depolarisation, with the majority of the foci located in the pulmonary veins and the other foci in the right and left atria. AF is maintained by multiple macro re-entrant circuits within both atria, which are responsible for its propagation (Fig. 18.2). For this to occur, AF requires a trigger, such as atrial ectopic foci and changes in atrial wall tension, secondary to atrial volume or pressure overload; an abnormal substrate, such as inflammation or fibrosis of the atrial wall; and modulating factors, such as the autonomic nervous system, including ganglionic plexi involvement and increased vagal activation.

The pathophysiological sequelae of AF include an irregular heartbeat, resulting in palpitations and patient anxiety; loss of synchronous atrio-ventricular contraction, which results in haemodynamic compromise; and stasis of atrial blood flow in the left atrium, which predisposes the patient to thromboembolism. Subsequently, AF is associated with significant morbidity and mortality, including being an independent risk factor for death (relative risk of 1.5–1.9) and stroke (relative risk 5.0).

Surgical Strategy

The principle of the surgical treatment of atrial fibrillation involves mechanical destruction of cardiac tissue to produce a transmural myocardial injury, resulting in a fibrotic reaction and the formation of scar tissue. As scar tissue does not conduct electrical impulses, it interrupts myocardial continuity and the propagation of electrical conduction. If the scar tissue lines are placed in a particular pattern, it can stop the induction pathways (focal areas of automaticity), with pulmonary vein isolation, and also prevent the formation of macro re-entrant circuits responsible for atrial fibrillation, with the atrial lesion sets.

Surgical treatment of atrial fibrillation has evolved through a variety of procedures, including left atrial isolation and the Guiraudon corridor procedure (Fig. 18.3). These procedures, however, leave the majority of atrial tissue still fibrillating, with the risk of systemic thromboembolism still present, as well as reduced cardiac output derived from the absence of atrioventricular synchrony and atrial contraction.

Earlier iterations of the Cox-Maze procedure isolated the sinoatrial (SA) node and interrupted its blood supply, causing chronotropic incompe-

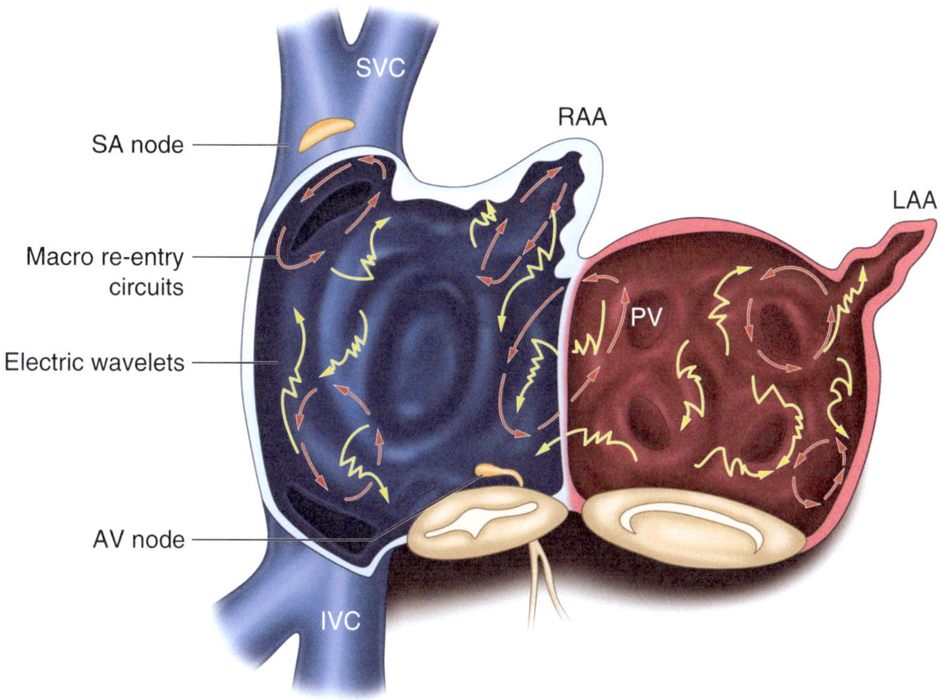

Fig. 18.2 Pathophysiology of atrial fibrillation, where macro re-entrant circuits (red) maintain the uncoordinated activity of the electric wavelets (yellow). RAA right atrial appendage, LAA left atrial appendage, SA sinoatrial, AV atrioventricular, PV pulmonary vein, SVC superior vena cava, IVC inferior vena cava

tence and the need for a permanent pacemaker, as well as affecting the Bachmann bundle, causing a conduction delay between the left and right atria and subsequent asynchronous contractions.

Cox-Maze III

The Cox-Maze III procedure also uses the concept of creating scar tissue to direct the electrical impulse from the SA node to the atrio-ventricular (AV) node and became the gold standard in the surgical treatment of AF. This 'cut-and-sew' technique involves making several incisions in the left and right atrial wall (Fig. 18.4) to create transmural lines of scar tissue that disrupt re-entrant circuits responsible for propagating the abnormal atrial fibrillation rhythm. Atrial transport function is preserved, as compared to previous iterations of the procedure, as the electrical impulse is directed from the SA node through a maze of scar in both atria to the AV node. The formation of macro re-entrant circuits is prevented by fixing the refractory period between areas of scar. By restoring sinus rhythm, atrial depolarisation and atrioventricular synchrony, the Cox-Maze III procedure significantly reduces the risk of thromboembolism, stroke and hemodynamic compromise. The procedure, however, significantly increases aortic cross-clamp and cardiopulmonary bypass times, and is technically demanding requiring a high level of surgical expertise, which has restricted its use.

Alternative Energy Sources

The invasive nature of the Cox-Maze III led to the development of a number of ablation devices, which use a variety of cold- or heat-based energy sources to recreate the transmural scar tissue produced by the 'cut-and-sew' technique, by

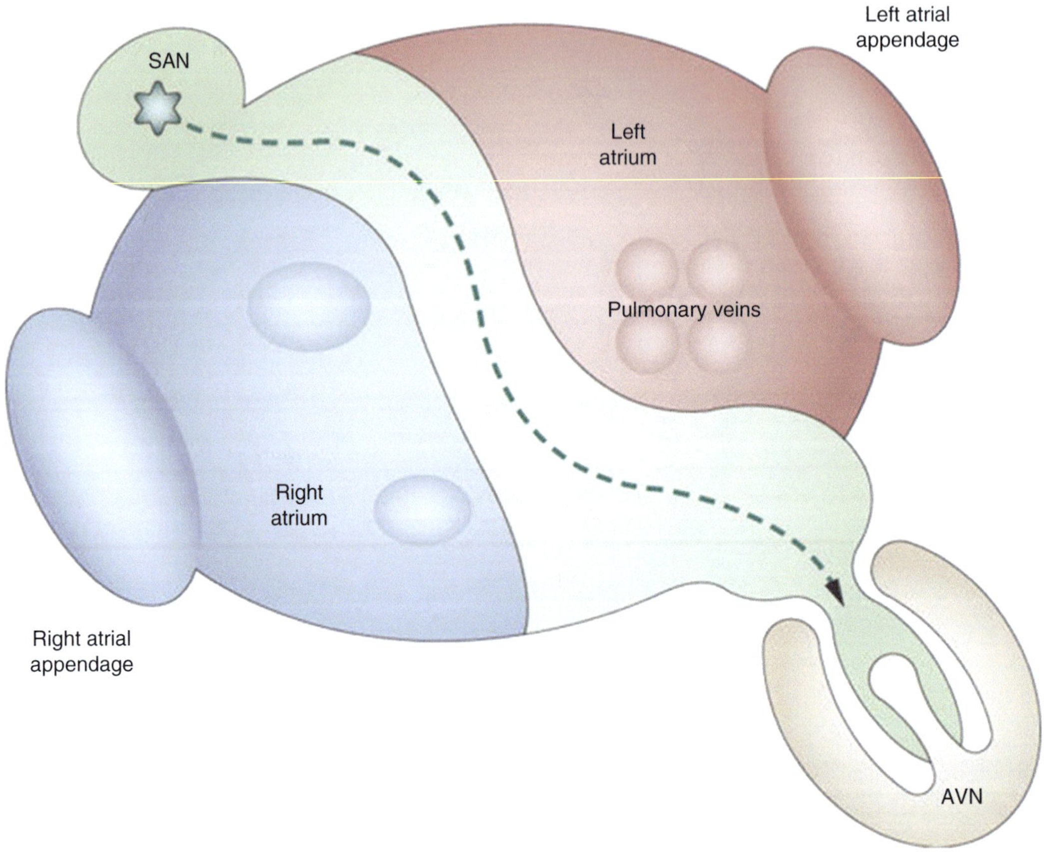

Fig. 18.3 The Guiraudon corridor procedure involves creating a pathway to guide the electrical impulse directly from the sinoatrial node (SAN) to atrioventricular node (AVN). The remainder of the left and right atrial tissue, however, continues to fibrillate, thereby maintaining the risk of thromboembolism and stroke. (Reproduced with permission from Lee R. Surgery for atrial fibrillation. *Nat Rev Cardiol*. 2009;6(8):505–13.)

replacing incisions with ablation lines. This simplified, more reproducible procedure, with reduced cross-clamp and bypass times and was termed the Cox-Maze IV. It has a similar but not identical lesion set to the Cox-Maze III but maintained the essential pre-requisites for success, including transmural lesions that are contiguous bilaterally (Fig. 18.5). Although laser, ultrasound and microwave energy has been used in the past, their ability to create transmural lesions has been questioned. This is especially important as partial thickness lesions leaves viable tissue and gaps as small as 1 mm have been shown to be capable of conduction and maintenance of macro re-entrant circuits. Hence, cryothermy and radiofrequency remain as the only reliable energy sources for creating consistent transmural lesions. They are associated with an approximately 90% freedom from atrial fibrillation at 12 months, offering a significant advantage over catheter-based ablation techniques.

Radiofrequency Ablation

Radiofrequency ablation conducts an alternating electrical current through the myocardial tissue, causing energy to be dissipated as heat, resulting in coagulative necrosis with irreversible protein denaturation and scar tissue formation that does not conduct electrical impulses. These lesions histologically resemble the healed incisions of the traditional Cox-Maze III operation. Although radiofrequency ablation can cause damage to

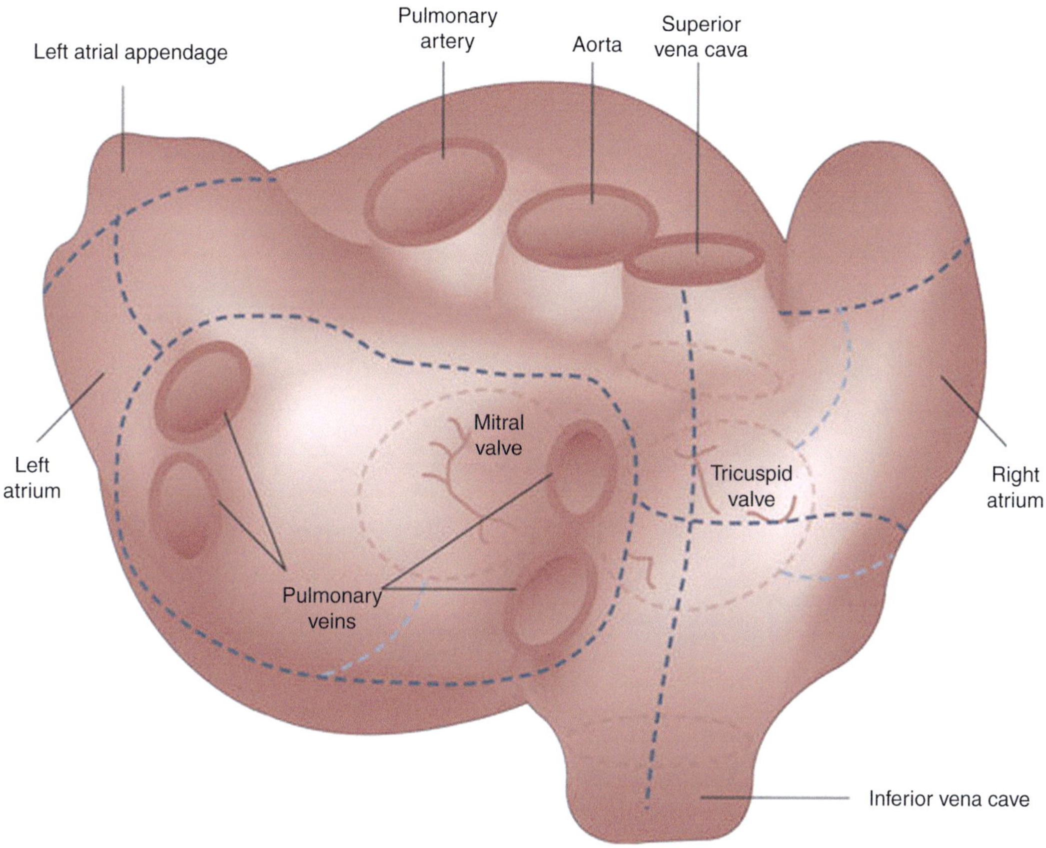

Fig. 18.4 Cox Maze III lesion set. (Reproduced with permission from Lee R. Surgery for atrial fibrillation. *Nat Rev Cardiol*. 2009;6(8):505–13.)

surrounding structures, such as the pulmonary veins, oesophagus or coronary arteries, the use of a bipolar radiofrequency ablation clamp device minimises collateral damage by ensuring that the energy stays between the two clamps. The duration of application of the bipolar radiofrequency clamp device is determined by tissue conductance or impedance, which indicate transmurality of the lesion. The device is applied two to three times to ensure complete conduction block. For the full Cox-Maze IV lesion set, however, it is not possible to create the mitral and tricuspid annuli lesions with bipolar radiofrequency, due to the proximity of the coronary arteries (right coronary artery with tricuspid valve annulus and circumflex coronary artery with mitral valve annulus). For these annular lesions, cryothermy is used.

Traditional unipolar radiofrequency ablation devices have limited use as they are unable to ensure transmurality and due to the spread of heat may cause damage to surrounding structures, including the oesophagus and coronary arteries. Saline irrigation of unipolar radiofrequency ablation pens have been used to achieve a more even distribution of the heat energy and minimise the production of surface char, both of which can improve the depth of penetration of the radiofrequency. In addition, newer suction-assisted unipolar devices may help to attach the atrial tissue to the device, thereby increasing the depth of penetration and helping to achieve a transmural lesion.

Cryoablation

Cryoablation uses cryothermal energy from pressurised liquid nitrous oxide that results in

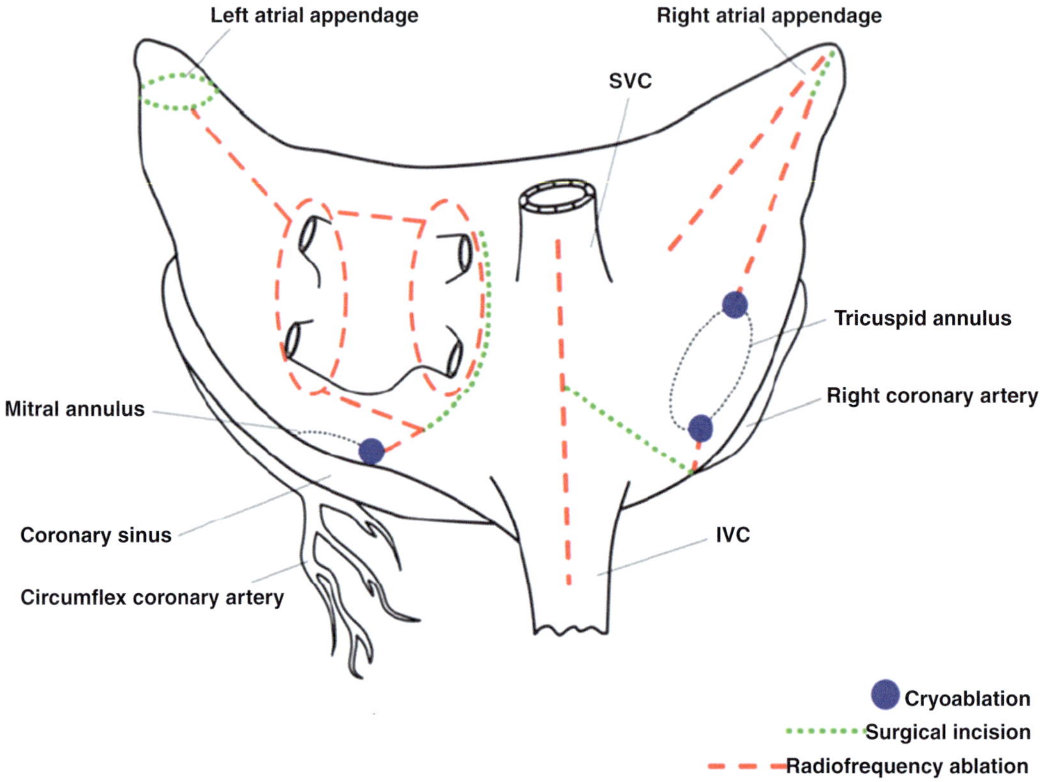

Fig. 18.5 Cox Maze IV lesion set. SVC superior vena cava, IVC inferior vena cava. (Reprinted with permission from Weimar et al. The Cox-maze IV procedure for lone atrial fibrillation: a single center experience in 100 consecutive patients. *J Interv Card Electrophysiol*. 2011;31(1):47–54.)

formation of ice crystals within the cells and microvascular disruption, resulting in cell death and scar tissue formation. Although there are no specific computed algorithms to demonstrate transmurality of a cryoablated lesion, the presence of a visible ice ball on the epicardial surface of the tissue, when the probe is applied to endocardial surface, serves as a reliable indicator of transmurality. The cryoprobe is usually applied for 2 min at −60 °C to create each lesion. The use of cryoablation, however, requires an arrested heart, as the warm blood of a beating heart would otherwise cause a heat sink effect and absorb the cryothermal energy, thereby making complete freezing of the myocardial tissue and attainment of a transmural lesion very difficult. Complications of cryoablation may include injury to nearby structures, including the phrenic nerve, oesophagus or coronary arteries. Argon gas can also be used as a cryothermal energy source.

Although cryothermy is the only energy modality that can create all the ablation lines in the Cox-Maze IV lesion set, it is often used in combination with bipolar radiofrequency ablation, where lesions to the mitral and tricuspid annulus are created with cryothermy and the remaining lesions created using bipolar radiofrequency. Cryothermy is an ideal energy source to complete lesions over annular tissues because it preserves the fibrous skeleton of the heart, thereby maintaining valvular function.

Lesion Sets

There are several different lesion sets used in current surgical practice, including:

(a) Isolated pulmonary vein isolation – with lesions:

   (i) Encircling the right superior and inferior pulmonary veins (Fig. 18.6)
   (ii) Encircling the left superior and inferior pulmonary veins (Fig. 18.7)
(b) Posterior left atrial box lesion set – with lesions:
   (i) Encircling the right superior and inferior pulmonary veins
   (ii) Encircling the left superior and inferior pulmonary veins
   (iii) From the right inferior pulmonary vein to left inferior pulmonary vein (Fig. 18.8)
   (iv) From the right superior pulmonary vein to left superior pulmonary vein (Fig. 18.9)
(c) Complete left atrial lesion set – with lesions:
   (i) Encircling the right superior and inferior pulmonary veins
   (ii) Encircling the left superior and inferior pulmonary veins
   (iii) From the right inferior pulmonary vein to left inferior pulmonary vein
   (iv) From the right superior pulmonary vein to left superior pulmonary vein
   (v) From the left atriotomy to the P2/P3 region of the posterior mitral valve annulus (Fig. 18.10) – which represents the mitral isthmus line that increases the chances of restoring sinus rhythm and reduces the risk of developing atrial flutter
   (vi) From the left atrial appendage to the left pulmonary veins (Fig. 18.11)

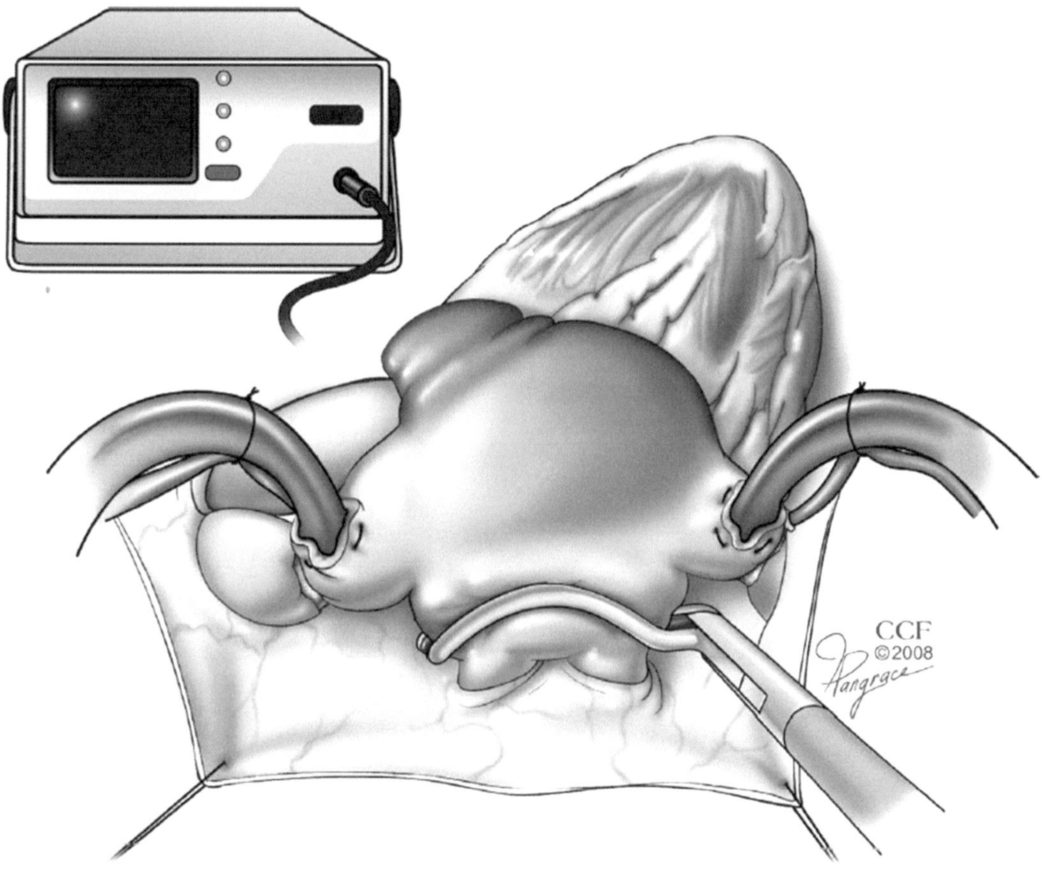

Fig. 18.6 Isolation of the right pulmonary veins using the bipolar radiofrequency clamp device. (Reproduced with permission from Gillinov M, Soltesz E. Surgical treatment of atrial fibrillation: today's questions and answers. *Semin Thorac Cardiovasc Surg*. 2013;25(3):197–205.)

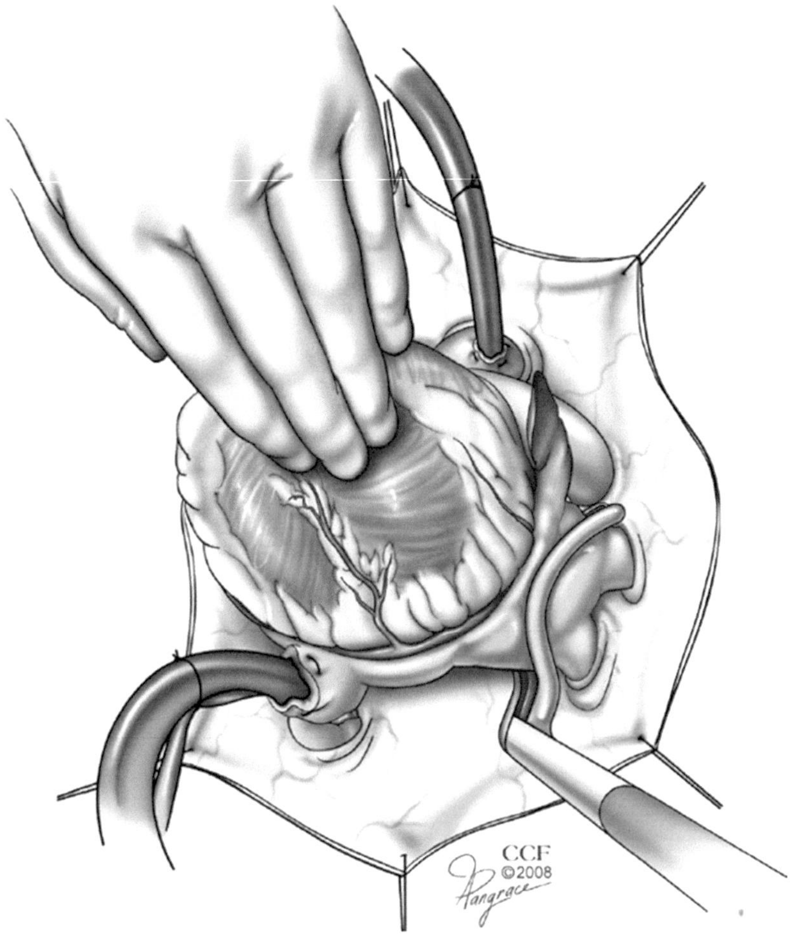

Fig. 18.7 After displacement of the heart towards the right, the left pulmonary veins are isolated using the bipolar radiofrequency clamp device. (Reproduced with permission from Gillinov M, Soltesz E. Surgical treatment of atrial fibrillation: today's questions and answers. *Semin Thorac Cardiovasc Surg*. 2013;25(3):197–205.)

(d) Complete left and right atrial lesion set (Cox-Maze IV) – with lesions:
   (i) Encircling the right superior and inferior pulmonary veins
   (ii) Encircling the left superior and inferior pulmonary veins
   (iii) From the right inferior pulmonary vein to left inferior pulmonary vein
   (iv) From the right superior pulmonary vein to left superior pulmonary vein
   (v) From the left atriotomy to the P2/P3 region of the posterior mitral valve annulus
   (vi) From the left atrial appendage to left pulmonary veins
   (vii) From the right atriotomy to the superior vena cava (Fig. 18.12)
   (viii) From the right atriotomy to the inferior vena cava (Fig. 18.13)
   (ix) From the right atriotomy to the 2 o'clock position on the tricuspid valve annulus (Fig. 18.14)
   (x) From the right atrial appendage to the 10 o'clock position on the tricuspid valve annulus (Fig. 18.15)

(e) Hybrid approaches – with epicardial pulmonary vein isolation and left atrial appendage excision performed through a minimally invasive off-pump approach, followed by the remaining lesions completed percutaneously by endocardial catheter ablation. Any lesions that are not transmural can be identified by electrophysiological mapping and completed as appropriate

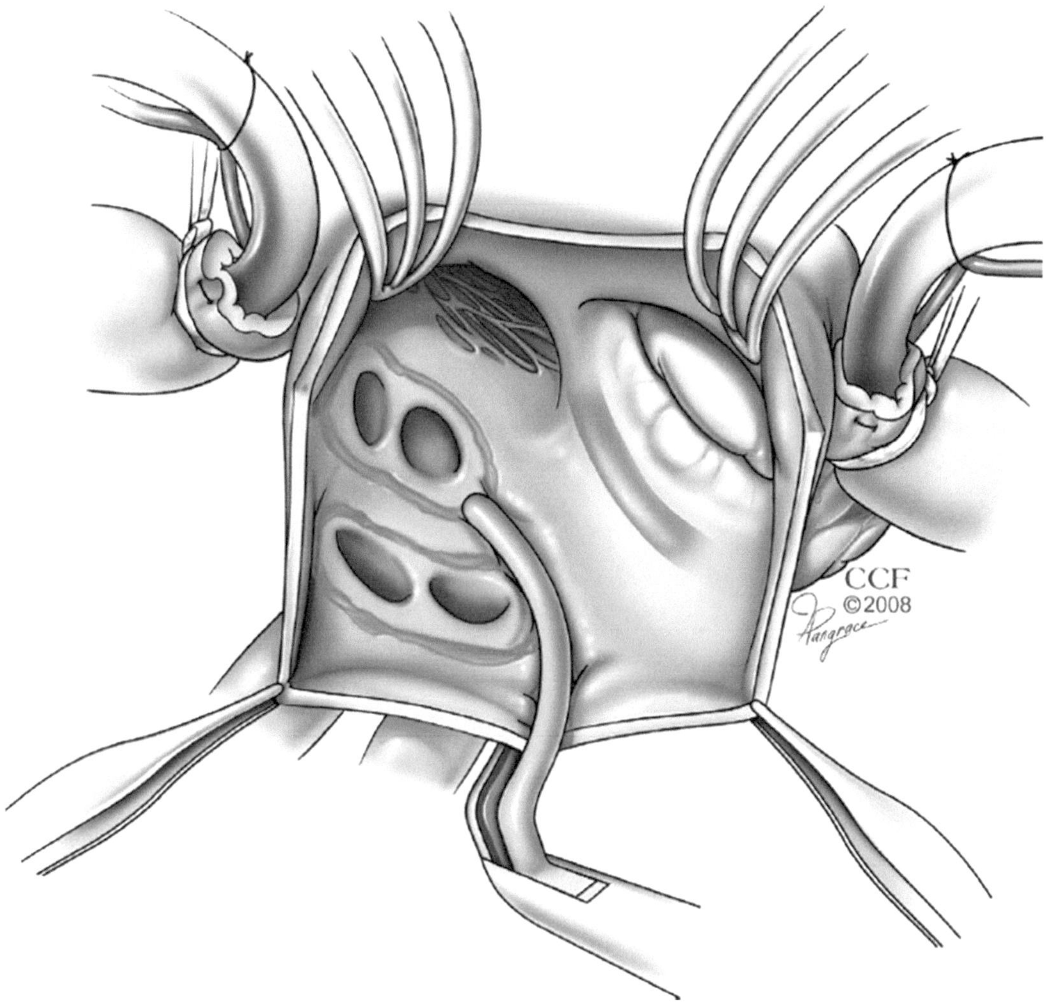

Fig. 18.8 Connecting lesion from the right inferior pulmonary vein to the left inferior pulmonary vein using the bipolar radiofrequency clamp device. (Reproduced with permission from Gillinov M, Soltesz E. Surgical treatment of atrial fibrillation: today's questions and answers. *Semin Thorac Cardiovasc Surg*. 2013;25(3):197–205.)

Some surgeons only perform the left or right atrial lesion sets when performing mitral and tricuspid valve surgery, respectively and in case of coronary artery bypass grafting or aortic valve replacement only perform pulmonary vein isolation. Ultimately, long-term freedom from AF will be determined by the lesion set used and the underlying type of atrial fibrillation (paroxysmal, persistent or long-standing persistent), with the best results achieved using the complete Cox-Maze IV lesion set. It is important to note that failure to isolate the pulmonary veins and entire posterior left atrium greatly increases the recurrence rate of atrial fibrillation.

Pulmonary Vein Isolation

Pulmonary vein isolation was developed following the discovery that 94% of the ectopic foci that act as the trigger of atrial fibrillation are located in the pulmonary veins. Hence, it would be expected than isolation of the pulmonary veins alone would result in a similar percentage of

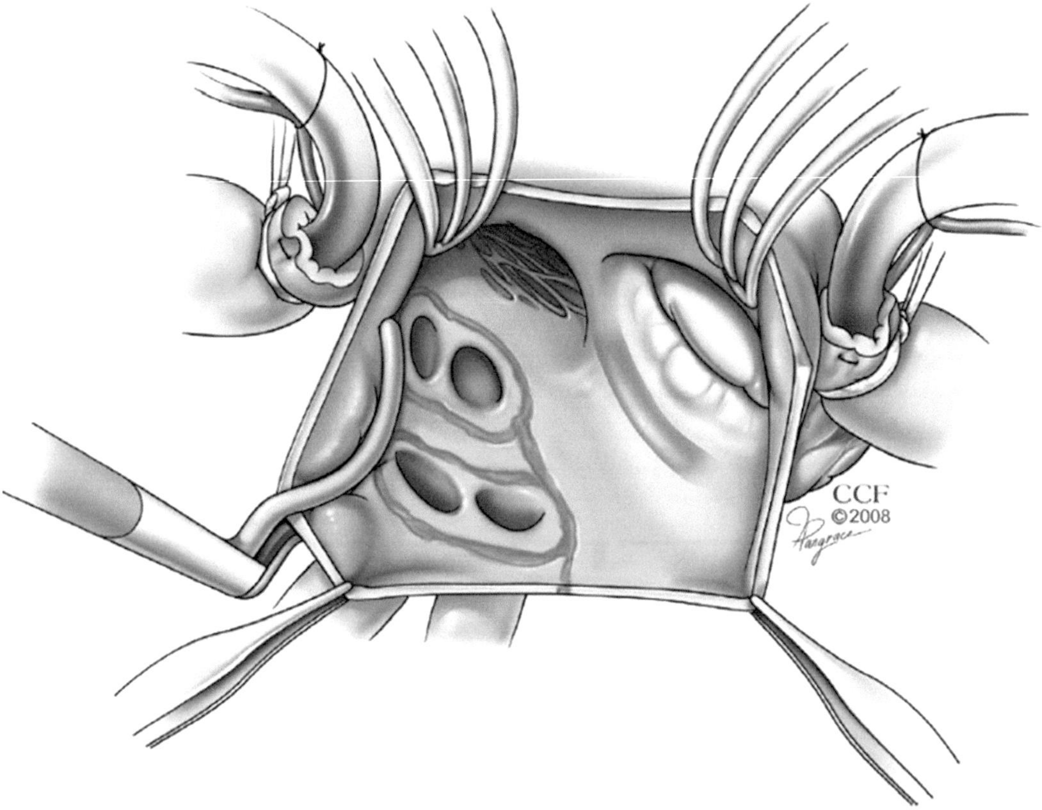

Fig. 18.9 Connecting lesion from the right superior pulmonary vein to the left superior pulmonary vein using the bipolar radiofrequency clamp device. (Reproduced with permission from Gillinov M, Soltesz E. Surgical treatment of atrial fibrillation: today's questions and answers. *Semin Thorac Cardiovasc Surg*. 2013;25(3):197–205.)

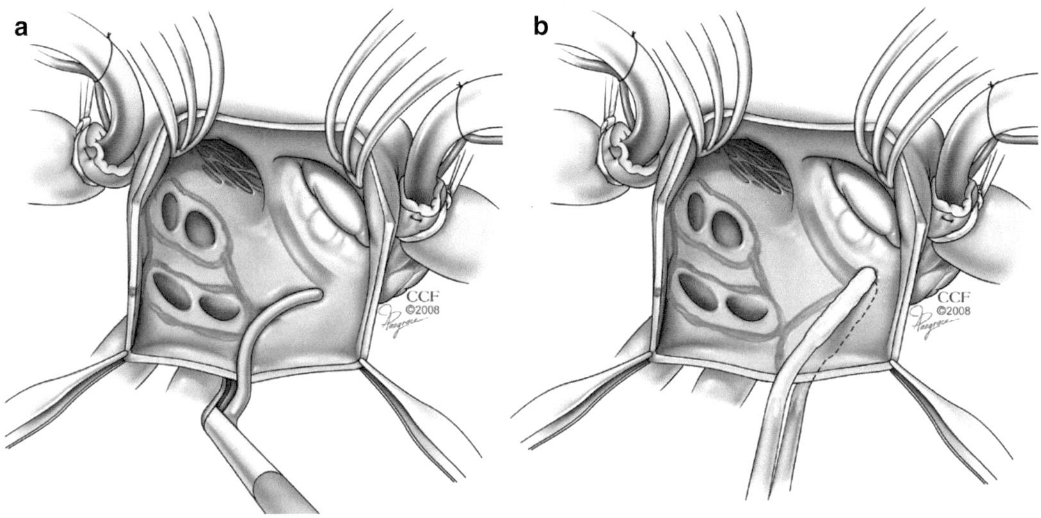

Fig. 18.10 Mitral isthmus line, (**a**) initially using the bipolar radiofrequency clamp device from the atriotomy towards the P2/P3 section of the posterior mitral valve annulus and (**b**) completed using the cryoprobe at the posterior mitral valve annulus. (Reproduced with permission from Gillinov M, Soltesz E. Surgical treatment of atrial fibrillation: today's questions and answers. *Semin Thorac Cardiovasc Surg*. 2013;25(3):197–205.)

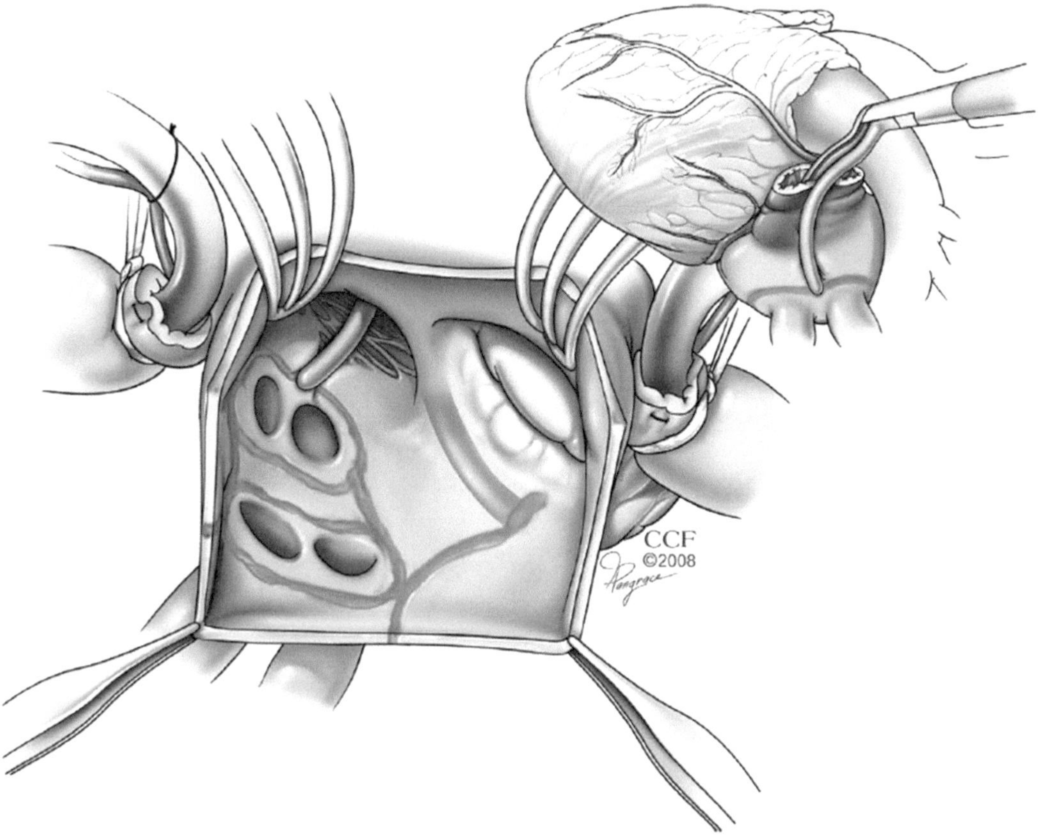

Fig. 18.11 Completion of the left atrial lesion set with the connecting lesion from the left atrial appendage to the encircling lesion around the left pulmonary veins, using the bipolar radiofrequency clamp device. (Reproduced with permission from Gillinov M, Soltesz E. Surgical treatment of atrial fibrillation: today's questions and answers. *Semin Thorac Cardiovasc Surg*. 2013;25(3):197–205.)

patients free from AF. Long-term studies, however, have shown that 5-year freedom from AF is approximately 50% following pulmonary vein isolation. Although acute conduction block at the level of the pulmonary veins can be demonstrated at the time of pulmonary vein isolation by pacing the pulmonary veins, this does not always result in long-term freedom from AF. It is thought that progressive atrial remodelling results in the atrial myocardium being capable of initiating and maintaining atrial fibrillation circuits independent of the pulmonary veins. Hence, although pulmonary vein isolation alone can be used successfully to treat paroxysmal AF, it may not be sufficient in patients with persistent or longstanding AF, where substrate modification of the atria is required using the complete Cox-Maze IV lesion set. Pulmonary vein stenosis is rare with surgical ablation, as it is performed on the antrum of the left atrium.

Left Atrial Appendage

The left atrial appendage has been shown to the site of thrombus in up to 90% of patients with atrial fibrillation who develop stroke. Although this would suggest that excluding the left atrial appendage from the circulation would reduce the incidence of stroke in patients with AF, the evidence for this is limited. Some of this is related to the technical aspects of the surgery. The left atrial appendage can be excluded from the circulation or excised completely, which can be achieved by

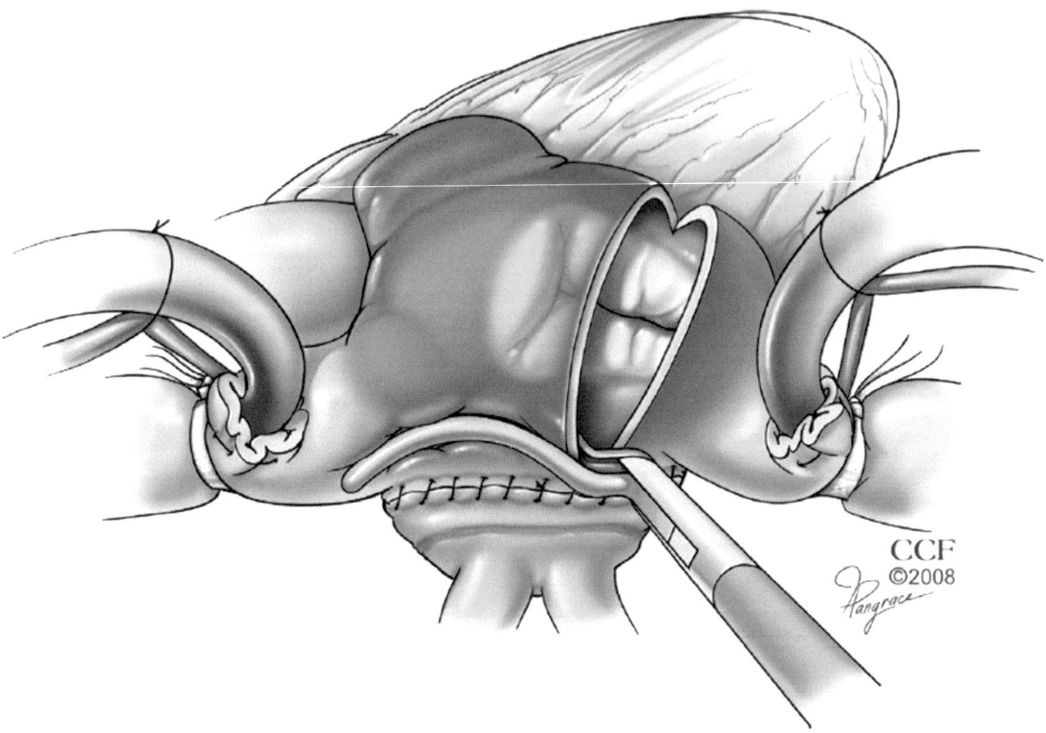

Fig. 18.12 Lesion from the lateral aspect of the right atriotomy to the superior vena cava using the bipolar radiofrequency clamp device. (Reproduced with permission from Gillinov M, Soltesz E. Surgical treatment of atrial fibrillation: today's questions and answers. *Semin Thorac Cardiovasc Surg*. 2013;25(3):197–205.)

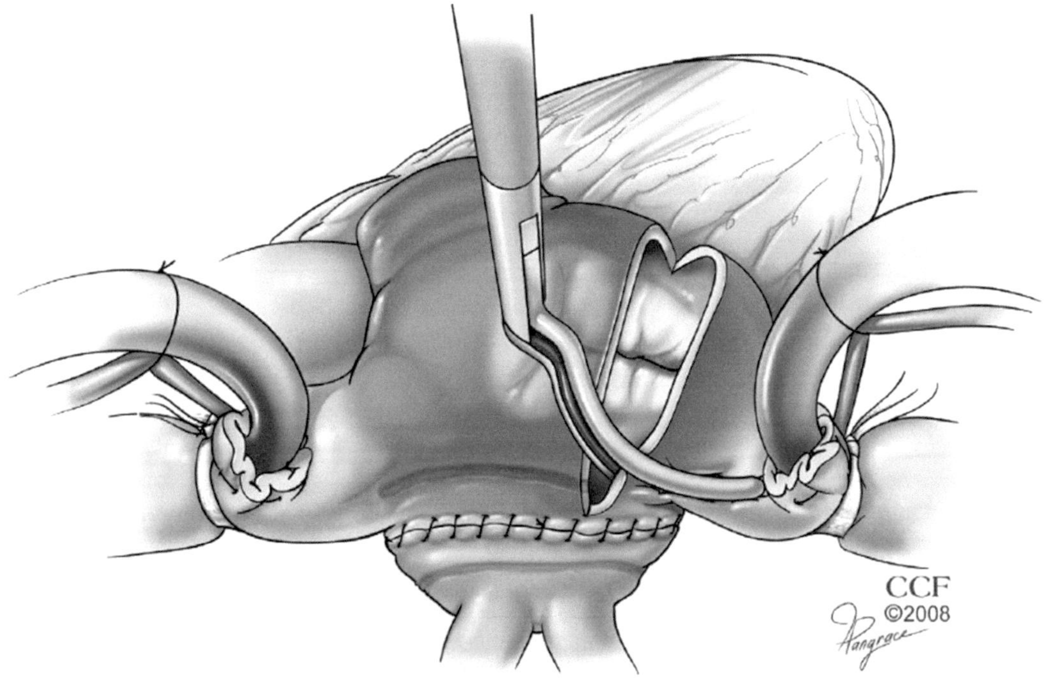

Fig. 18.13 Lesion from the lateral aspect of the right atriotomy to the inferior vena cava using the bipolar radiofrequency clamp device. (Reproduced with permission from Gillinov M, Soltesz E. Surgical treatment of atrial fibrillation: today's questions and answers. *Semin Thorac Cardiovasc Surg*. 2013;25(3):197–205.)

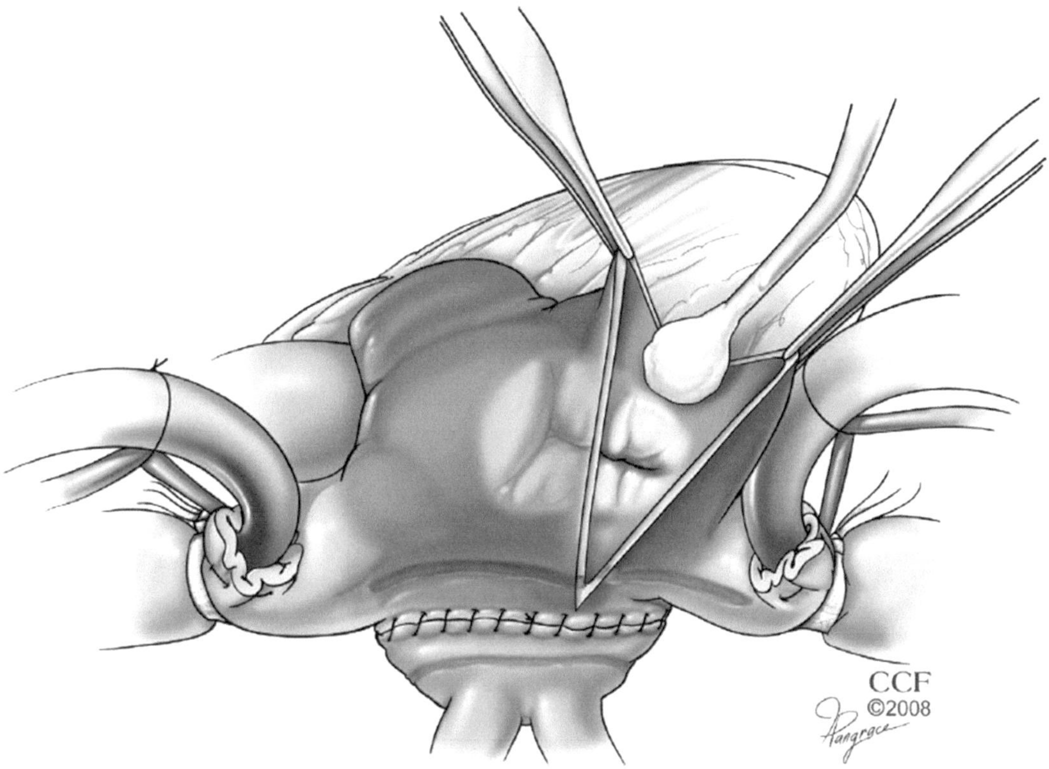

Fig. 18.14 Lesion from the medial aspect of the right atriotomy to the 2 o'clock position of the tricuspid valve annulus using the cryoprobe. (Reproduced with permission from Gillinov M, Soltesz E. Surgical treatment of atrial fibrillation: today's questions and answers. *Semin Thorac Cardiovasc Surg*. 2013;25(3):197–205.)

suture ligation or the use of mechanical devices, such as a stapling device (Fig. 18.16) or specifically designed atrial appendage clips. Techniques that exclude the left atrial appendage from the circulation, as opposed to those that excise the left atrial appendage, especially with internal suturing of the orifice of the left atrial appendage, have been shown to be incomplete in a significant proportion (up to 50%) of cases. In fact, the residual communication with a small orifice may even increase the risk of thrombus formation and subsequent stroke. If the left atrial appendage is excluded but not resected, any residual flow should be checked using intra-operative trans-oesophageal echocardiography. For patients undergoing excision of the left atrial appendage, it is important not to leave a residual stump greater than 1 cm in size. Although there is insufficient evidence to prove that LAA exclusion has a benefit in terms of stroke reduction or mortality, the current guidelines comment that exclusion/excision of the left atrial appendage may be considered in patients undergoing cardiac surgery with AF, as a class IIb indication.

The main risk factors for failure to restore sinus rhythm include left atrial enlargement, longer duration of AF and increased patient age. These factors, however, should not be considered as contra-indications, as restoration of sinus rhythm remains possible in these patients. Although some patients only require pulmonary vein isolation and others a complete Cox-Maze IV procedure to restore sinus rhythm, there are no specific investigations that have the ability to tailor the AF ablation strategy to each individual patient. In view of this, to achieve the best results, a full Cox-Maze IV procedure is recommended in all patients undergoing cardiac surgery with concomitant symptomatic atrial fibrillation, irrespective of whether it is paroxysmal, persistent or

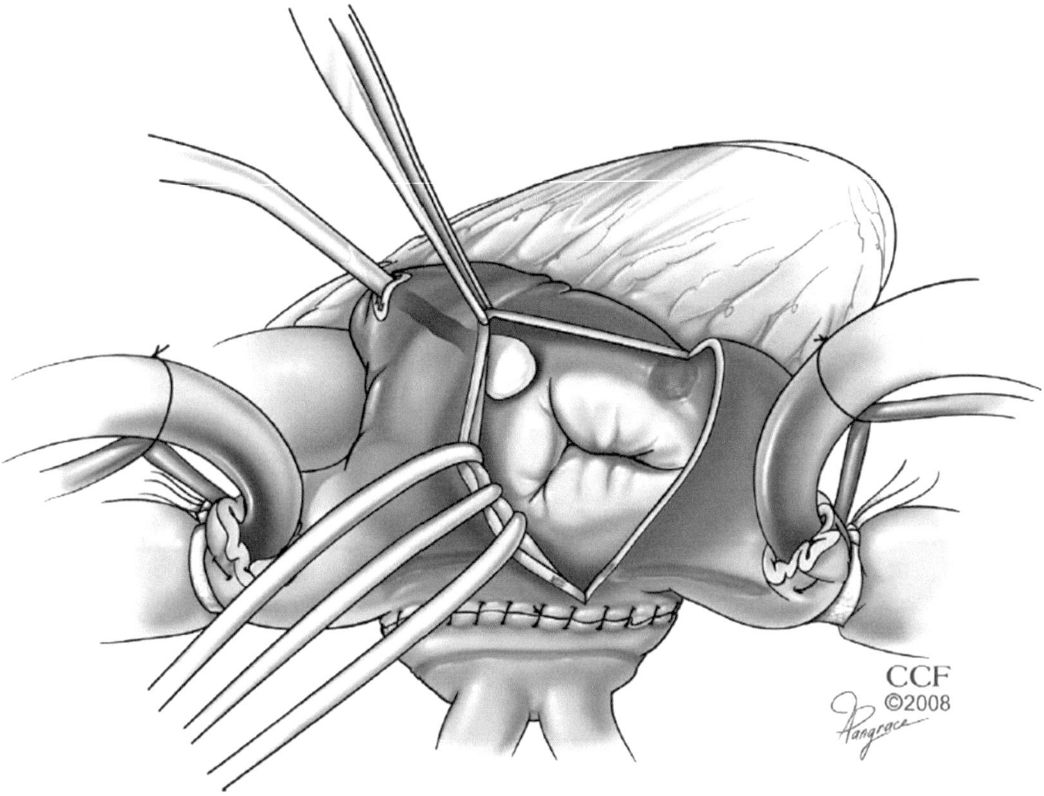

Fig. 18.15 Lesion from the right atrial appendage to the 10 o'clock position of the tricuspid valve annulus using the cryoprobe. (Reproduced with permission from Gillinov M, Soltesz E. Surgical treatment of atrial fibrillation: today's questions and answers. *Semin Thorac Cardiovasc Surg*. 2013;25(3):197–205.)

long-standing persistent. In patients with asymptomatic atrial fibrillation, the ablation procedure should be added if it is not expected to increase the operative risks.

Post-operative Management

Approximately 50% of patients who undergo surgical ablation develop atrial fibrillation in the post-operative period. In these patients, anti-arrhythmic medication, most commonly amiodarone, is commenced and if the patient fails to chemically cardiovert, an electrical cardioversion is attempted in hospital, prior to discharge. The anti-arrhythmic medication is continued for 2 months. If at this stage, atrial fibrillation is absent on long-term monitoring, then the anti-arrhythmic medication can be stopped. Anticoagulation should be continued for 3 months following the ablation procedure and can be stopped if the patient has sustained sinus rhythm, echocardiography demonstrates the absence of left atrial smoke and a left atrial appendage stump, and that their stroke risk is deemed to be low. Electrical cardioversion is attempted for patients who remain in atrial fibrillation at 3 months post-operatively. A simple ECG is not sufficient to demonstrate absence of AF, as approximately 50% of all AF episodes are asymptomatic. Hence, monitoring over a longer period is necessary to make appropriate decisions regarding the cessation of antiarrhythmic and anticoagulation mediations. The recent guidelines recommend follow-up of at least 1 year with a minimum of 24–72 h Holter monitoring, trans-telephonic monitoring, 30-day auto event triggered monitoring or outpatient telemetry. Success is defined as freedom

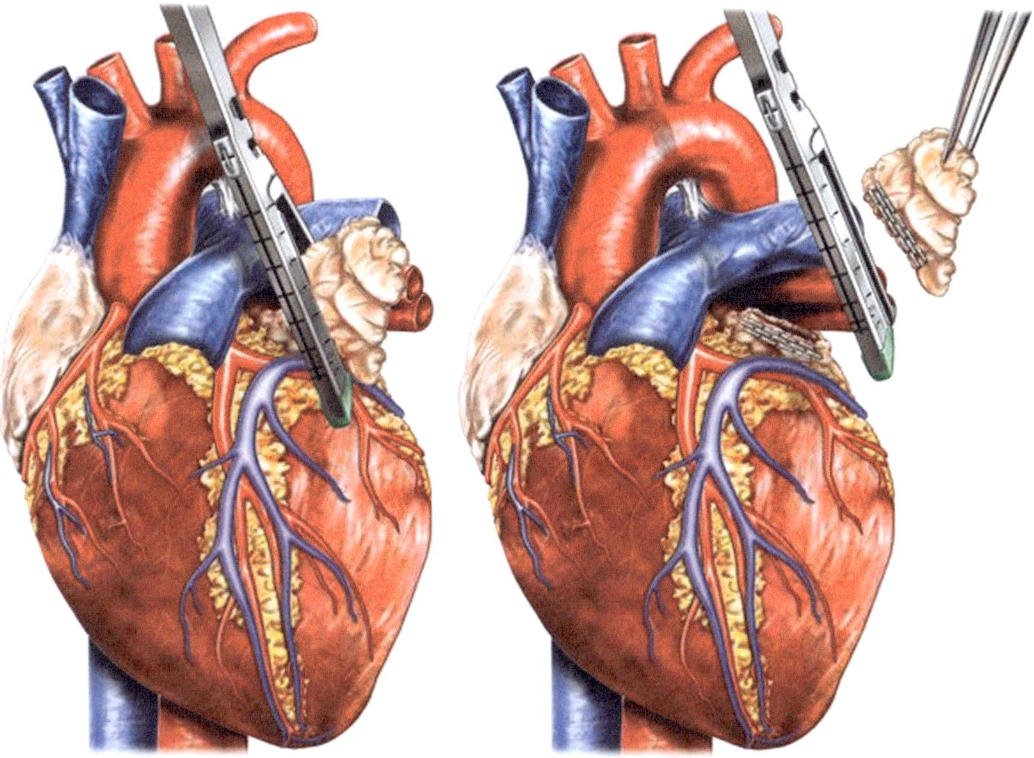

Fig. 18.16 Left atrial appendage excision using a stapling device. (Reproduced with permission from Chatterjee S. Left atrial appendage occlusion: lessons learned from surgical and transcatheter experiences. *Ann Thorac Surg*. 2011;92(6):2283–92)

from any atrial arrhythmia (AF, atrial flutter or atrial tachycardia) lasting longer than 30 s, documented by an ECG or device recording system more than 3 months after the procedure.

Surgical Technique

Intra-operative trans-oesophageal echocardiography was used to ensure the absence of thrombus in the left atrium, especially left atrial appendage. Following median sternotomy and initiation of cardiopulmonary bypass, the superior vena cava and inferior vena cava were mobilised.

Pulmonary vein isolation was performed on cardiopulmonary bypass with a decompressed beating heart to allow exit block to be determined by pulmonary vein pacing. The area between the right pulmonary artery and right superior pulmonary vein was then developed into the oblique sinus. Blunt dissection of the right superior and inferior pulmonary veins was performed to enable an umbilical tape to be passed around both veins together. Pacing thresholds were then measured from each pulmonary vein using a bipolar pacing probe. A bipolar radiofrequency clamp device (Atricure Inc., West Chester, OH) was placed onto the left atrial tissue immediately adjacent to the junction with right pulmonary veins (Fig. 18.17a). By placing the clamp on atrial tissue, it reduced the risk of developing pulmonary vein stenosis. The duration of the ablation was determined by the computed algorithms calculated from the impedance monitoring. The lesion was repeated a second time by moving the clamp slightly to produce a parallel ablation line, thereby ensuring complete electrical isolation of the left atrium from the pulmonary veins had been achieved. Isolation was confirmed by demonstrating exit block, which was evidenced by

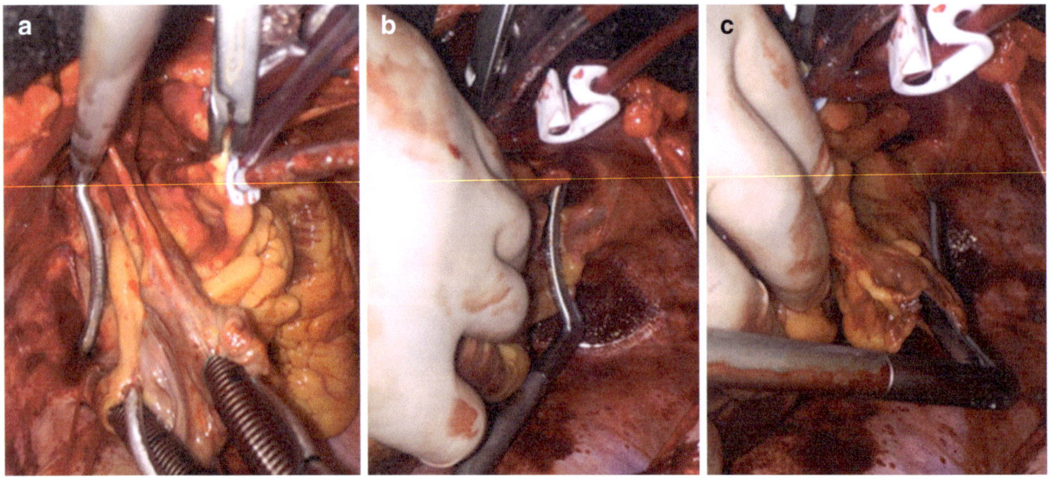

Fig. 18.17 (**a**) Right and (**b**) left pulmonary vein isolation using a bipolar radiofrequency clamp device, followed by (**c**) the lesion connecting the left atrial appendage to the lesion encircling the left pulmonary veins

the inability to pace the atrium from either of the pulmonary veins. If exit block had not been demonstrated, additional ablations would have been performed, as required.

Access to the left pulmonary veins was achieved by retracting the heart towards the right. Blunt dissection of the left superior and inferior pulmonary veins was performed, including dissection of the ligament of Marshall, again to enable a tape to be passed around both veins together. Once pacing thresholds were measured from each vein, the bipolar radiofrequency clamp device was passed onto the left atrial tissue immediately adjacent to the junction with left pulmonary veins (Fig. 18.17b). The lesion was repeated with a second parallel ablation line and again isolation was confirmed by demonstrating exit block when pacing the pulmonary veins.

A small incision is then made in the left atrial appendage. With the heart elevated, the left atrial appendage was incised. The bipolar radiofrequency clamp device was placed into the left atrial appendage stump to create an ablation line to connect with the one encircling the left pulmonary veins (Fig. 18.17c).

The left atrial appendage stump was excised using a stapling device (Fig. 18.18).

Following mobilisation of Sondergaard's interatrial groove anterior to the right pulmonary veins, a standard left atriotomy was then performed. To achieve isolation of the entire posterior left atrium, the bipolar radiofrequency clamp device was first placed at the inferior aspect of the left atriotomy next to the right inferior pulmonary vein orifice across the floor of the left atrium towards the orifice of left inferior pulmonary vein (Fig. 18.19a), and then at the superior aspect of the left atriotomy next to the right superior pulmonary vein orifice across the roof of the left atrium towards the orifice of left superior pulmonary vein (Fig. 18.19b), to complete the box lesion set.

The next step of the left atrial lesion set was the mitral isthmus line, which required a combination of bipolar radiofrequency and cryothermy, as the bipolar radiofrequency clamp device is unable to create a transmural lesion up to the mitral valve annulus due to the thickness of the tissue at that level. The bipolar radiofrequency clamp device was used to create an ablation line from the inferior aspect of the left atriotomy across the floor of the left atrium towards the mitral valve annulus (Fig. 18.19c). It is important to avoid the circumflex coronary artery, which runs parallel to the posterior mitral valve annulus, when creating this ablation line. The final 1–2 cm

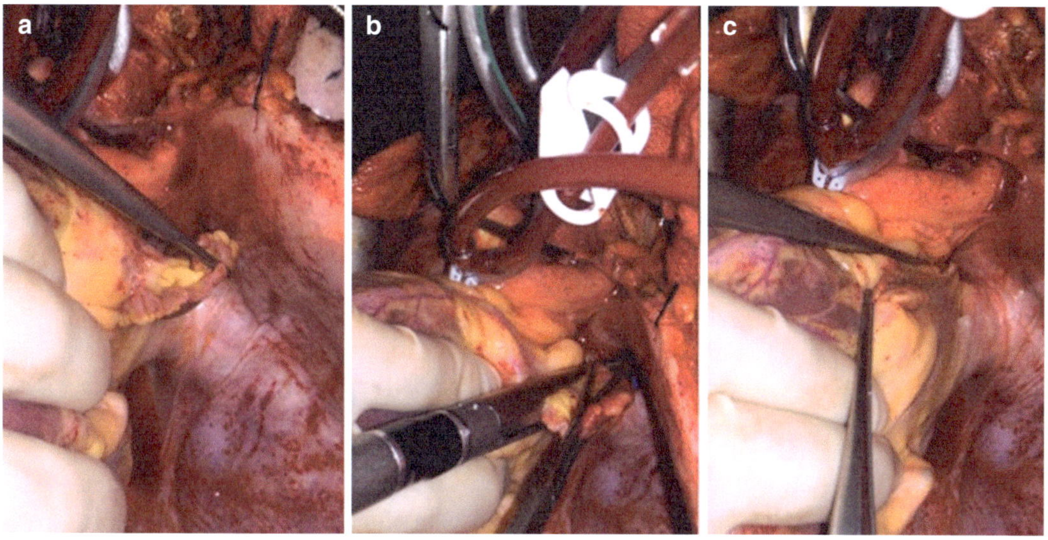

Fig. 18.18 Operative images illustrating (**a**) stretching of the left atrial appendage, (**b**) excision of the appendage using a stapling device, and (**c**) the residual stump, which is <1 cm in height

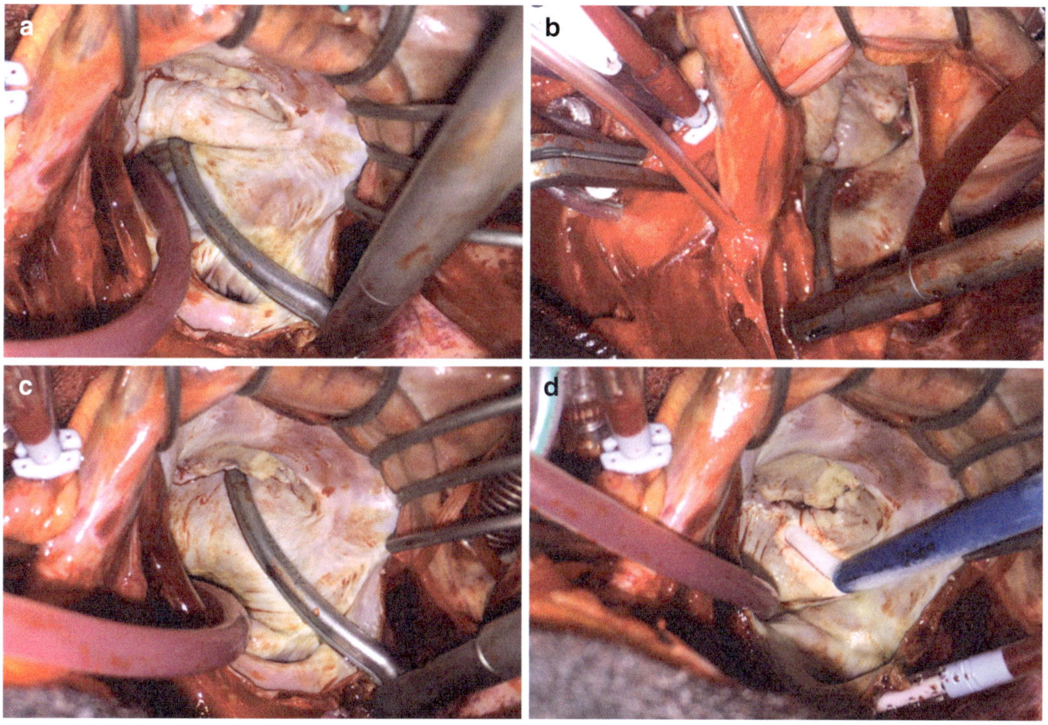

Fig. 18.19 Completion of the left atrial lesion set, including (**a**) connecting lesion from the right inferior pulmonary vein to left inferior pulmonary vein across the floor of the left atrium using a bipolar radiofrequency clamp device, (**b**) connecting lesion from the right superior pulmonary vein to left superior pulmonary vein across the roof of the left atrium using a bipolar radiofrequency clamp device, (**c**) lesion from the left atriotomy to the P2/P3 region of the posterior mitral valve annulus (mitral isthmus line) using a bipolar radiofrequency clamp device, and (**d**) completion of the mitral isthmus line for the final 1–2 cm up to the mitral annulus using a cryoprobe

up to the mitral annulus was then completed using a cryoprobe (Fig. 18.19d), followed by a separate application of the cryoprobe on the epicardial surface of the coronary sinus. The cryoprobe was applied for 2 min at −60 °C and thawed before removal, to avoid tearing of attached tissue. As the patient had a right-dominant coronary artery system, the isthmus line was directed towards the junction of the P2 and P3 scallops of the posterior leaflet. In patients with a left-dominant coronary artery system, the isthmus line is directed towards the posteromedial commissure to avoid injury to the circumflex coronary artery. The left atriotomy was then closed with a single-layer 3/0 non-absorbable monofilament polypropylene suture.

After snaring the cavae with tapes, a vertical right atriotomy was made from the intra-atrial septum up towards the right atrioventricular groove, at a level with the 2 o'clock position of the tricuspid valve. The bipolar radiofrequency clamp device was used to create ablation lines from the lateral aspect of the atriotomy towards the superior (Fig. 18.20a) and inferior venae cavae (Fig. 18.20b) onto caval tissue. The cryoprobe was then used to create a lesion from the medial aspect of the atriotomy towards the 2 o'clock position of the tricuspid valve annulus (Fig. 18.20c). A small incision was made in the right atrial appendage and the cryoprobe was placed to create a lesion from the appendage towards the 10 o'clock position of the tricuspid valve annulus (Fig. 18.20d). The right atriotomy and right atrial appendage incision were closed with a double-layer 4/0 non-absorbable monofilament polypropylene suture.

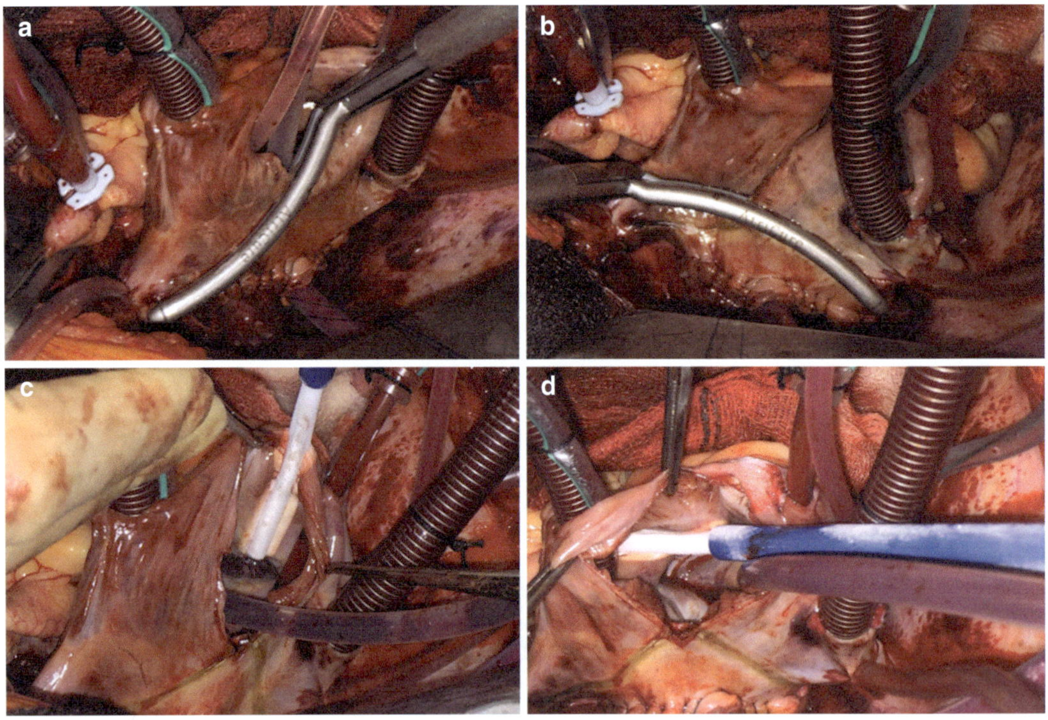

Fig. 18.20 Right atrial lesion set, including (**a**) lesion from the lateral aspect of the atriotomy towards the superior vena cava using a bipolar radiofrequency clamp device, (**b**) lesion from the lateral aspect of the atriotomy towards the inferior vena cava using a bipolar radiofrequency clamp device, (**c**) lesion from the medial aspect of the atriotomy towards the 2 o'clock position of the tricuspid valve annulus using a cryoprobe, and (**d**) lesion from the right atrial appendage towards the 10 o'clock position of the tricuspid valve annulus using a cryoprobe

Surgical Tips

1. Concomitant ablation should be performed in patients with paroxysmal or persistent atrial fibrillation undergoing cardiac surgery, using a complete right and left atrial lesion set (Cox-Maze IV)
2. The majority of the lesions should be performed with bipolar radiofrequency because of the ease of use and in determining transmurality by impedance monitoring
3. Cryothermy is an ideal energy source to complete the lesions over mitral and tricuspid annuli because it preserves the fibrous skeleton of the heart, thereby maintaining valvular function
4. Pulmonary vein isolation should be confirmed by demonstrating exit block, which is evidenced by the inability to pace the atrium from any of the pulmonary veins.

Comment

For patients undergoing cardiac surgery, concomitant ablation of atrial fibrillation is recommended in patients with paroxysmal, persistent or long-standing persistent atrial fibrillation, and can be performed without increased risk of morbidity and mortality. It has been shown to be associated with a significantly increased incidence of sinus rhythm at short- and long-term follow-up, improved ejection fraction and exercise tolerance, reduced risk of thromboembolic events and stroke, and improved long-term survival. The reduction in thromboembolic events after the ablation procedure is thought to be secondary to restoration of atrial contraction, as well as removal of the left atrial appendage. At 1 year, the complete Cox-Maze IV bi-atrial lesion set results in up to 90% freedom from AF in patients with paroxysmal AF and 80% freedom from AF in those with persistent AF. This effect has been shown to be sustained at 5 years.

Pre-operative risk factors for recurrence of AF include older age, lesion set (for patients in long-standing persistent atrial fibrillation), longer atrial fibrillation duration (>5 years), larger left atrial diameter (>8 cm) and persistent atrial fibrillation. The absence of the right atrial lesion set is thought to decrease the effectiveness of the ablation procedure by 10–15%. Pulmonary vein isolation is thought to further decrease the effective of the ablation procedure, especially for patients with persistent AF. In association with the freedom from AF, there is a 90% freedom from anticoagulation and 70–80% freedom from anti-arrhythmic therapy. In patients undergoing cardiac surgery with atrial fibrillation, the addition of surgical ablation does not seem to increase the incidence of post-operative permanent pacemaker requirement (4–5%).

Recommended Reading

Cox JL. The surgical treatment of atrial fibrillation. IV. Surgical technique. J Thorac Cardiovasc Surg. 1991;101:584–92.

Damiano RJ Jr, Schwartz FH, Bailey MS, Maniar HS, Munfakh NA, Moon MR, Schuessler RB. The Cox maze IV procedure: predictors of late recurrence. J Thorac Cardiovasc Surg. 2011;141:113–21.

Dunning J, Nagendran M, Alfieri OR, Elia S, Kappetein AP, Lockowandt U, Sarris GE, Kolh PH. Guideline for the surgical treatment of atrial fibrillation. Eur J Cardiothorac Surg. 2013;44:777–91.

Gillinov AM, Gelijns AC, Parides MK, DeRose JJ, Moskowitz AJ, Voisine P, Ailawadi G, Bouchard D, Smith PK, Mack MJ, Acker MA, Mullen JC, Rose EA, Chang HL, Puskas JD, Couderc JP, Gardner TJ, Varghese R, Horvath KA, Bolling SF, Michler RE, Geller NL, Ascheim DD, Miller MA, Bagiella E, Moquete EG, Williams P, Taddei-Peters WC, O'Gara PT, Blackstone EH, Argenziano M, CTSN Investigators. Surgical ablation of atrial fibrillation during mitral-valve surgery. N Engl J Med. 2015;372:1399–409.

January CT, Wann LS, Alpert JS, Calkins H, Cigarroa JE, Cleveland JC Jr, Conti JB, Ellinor PT, Ezekowitz MD, Field ME, Murray KT, Sacco RL, Stevenson WG, Tchou PJ, Tracy CM, Yancy CW, ACC/AHA Task Force Members. 2014 AHA/ACC/HRS guideline for the management of patients with atrial fibrillation: a report of the American College of Cardiology/American Heart Association Task Force on practice guidelines and the Heart Rhythm Society. Circulation. 2014;130(23):e199–267.

Kanderian AS, Gillinov AM, Pettersson GB, Blackstone E, Klein AL. Success of surgical left atrial appendage closure: assessment by transesophageal echocardiography. J Am Coll Cardiol. 2008;52:924–9.

Kirchhof P, Benussi S, Kotecha D, Ahlsson A, Atar D, Casadei B, Castella M, Diener HC, Heidbuchel H, Hendriks J, Hindricks G, Manolis AS, Oldgren J, Popescu BA, Schotten U, Van Putte B, Vardas P, Agewall S, Camm J, Baron Esquivias G, Budts W, Carerj S, Casselman F, Coca A, De Caterina R, Deftereos S, Dobrev D, Ferro JM, Filippatos G, Fitzsimons D, Gorenek B, Guenoun M, Hohnloser SH, Kolh P, Lip GY, Manolis A, McMurray J, Ponikowski P, Rosenhek R, Ruschitzka F, Savelieva I, Sharma S, Suwalski P, Tamargo JL, Taylor CJ, Van Gelder IC, Voors AA, Windecker S, Zamorano JL, Zeppenfeld K. 2016 ESC guidelines for the management of atrial fibrillation developed in collaboration with EACTS. Eur J Cardiothorac Surg. 2016;50(5):e1–e88.

Shemin RJ, Cox JL, Gillinov AM, Blackstone EH, Bridges CR. Guidelines for reporting data and outcomes for the surgical treatment of atrial fibrillation. Ann Thorac Surg. 2007;83:1225–30.

Soltesz E, Gillinov M. Ablation of atrial fibrillation with concomitant surgery. Op Tech Thorac Cardiovasc Surg. 2009;14(3):193–207.

Index

N. Moorjani et al., *Operative Mitral and Tricuspid Valve Surgery*,
https://doi.org/10.1007/978-1-4471-4204-1